A Quick Guide on How to Conduct Medical Research

Marieke M. ter Wee
Birgit I. Lissenberg-Witte

A Quick Guide on How to Conduct Medical Research

From Set-Up to Publication

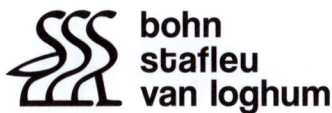

bohn
stafleu
van loghum

Houten 2019

ISBN 978-90-368-2247-3   ISBN 978-90-368-2248-0 (eBook)
https://doi.org/10.1007/978-90-368-2248-0

NUR 871
Ontwerp illustratie omslag: Birgit I. Lissenberg-Witte & Marieke M. ter Wee
Basisontwerp omslag: Studio Bassa, Culemborg
Automatische opmaak: Scientific Publishing Services (P) Ltd., Chennai, India

Bohn Stafleu van Loghum
Walmolen 1
Postbus 246
3990 GA Houten

www.bsl.nl

If we knew what it was we were doing, it would not be called research, would it?

-Albert Einstein-

Foreword

We make thousands of decisions every day, of which a considerable part unconscious, often based on intuition. Also, in clinical practice, the care of a doctor for a patient is greatly supported by fast recognition of patterns that safely guide the choice of therapy. And how often was a discovery not revealed just by serendipity? It was on the 28th of September in 1928 that Alexander Fleming, a scientist investigating staphylococcus species, noticed that around a contamination of mold on the culture plate all bacteria died. From that mold the antibiotic penicillin was isolated.

However, outstanding medical practice needs more than that. The complexity of diseases, the fortunate, but enormous increase in diagnostic and therapeutic possibilities, and the wish of patients to be informed about the motives behind medical choices, requires thorough weighing of evidence.

This cannot be implemented without knowledge about good methodology and proper statistical analyses, or with other words 'to know what is good medical research'. Not only as an investigator, even as a reader of medical science you need to know the basics of research methodology to weigh the evidence in a correct way.

While theory on research methodology and statistical analyses are part of (bio)medical education, the actual experience of junior doctors, or life sciences students with the initiation and execution of research projects, is limited. The complex procedure of medical research, which starts with the right research question and ends with the submission of a high-quality scientific paper, requires curiosity and perseverance, but not to forget education and guidance. The lack of concise and simple practical guides describing the total process from the formulation of a research hypothesis to the analyses of available data, may be experienced as a hurdle by young professionals.

The 'Quick Guide on How to Conduct Medical Research' is a simple and clear guide leading you through all the steps of medical research. The simple illustrations are helpful in understanding concepts of research methodology and statistical analyses.

We are convinced, although not tested statistically, that this guide will help young and older professionals to overcome the methodological and technical challenges during their scientific journey. Furthermore, this guide will also contribute to get data into the public domain for the benefit of patients and doctors. That brings us back to the first lines: reading this book is a decision you will not regret.

Prof.dr. Sonja Zweegman, MD PhD
Head of the Department of Hematology Amsterdam UMC

Prof.dr. Christa Boer, MSc PhD
Director VUmc School of Medical Sciences Amsterdam UMC

Preface

Since the foundation of medicine, by Hypocrates around 400 BC, the performance of medicine is mainly driven by evidence based medicine for treatments and evidence based practice of applied therapies and diagnostic tests that are used. This evidence is mostly provided by medical scientific research. Although medical students are taught the importance of evidence based medicine, they receive limited education on how to set-up, conduct and analyze medical research. Epidemiologists are medical researchers with a health care (or medical) background, and will have received more statistical training. Epidemiologists are needed to conduct medical research in the best methodological way, and can help with the more common and some of the advanced statistical techniques. However, nowadays, more complex research designs are required to investigate complicated medical research questions which require advanced statistical methods to analyze the extensive data. As a result biostatisticians have become more involved in medical research. Biostatisticians have a mathematical background, but lack the medical background which is needed to translate the statistical results into daily practice. The ideal collaboration in medical research, therefore consists of a medical researcher, an epidemiologist and a biostatistician.

In our work as an epidemiologist and a biostatistician in an academic medical research center, we often see medical doctors conducting medical research. In our experience, the problems researchers encounter in their research are caused by poorly defined research questions and the limited statistical training in their educational program. Moreover, any training they have received was usually based on artificial examples. Once they begin conducting their own research, they find themselves needing appropriate statistical and methodological knowledge, as terminology is often confusing, for example, the terms association and prediction. There is a need for simple and clear references that a researcher could use to refresh his/her statistical foundation as well as to enhance his/her methodological knowledge. Many statistical textbooks exist, but these are either too technical or ignore the starting point of conducting research: formulating the research question and choosing the appropriate research design. We felt that a quick guide that serves as a reference for junior researchers (who have just begun their careers), as well as for senior researchers supervising the junior researchers, was missing.

In this quick guide, we cover all steps in conducting research: from the set-up, through data analyses to publication of the results in a scientific paper. All research begins with writing a solid research proposal. The research question and the analyses plan are two important elements of such a proposal. In ▶Chap. 1, we describe all elements of the research proposal. In ▶Chap. 2, we introduce basic statistical terminology and concepts, such as descriptive statistics, effect sizes, confidence intervals and p-values. In ▶Chaps. 3–5, we explain several fundamental statistical methods for three different types of outcome variables, continuous, dichotomous and time to event, and illustrate how to compare two or more groups. We also introduce the linear, logistic and Cox regression model, to investigate the association between the outcome variable and a continuous determinant. In ▶Chap. 6, we describe three different types of influencing factors that could act on an association: confounding, effect modification and mediation. We explain how to deal with influencing variables and how to interpret the corrected results. In ▶Chap. 7, we focus on prediction models; how do they differ from association models, how are they built and how good are they? All examples of the statistical analyses in ▶Chaps. 3–7 are preceded by a research question. In ▶Chap. 8, we cover missing data, an important topic that every researcher encounters. And last, in ▶Chap. 9, we consider all the steps that need to be taken to publish the results of the research as a scientific paper in a peer reviewed journal. Additionally, we explain how to critically appraise existing literature. It is a common misconception that published papers in high impact factor journals are always of good quality, unfortunately this is often not the case.

We aim to provide a complete overview that covers all steps of conducting research, but also aim to be a quick guide that summarizes the fundamental concepts of the statistical analyses. This appears to be contradictory to the complete overview. We therefore end each chapter with a further reading section, which refers to more in-depth information on the topics covered in each chapter as well as on more specialized topics. We have tried to limit the number of mathematical equations, but we cannot explain statistics without them. In the Supplementary Information 'Mathematical Equations and Models', the important equations and models are summarized, with references to the sections they were introduced in.

Information endures better when knowledge is applied in practice. Therefore, we illustrate the methods described in this quick guide using two studies. The first study is the COmbinatie Behandeling bij Reumatoïde Artritis (COBRA)-light trial. The primary objective of this randomized controlled trial was to assess non-inferiority of the COBRA-light strategy compared to the COBRA strategy after 26 and 52 weeks of treatment [1, 2] (© BMJ and EULAR 2018). Patients who had been recently diagnosed with rheumatoid arthritis (RA), were included in this trial, and randomized to receive either the COBRA strategy or the COBRA-light strategy. Patients randomized to the COBRA strategy received 7.5 mg/week methotrexate, 2 g/day sulfasalazine and initially high-dose prednisolone (60 mg/day) which was tapered to 7.5 mg/day in 7 weeks. Patients randomized to the COBRA-light strategy received 25 mg/week methotrexate and initially 30 mg/day prednisolone tapered to 7.5 mg/day in 9 weeks. Etanercept was added to both strategies after 26 or 39 weeks if the patient did not reach minimal disease activity. The primary outcome variable of this trial was reaching a disease activity score of 44 joints (DAS44) of below 1.6. Patients were seen three-monthly and medication was protocolized up to 1 year.

The second study is the prospective cohort study of van de Stadt et al. [3] (© BMJ and EULAR 2018), which we refer to as the RA-cohort. The primary objective of this study was to develop a prediction model for the development of arthritis in arthralgia patients who are IgM rheumatoid factor positive and/or anticyclic citrullinated peptide positive. These patients are at risk of developing RA, but it was unknown which patients would develop RA and within which time frame. At study entry, medical history and disease related details were recorded. Patients were seen every half year during the first year of follow-up and every year thereafter. The main outcome variable of the RA cohort study was the time that elapsed to the development of RA.

We illustrate all statistical analyses with output of the Statistical Package for the Social Sciences (SPSS, version 22; IBM Corp., Armonk, NY, USA). SPSS produces more output than we include in this quick guide, we only use the relevant part(s) of the output. A quick guide on how to perform these analyses in SPSS can be found in the Supplementary Information 'SPSS Quick Guide'. In all analyses, we set the significance level α of the statistical tests to 0.05, unless stated otherwise.

This book could not have been established without the help of others. We would therefore like to thank first of all Lydia Nieuwendijk and Hester Presburg of Bohn Stafleu van Loghum, part of Springer Nature, for having the confidence in us to write this book. We really appreciated that we were able to use the data of the COBRA-light trial and the RA-cohort as examples. We are grateful to the research groups from these two studies, specifically Prof. Willem Lems and Prof. Dirkjan van Schaardenburg. We would like to thank Federica Inturissi for pre-reading some chapters to provide us with valuable comments and Prof. Sonja Zweegman and Prof. Christa Boer for taking their time to write the foreword. We are grateful to work at the department of Epidemiology and Biostatistics at the Amsterdam UMC, location VUmc, which provided us with the knowledge, expertise and experience that enabled us to write this book. Special thanks to Prof. Jos Twisk who is our role model on how to apply statistics in practice.

And last but not least, we would like to thank our family: our parents for their constant support and belief in our capabilities, and our spouses Christiaan Zaal and Yoeri Lissenberg for making it possible for us to write this book. Without your help, we would not have been able to make this all happen. We love you!

We truly hope that many researchers – student, junior and senior – feel more confident in conducting medical research with this quick guide at hand.

Dr. Marieke M. ter Wee
Dr. Birgit I. Lissenberg-Witte
Amsterdam, The Netherlands, October 15, 2018

References

1. den Uyl D, et al. A non-inferiority trial of an attenuated combination strategy ('COBRA-light') compared to the original COBRA strategy: clinical results after 26 weeks. Ann Rheum Dis. 2014;73(6):1071–8.
2. ter Wee MM, et al. Intensive combination treatment regimens, including prednisolone, are effective in treating patients with early rheumatoid arthritis regardless of additional etanercept: 1-year results of the COBRA-light open-label, randomised, non-inferiority trial. Ann Rheum Dis. 2015;74(6):1233–40.
3. van de Stadt LA, et al. A prediction rule for the development of arthritis in seropositive arthralgia patients. Ann Rheum Dis. 2013;72(12):1920–6.

Contents

About the authors

Marieke M. ter Wee studied Occupational Therapy (BSc) at the Hogeschool van Amsterdam, Health Sciences (MSc) at the VU University of Amsterdam, Epidemiology (postgraduate, MSc) at the VU University Medical Center, and obtained her PhD in Medicine at the VU University Amsterdam. She worked as a clinical research associate at Quintiles Transnational, and since October 2015 she has been working as an education coordinator and science lector at the Department of Epidemiology and Biostatistics of the VU University Medical Center in Amsterdam (as of June 2018: Amsterdam UMC, location VUmc). She coordinates and teaches in several courses on methodology and statistics at the VUmc School of Medical Sciences. Since May 2017, she also has been working as a senior researchers at the Department of Rheumatology of Amsterdam UMC, location VUmc. Her research focusses on the impact of inflammatory arthritis on work participation as well as on other patient reported outcomes (PROs).

Birgit I. Lissenberg-Witte studied Mathematics (MSc) at the VU University Amsterdam, and obtained her PhD in Mathematical Statistics at the Delft University of Technology. Since November 2010, she has been working as a scientific researcher at the Department of Epidemiology and Biostatistics of the VU University Medical Center in Amsterdam (as of June 2018: Amsterdam UMC, location VUmc). Her research focusses on developing new methodology in health science. Besides, she coordinates the requests of medical researchers for statistical help through the statistical helpdesk. Moreover, she works as a statistical consultant with junior and senior medical researchers and physicians, teaches a course on Biostatistics for research master students in the area of cardiovascular diseases and oncology, and is member of the Medical Ethical Review Board of Amsterdam UMC, location VUmc.

Abbreviations and acronyms

aCCP	anticyclic citrullinated peptide
ANOVA	analysis of variance
AUC	area under the curve
BC	Before Christ
BMI	body mass index
CEA	cost-effectiveness analysis
CHEERS	Consolidated Health Economic Evaluation Reporting Standards
CI	confidence interval
CRP	C reactive protein
COBRA	COmbinatie Behandeling bij Rheumatoïde Artritis
CONSORT	CONsolidated Standards Of Reporting Trials
COREQ	COnsolidated criteria for Reporting Qualitative research
COSMIN	COnsensus-based Standards for selection of health Measurement INstruments
DAS44	Disease Activity Score of 44 joints
DAS28	Disease Activity Score of 28 joints
e.g.	exempli gratia
ESR	erythrocyte sedimentation rate
etc.	etcetera
exp	exponential
FDR	first-degree relative
GCP	Good Clinical Practice
H0	null hypothesis
H1	alternative hypothesis
HAQ	(Health Assessment) Questionnaire
HR	hazard ratio
(HR)-PROM	(Health-Related) Patient-Reported Outcome Measure
ICMJE	International Committee of Medical Journal Editors
i.e.	id est
IgM-RF	rheumatoid factor type immunoglobulin M
IQR	interquartile range
kg	kilograms
L	liter
ln	natural logarithm
LP	linear predictor
LR	likelihood ratio
MAR	missing at random
MCAR	missing completely at random
MERB	Medical Ethical Review Board
mg	milligram

mmHg	millimeters of mercury
MNAR	missing not at random
MOOSE	Meta-analyses Of Observational Studies in Epidemiology
NOS	Newcastle-Ottawa Scale
NSAID	non-steroid anti-inflammatory drug
OR	odds ratio
PICO(t)	patient/population; intervention; comparison; outcome measure; time
PRISMA	Preferred Reporting Items for Systematic reviews and Meta-Analyses
QQ-plot	quantile-quantile plot
RA	rheumatoid arthritis
RCT	randomized controlled trial
RD	risk difference
RECORD	REporting of studies Conducted using Observational Routinely collected health Data
ROC	receiver operating characteristic (curve)
RR	relative risk
SD	standard deviation
SE	standard error
SJC44	swollen joint count in 44 joints
SPSS	Statistical Package for the Social Sciences
STARD	STAndards for Reporting of Diagnostic accuracy
STROBE	STrengthening the Reporting of OBservational studies in Epidemiology
TJC53	tender joint count in 53 joints
TSJC	total swollen joint count
TREND	Transparent Reporting of Evaluations with Nonrandomized Designs
TRIPOD	Transparent Reporting of a multivariable prediction model for Individual Prognosis Or Diagnosis
VAS	visual analogue scale

The Start – Steps to Set-up a Research

Abstract

Translating a research idea into high quality research is not always easy. Many steps need to be taken. The best way to start off is to write a research proposal. Often, a proposal is required to apply for research funding and to obtain the approval of the Medical Ethical Review Board. A research proposal will lay out all the ideas and plans for the research. In this chapter, we provide an overview of all elements of the research proposal.

© Bohn Stafleu van Loghum is een imprint van Springer Media B.V., onderdeel van Springer Nature 2019
M. M. ter Wee and B. I. Lissenberg-Witte, *A Quick Guide on How to Conduct Medical Research*,
https://doi.org/10.1007/978-90-368-2248-0_1

1.1   Research Proposal

Within a research proposal, every step of the research that is to be conducted is laid out. Each activity that will be carried out through every stage of the research is described. For the researcher him-/herself, the proposal provides the structure of their research to ensure they won't lose focus. Other researchers can understand and judge what the intention of the research is by reviewing the proposal. ◻Table 1.1 lists all the important items within the research proposal, from the title to the potential results that the researcher might expect.

1.2   Title of Research

Although the title of the research seems the least important, a good title creates a positive attitude towards the research. It is the first introduction to the research and should therefore grab the reader's attention. An effective title covers the main topic of the study and is concise. To come up with a title, list all important topics of the idea, and write down the most important message. Combine the important topics and the message into a title. Select several options and ask for the opinion of colleagues. Let them explain what they think the research is about, based on the title. Fine-tune the title for a final version. The title of the research also forms the basis of the title of the scientific paper which will be written at the end of the research.

1.3   Scientific Background

The scientific background of the research is used to position the research idea in the current available literature. The hourglass template can be used to write the scientific background of the research idea (◻Fig. 1.1). First, the importance of the topic is established. The existing research is then reviewed. Finally, the research gap addressed by the new research idea is discussed. Read all existing relevant literature regarding the health-care problem and/or the possible interventions used. The hourglass template could be used to write a research proposal as well as a scientific paper (▶Chap. 9).

1.4   Research Question/Aim

The primary research question (or research aim) results from the existing research gap in the scientific background. The main focus of the research is to answer this question. Sometimes secondary and even tertiary research questions (or aims) are investigated as well. All research questions/aims should be described in the research proposal. A proper research question is developed according to the PICO(t) model:

◻ **Table 1.1**   Overview of all required items in the research proposal

Title of research	• Informative and relevant to the research project proposed
Scientific background of the research	• Description of the health-care problem/ disease state • Scientific background, i.e., relevant knowledge, theories and/or concepts supported by up-to-date literature • Scientific and societal relevance of the research question • Structure goes from general to specific
Research question/aim	• Well-defined research question/aim, translated to a null and alternative hypothesis • Needs to be relevant for the presented health-care problem • Possibly secondary and tertiary research questions
Research design, study population and methods	• Description of research design • Description of the study population • In- and exclusion criteria • Sample size calculation • Description of variables to be measured • Validity and reliability of the measurement instruments • Statistical analyses plan • Expected tables and figures
Feasibility and planning	• Planning of the work, with enough time for reading and summarizing the literature, data collection, analyses, and interpretation
Reference list	

PICO(t)

P   the patient, the research population, or the research problem;
I   the intervention, the determinant (also referred to as the exposure), or a prognostic factor;
C   the comparison;
O   the outcome variable;
(t)   the time period, which is sometimes added to a question. This is not a necessity.

Note that the order of these items in the research question does not necessarily follow PICO(t): the outcome variable is usually mentioned first, then the intervention. ▶ Example 1.1 shows an exemplary research question for the COmbinatie Behandeling Reumatoïde Artritis (COBRA)-light trial [1].

Example 1.1

Possible research question COBRA-light trial

Is there a difference in the decrease of the disease activity (the outcome, O) between the COBRA-light strategy (the intervention, I) and the COBRA strategy (the comparison, C) in patients with early rheumatoid arthritis (the patient, P) after 52 weeks of treatment (the time, T)?

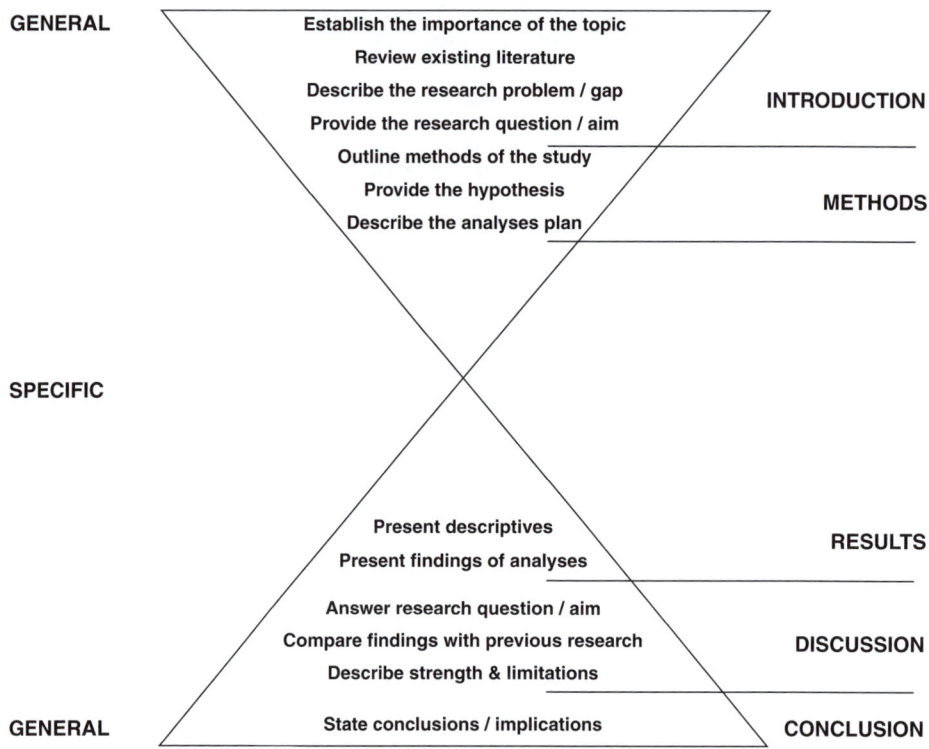

☐ Fig. 1.1 Hourglass template for writing a research proposal and scientific paper

The research question is then translated in two hypotheses: the null hypothesis and the alternative hypothesis. All statistical analyses considered in ►Chaps. 3–7 test whether the null hypothesis is true or not. The alternative hypothesis (denoted by H1 or Ha) is the hypothesis that is expected to be true, but until proven otherwise, the null hypothesis (denoted by H0) is the working hypothesis. In general, the alternative hypothesis states that there is a difference between the groups or that there is an association between two variables. The null hypothesis states the opposite, i.e., that there is no difference or no association.

Example 1.2

Possible null and alternative hypothesis COBRA-light trial
H0: there is no difference in decrease of the disease activity between the COBRA-light and the COBRA strategy;
H1: there is a difference in decrease of the disease activity between the COBRA-light and the COBRA strategy.

The alternative hypothesis of ►Example 1.2 aims to prove superiority of one treatment over the other. Sometimes, the alternative hypothesis aims to prove non-inferiority of one treatment compared to the other or equivalence between two treatments, because, for example, one treatment has less side effects or is less expensive [1, 2]. The COBRA-light trial was designed to prove non-inferiority of the COBRA-light strategy compared to the COBRA-strategy. The corresponding research question is stated in ▶Example 1.3.

Example 1.3

Actual research question COBRA-light trial
Is the change in the disease activity (the outcome, O) in the COBRA-light strategy (the intervention, I) non-inferior compared to the COBRA strategy (the comparison, C) in patients with early rheumatoid arthritis (the patient, P) after 26 weeks of treatment (the time, T)?

1.5 Research Designs, Study Population and Methods

1.5.1 Research Designs

The next step is to choose a research design. Many types of research designs exist, each with advantages and disadvantages. Knowing what these are, will help you to choose the most suitable design. A major distinction is made between fundamental, quantitative and qualitative research.

Fundamental research focuses on basic principles, basic mechanisms and theoretical understandings. For example, how does a normal cell turn into a cancer cell or what is the effect of certain types of endothelial and smooth muscle cells on cardiac explants [3]. Fundamental medical research is often called translational research, and aims to find new practical uses for new discoveries [4].

In quantitative research, a specific outcome variable is measured to investigate, for example, how often a certain outcome occurs within the population or how much a certain measure changes after a fixed time period or intervention [5, 6]. Advantages of quantitative research is that a lot of data can be collected in a short time period. And it is easily quantifiable. A disadvantage of quantitative research is that only data is collected on what is investigated, providing no information on, for example, opinions or emotions [5].

With qualitative research, in-depth information on phenomena is gathered, for example on opinions, emotions or problems that participants encounter. Questions such as "what", "how" or "why" are studied, instead of questions such as "how much" and "how often". Participants are studied in their natural setting (if possible), attempting to interpret phenomena in terms of meanings people bring to them [7]. With qualitative research, findings of quantitative studies could be explained or the treatment impact on the patient as seen by the patient him- or herself could be monitored. An example of qualitative research is a study on the impact of rheumatoid arthritis (RA) on patients' life as seen by the patients themselves [8]. A disadvantage of qualitative research is that it only provides information on the subjects under study and is not generalizable to the research population as a whole. Qualitative research produces hypotheses that can be verified by quantitative research.

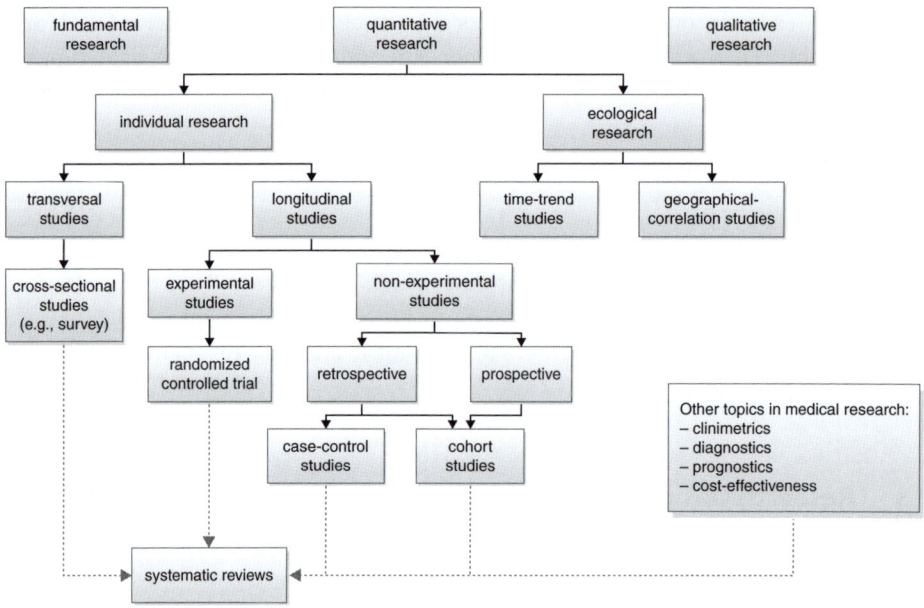

■ **Fig. 1.2**   Overview of research designs, parts used from Bouter et al. [5]

Most of the research worldwide is quantitative research. Many different types of quantitative research are distinguished (■Fig. 1.2).

Ecological Versus Individual Research

In ecological research, individuals are compared to each other at the population level, such as countries, hospitals, or schools. Populations are compared over time in time-trend studies or between geographical sites in geographical-correlation studies. An example of a time-trend study is a study on the change in long-term treatment response of patients with hematological malignancies over time [9]. An example of a geographical-correlation study is a study on global geographical variations in myocardial infarction management [10].

In individual research, individuals are compared to each other at the individual level. Individual research is either transversal or longitudinal. In transversal studies, also known as cross-sectional studies, all variables are measured at once, at the same point in time, such as in a survey. Transversal studies aim to establish the prevalence of a disease or an event, or the variation between patients. For example, a study assessing the anxiety of parents whose children will undergo cardiac surgery [11]. Advantages are that a large population is studied at once and it is less costly in comparison to other study designs. A disadvantage is that it is not possible to make causal inference, i.e., establish an association between cause and effect. In longitudinal research the outcome variable and the determinant are measured repeatedly over time. Longitudinal research is divided into experimental and non-experimental research.

Experimental Versus Non-Experimental Studies

In experimental studies, such as randomized controlled trials (RCTs), the allocation of the determinant (e.g., therapy or placebo) is determined by randomization. These type of trials are highly controlled, and therefore lead to less bias in the study population, the determinant, and the results. The COBRA-light trial is an example of an RCT. Experimental studies provide the highest level of evidence and intend to find a causal association between the outcome variable and the determinant. However, external validity is low because the study population is highly selected, based on in- and exclusion criteria. Moreover, these type of studies can be very expensive and it may be difficult to recruit patients. After all, the type of treatment they will receive depends on chance.

In non-experimental studies, further divided into prospective and retrospective studies, allocation of the determinant is not determined by randomization. In prospective studies, the study population is followed over time to assess the outcome in the future, for example, the incidence of a certain disease or event, or to assess changes over time within the subjects. In retrospective studies, the outcome is assessed at the time of the study while the exposure of interest is assessed by looking back in time.

Retrospective Versus Prospective Cohort Studies

Both retrospective and prospective studies are a form of cohort studies. That is, participants with similar exposures or similar characteristics are included. An example of a prospective cohort study is a study on the effect of undergoing a coronary artery bypass grafting on work participation [12], as well as the study of van de Stadt et al. [13]. An example of a retrospective cohort study is the assessment of the safety and risk factors of revision adenoidectomy in children and adolescents, through a nationwide retrospective population-based cohort study [14]. An advantage of a prospective cohort study is that it could be performed when an RCT is not ethical to perform. Furthermore, the only way to establish the incidence of a certain disease or event is through prospective or retrospective cohort studies. Some causality could also be established with cohort studies. After all, the outcome variable is always measured after the exposure to the determinant occurred. An important disadvantage is that cohort studies are especially prone to selection bias (e.g., for a specific treatment) and confounding. Selection bias is bias arisen through the selection procedure of the study population resulting in a non-representative sample of the research population. Moreover, if a disease is rare, many patients are required and follow-up time needs to be sufficiently long for the event to occur. As a consequence, prospective cohort studies can be quite expensive to perform, contrary to retrospective cohort studies.

A special type of retrospective cohort studies are case-control studies. In such studies, a group of patients with the disease state of interest (called the cases) are compared to a group of patients without the disease state of interest (called the controls). In both the cases and the controls, the determinant of interest is assessed in the past. An example of a case-control study, is a study on the benefit of an operating vehicle preventing peritonitis in peritoneal dialysis patients [15]. An advantage of a case-control study is that the outcome is already assessed, leading to a shorter study time and lower costs. A disadvantage is the high susceptibility to several kinds of bias such as selection bias and recall bias. Recall bias is a systematic error caused by differences in the accuracy or completeness of the recollections retrieved (recalled) by study participants regarding events or experiences from the past [16].

Systematic Reviews

A final type of research is a systematic review. As many researchers publish their work, multiple scientific papers on a specific topic are available. Systematic reviews summarize the existing literature, based on a specific clinical research question. A systematic plan has to be followed to provide the strengths and weaknesses of the evidence that is presented on the specific topic. In- and exclusion criteria are used to select relevant scientific papers. For each paper the risk of bias is assessed by several checklists. A meta-analysis of all included scientific papers could be performed if the heterogeneity between the papers is not too big, i.e., they used similar selection criteria for the study population and the same instruments to measure the outcome. A meta-analysis is a statistical analysis that combines the results of the included studies to estimate an overall (pooled) effect. In case of high heterogeneity, a meta-analysis might not be possible, but a systematic overview of the separate results could give a reliable overall conclusion. The Cochrane Library is a database consisting of many systematic reviews on a wide variety of topics, and also provides guidelines on how to conduct a systematic review [17, 18].

Research Topics within Research Designs

RCTs, and cohort or case-control studies are the most commonly chosen research designs in medical research. However, these designs could also be used to assess specific topics as well, such as clinimetrics, prognostic outcomes, and cost-effectiveness. In a study with a clinimetric topic, new measurement instruments are developed and their psychometric properties, i.e., reliability and validity, are determined. Also the psychometric properties of existing measurement instruments are studied. Reliability (of the instrument) refers to the overall consistency of the measurement instrument: if nothing changes at all, the measurement value should be the same as well. It is the degree to which the instrument is free from measurement error. Validity is the degree to which the instrument measures the construct it is intended to measure [19]. Many measurement instruments exist, often assessing the same outcome variable. Selecting the most reliable and valid instrument to measure the determinant and the outcome variable could be quite difficult. Therefore, a critical appraisal of existing instruments according to a standardized checklist, such as the COnsensus-based Standards for the selection of health Measurement Instruments (COSMIN), is advised. The COSMIN initiative aims to improve the selection of instruments, to evaluate the methodological quality of studies on measurement properties, and to serve as a guide for designing or reporting research on measurement properties [19–21].

In prognostic research/studies, or prediction studies, the outcome is predicted by other variables measured prior to assessment of the outcome, for example baseline variables. Prognostic studies are in fact also cohort studies. The only difference is that several risk factors (multiple determinants) are selected to predict the outcome variable, instead of investigating the association between the outcome variable and a single determinant (►Chap. 7). The RA-cohort of van de Stadt et al. was set up as a prediction study [13].

Finally, in a study with an economic evaluation focus, medical research is combined with cost evaluation analyses. In these analyses the costs of new treatment modalities and their efficacy are compared to the cost and efficacy of existing treatment options. Data on patients' expenses are collected, as well as costs for hospital and primary care expenses whilst monitoring or treating the patient. To authorize the use of new treatment, national public health agencies require such type of research.

We provide references with more detailed information on various designs in the further readings (▶Sect. 1.8).

1.5.2 Study Population

Ideally, one would include every individual of the population of interest (also referred to as the research population) to obtain an accurate estimate of the effect in this population. However, this is not feasible, so a selection has to be made. Different terms are used to describe the group of selected study participants as well as the individuals within this group: study population or (study) sample, and patients, participants, or subjects, amongst others. As long as the same terminology is used throughout the proposal (or scientific paper), the reader knows to which group is being referred to. In this book, individuals are referred to as patients, the group of patients under study is called the study population and the general population is called the research population.

Individuals are selected for the study population based on in- and exclusion criteria to establish a homogenous population. This allows for generalization of the results to the research population. The inclusion criteria describe all criteria a patient has to meet to be included in the study. The exclusion criteria describe all criteria a patient cannot meet.

Example 1.4

In- and exclusion criteria COBRA-light trial

Inclusion criteria
- Active rheumatoid arthritis according to American college of Rheumatology 1987 criteria;
- $\geq$ 6 swollen joints or $\geq$ 6 painful joints;
- Disease duration < 2 years;
- Erythrocyte sedimentation rate $\geq$ 28 mm and/or general health score of $\geq$ 20 measured by a visual analogue scale;
- Age $\geq$ 18 years.

Exclusion criteria
- Prior treatment with disease modifying anti-rheumatic drugs except hydroxychloroquine;
- Insulin-dependent diabetes mellitus;
- Uncontrollable non-insulin dependent diabetes mellitus;

- Heart failure based on the New York Heart Association classification class 3–4;
- Uncontrollable hypertension;
- Alanine-aminotransferase or aspartate transaminase > 3 times the normal values;
- Reduced renal function (serum creatinine > 15 mmol/L);
- Contra-indications for methotrexate, sulphasalazine or prednisolone;
- Indications of probable tuberculosis.

To avoid selection bias, it is important to keep track of the number of patients that were invited to participate. If possible, also collect the reasons for not participating. In the research proposal, the selection procedure of the study population always has to be described, ideally including a flowchart illustrating the selection procedure. ■Figure 1.3 shows an exemplary flowchart.

Sample Size Calculation

A sample size calculation (or power calculation) is mandatory in every research proposal. The more patients included, the more certain one will be about the conclusion of the research question. Time and money constraints may limit the number of patients to be included. And it may be unethical to withhold an effective new treatment from patients, by randomizing them to receive a placebo or standard treatment. On the other hand, too few patients may limit the statistical funding for a solid conclusion. When testing a null hypothesis, the probability that it is falsely rejected (i.e., it is actually true) should be as small as possible while the probability that it is truly rejected (i.e., it is actually false) should be as high as possible. The first probability is the significance level (denoted by α, alpha), the second probability is one minus the power (denoted by β, beta) of a statistical test (see also ► Chap. 2). At a given expected (or clinical relevant) effect, the required sample size is calculated for a fixed significance level and power. The sample size is a trade-off between a low significance level and a high power. The higher the power, the larger the sample size. On the other hand, the lower the significance level, the larger the sample size. However, a significance level of zero and a power of one is impossible. Moreover, the larger the expected effect, the smaller the sample size. Once the significance level is fixed in the sample size calculation, that significance level is also used for the statistical analyses. It is usually set at 0.05 whereas the power β is usually set at 0.8. A wide variety of statistical software, such as G*Power and PASS, is available to compute the sample size.

In the sample size calculation, one must also take into account possible dropout of patients. A common mistake in accounting for dropout, is to calculate the anticipated number of drop-out patients from the result of the sample size calculation. This is incorrect, the sample size calculation provides the number of patients that do not drop out. So to account for dropout, always multiply the result of the sample size calculation by $\frac{100}{(100 - \text{drop out rate})}$.

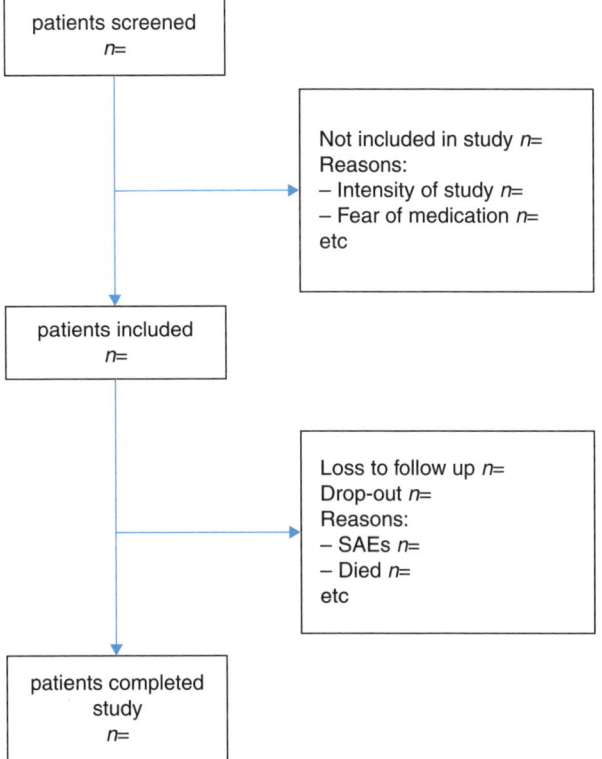

■ **Fig. 1.3**   An example of a flowchart

Example 1.5

Sample size calculation of the COBRA-light trial
The primary outcome variable of the COBRA-light trial was the change in disease activity score in 44 joints after 26 weeks. The sample size calculation for this trial was as follows. To detect non-inferiority between the COBRA-light and the COBRA strategy of at most 0.5 points, with a standard deviation of 1.05, 71 patients per arm were needed with a two-sided significance level of 0.05 (which is equivalent to a one-sided significance level of 0.025) and a power of 0.8.
Taking a dropout rate of 10 % into account, the minimum number of patients needed was $71 \times \frac{100}{100 - 10} = 78.8$. Therefore 79 patients per arm, and 158 patients in total, were required.
Note that the study was not designed to prove superiority of COBRA–light strategy.

Informed Consent

Patients participating in medical research always have to be informed about the study before they are included. They need to know what the aim of the study is and what the possible risks and benefits are. Therefore, each patient participating in medical research has to sign an informed consent form. This form needs to be approved by a Medical Ethical Review Board (MERB). An MERB reviews research proposals and decides whether the study can be conducted. In making their decision, the review board keeps the burden for participants, the ethics and the possible revenue of the study in mind. Also, all research has to be conducted in agreement with the Declaration of Helsinki [22], and Good Clinical Practice (GCP) guidelines

1.5.3 Methods

The research proposal also requires a description of the study methods. These methods include all data that will be collected, such as laboratory tests, radiological images and questionnaires, and the frequency of visits. For every measurement instrument, the psychometric properties need to be provided, to avoid measurement bias. This provides insight in the quality of the measurement instruments and hence on the quality of the results.

At last, a short analyses plan needs to be worked out. This plan contains all steps that will be taken to analyze the data:

- What is the outcome variable, what is, or are the determinant(s), and of what type are they?
- What are the characteristics of the study population (e.g., mean age, disease duration, etc.)?
- Which statistical tests are used, and what is the significance level?
- What assumption are checked, and how?
- Which potential influencing factors, i.e., confounders, effect modifiers and mediators, are checked and corrected for (if necessary)?
- How is missing data handled?
- Which patients are included in the intention-to-treat analysis (i.e., all randomized patients) and which in the per-protocol analysis (i.e., exclusion of patients with protocol deviations due to, for example, intake of concomitant medication or non-sufficient exposure)?

Ideally, one also works out how the results will be presented in the scientific paper. All these steps are described in detail in ▶ Chaps. 2–8.

1.6   Feasibility and Planning

The last part of the proposal contains the feasibility and planning. Although this part may speak for itself, especially for the MERB and the sponsor of the study, the planning is essential. This includes the inclusion period, end date of the study, and expected submission of the scientific paper(s). It provides clarity on how long the study will take before the results are published.

1.7 Preparing the Database

As soon as the research proposal has been written, and is approved by the MERB, patients are included and data collection starts. A lot of data will be collected and saved into a database (or dataset) that is analyzed after the study has finished. Before analyzing the data, the data needs to be validated. Possible outliers need to be checked, missing data needs to be established and confirmed if truly missing (▶Chap. 8), and privacy data needs to be deleted. If not screened carefully, incorrect conclusions could be drawn since all results (and hence conclusions) are determined by the quality of the prepared data. Although this step is time consuming, it is really necessary to assure valid data.

1.8 Further Readings

We did not pay detailed attention to writing a study protocol, which is the document the MERB actually reviews. The study protocol mainly consists of the same topics as a research proposal. The Standard Protocol Items: Recommendations for Interventional Trials (SPIRIT) statement provides recommendations for a minimum set of scientific, ethical, and administrative elements that should be addressed in a clinical trial protocol [23–25].

Some general and specific textbooks are available for the different study designs, such as the books written by Bouter et al. and Ahrens & Pigeot (general) or Jadad & Enkin (for RCTs) [5, 26, 27]. There are a limited number of books and papers on time-trend studies, but the book written by Dragt is noteworthy [28]. For more information on geographical-correlation studies, read the books written by Elliot et al. and Ahrens & Pigeot [26, 29]. Two good basic books on qualitative research are written by Flick and by Maxwell [30, 31]. For a good book on translational science, we advise the book written by Wehling [32]. For more information on clinimetric research, read the book written by de Vet et al. [33]. For information on systematic reviews, we refer to the Cochrane handbook [34], and on meta-analysis to the book written by Cleophas & Zwinderman [35]. Two basic books on cost-effectiveness analyses are written by Muennig and by Nuemann et al. [36, 37]. Elashoff & Lemeshow wrote a good chapter on sample size determination in the Handbook of epidemiology [26, 38]. Non-inferiority and equivalence trials have received increasing attention during the last decades. The basic concepts of these trials, with illustrative figures explaining the differences between such study designs and 'classical' superiority designs, are explained well, for example, by Siegel and Walker & Nowacki [39, 40].

References

1. ter Wee MM, den Uyl D, Boers M, Kerstens P, Nurmohamed M, van Schaardenburg D, et al. Intensive combination treatment regimens, including prednisolone, are effective in treating patients with early rheumatoid arthritis regardless of additional etanercept: 1-year results of the COBRA-light open-label, randomised, non-inferiority trial. Ann Rheum Dis. 2015;74(6):1233–40. ▶ https://doi.org/10.1136/annrheumdis-2013-205143.

2. den Uyl D, ter Wee MM, Boers M, Kerstens P, Voskuyl A, Nurmohamed M, et al. A non-inferiority trial of an attenuated combination strategy ('COBRA-light') compared to the original COBRA strategy: clinical results after 26 weeks. Ann Rheum Dis. 2014;73(6):1071–8. ► https://doi.org/10.1136/annrheumdis-2012-202818.

3. Zakharova IS, Zhiven MK, Saaya SB, Shevchenko AI, Smirnova AM, Strunov A, et al. Endothelial and smooth muscle cells derived from human cardiac explants demonstrate angiogenic potential and suitable for design of cell-containing vascular grafts. J Transl Med. 2017;15(1):54. ► https://doi.org/10.1186/s12967-017-1156-1.

4. Mahla RS. Stem cells applications in regenerative medicine and disease therapeutics. Int J Cell Biol. 2016;2016:6940283. ► https://doi.org/10.1155/2016/6940283.

5. Bouter LM, van Dongen MJCM, Zielhuis GA. Textbook of epidemiology. Houten: Bohn Stafleu van Loghum; 2017.

6. McCusker K, Gunaydin S. Research using qualitative, quantitative or mixed methods and choice based on the research. Perfusion. 2015;30(7):537–42. ► https://doi.org/10.1177/0267659114559116.

7. Kvrgic Z, Asiedu GB, Crowson CS, Ridgeway JL, Davis JM, 3rd. "Like no one is listening to me": a qualitative study of patient-provider discordance between global assessments of disease activity in rheumatoid arthritis. Arthritis Care Res (Hoboken). 2017. ► https://doi.org/10.1002/acr.23501.

8. ter Wee MM, van Tuyl LH, Blomjous BS, Lems WF, Boers M, Terwee CB. Content validity of the Dutch Rheumatoid Arthritis Impact of Disease (RAID) score: results of focus group discussions in established rheumatoid arthritis patients and comparison with the international classification of functioning, disability and health core set for rheumatoid arthritis. Arthritis Res Ther. 2016;18:22. ► https://doi.org/10.1186/s13075-015-0911-z.

9. de Vries VA, Muller MCA, Sesmu Arbous M, Biemond BJ, Blijlevens NMA, Kusadasi N, et al. Time trend analysis of long term outcome of patients with haematological malignancies admitted at dutch intensive care units. Br J Haematol. 2018. ► https://doi.org/10.1111/bjh.15140.

10. Rossello X, Huo Y, Pocock S, van de Werf F, Chin CT, Danchin N, et al. Global geographical variations in ST-segment elevation myocardial infarction management and post-discharge mortality. Int J Cardiol. 2017;245:27–34. ► https://doi.org/10.1016/j.ijcard.2017.07.039.

11. Kobayashi D, Turner DR, Forbes TJ, Aggarwal S. Parental anxiety among children undergoing cardiac catheterisation. Cardiol Young. 2017:1–7. ► https://doi.org/10.1017/s1047951117002074.

12. Butt JH, Rorth R, Kragholm K, Kristensen SL, Torp-Pedersen C, Gislason GH, et al. Return to the workforce following coronary artery bypass grafting: a Danish nationwide cohort study. Int J Cardiol. 2017. ► https://doi.org/10.1016/j.ijcard.2017.10.032.

13. van de Stadt LA, Witte BI, Bos WH, van Schaardenburg D. A prediction rule for the development of arthritis in seropositive arthralgia patients. Ann Rheum Dis. 2013;72(12):1920–6. ► https://doi.org/10.1136/annrheumdis-2012-202127.

14. Lin DL, Wu CS, Tang CH, Kuo TY, Tu TY. The safety and risk factors of revision adenoidectomy in children and adolescents: a nationwide retrospective population-based cohort study. Auris Nasus Larynx. 2018;45(6):1191–8. ► https://doi.org/10.1016/j.anl.2018.03.002.

15. Fang P, Lu J, Liu YH, Deng HM, Zhang L, Zhang HQ. Benefit of an operating vehicle preventing peritonitis in peritoneal dialysis patients: a retrospective, case-controlled study. Int Urol Nephrol. 2018. ► https://doi.org/10.1007/s11255-018-1823-z.

16. Last JM, editor. A dictionary of epidemiology. New York: Oxford University Press; 2001.

17. Cochrane. Cochrane Library. ► http://www.cochranelibrary.com. Accessed 2 Oct 2018.

18. Higgins JPT, Green S, editors. Cochrane handbook for systematic reviews of interventions version 5.1.0 [updated March 2011]. The Cochrane Collaboration; 2011. Available from ► http://handbook.cochrane.org.

19. Mokkink LB, Terwee CB, Knol DL, Stratford PW, Alonso J, Patrick DL, et al. Protocol of the COSMIN study: COnsensus-based Standards for the selection of health Measurement INstruments. BMC Med Res Methodol. 2006;6:2. ► https://doi.org/10.1186/1471-2288-6-2.

20. Mokkink LB, Prinsen CA, Bouter LM, de Vet HCW, Terwee CB. The COnsensus-based Standards for the selection of health Measurement INstruments (COSMIN) and how to select an outcome measurement instrument. Braz J Phys Ther. 2016;20(2):105–13. ► https://doi.org/10.1590/bjpt-rbf.2014.0143.

21. Mokkink LB, Terwee CB, Knol DL, Stratford PW, Alonso J, Patrick DL, et al. The COSMIN checklist for evaluating the methodological quality of studies on measurement properties: a clarification of its content. BMC Med Res Methodol. 2010;10:22. ► https://doi.org/10.1186/1471-2288-10-22.

22. World Medical Association. World medical association declaration of Helsinki: ethical principles for medical research involving human subjects. JAMA. 2013;310(20):2191–4. ► https://doi.org/10.1001/jama.2013.281053.

23. Chan AW, Tetzlaff JM, Altman DG, Dickersin K, Moher D. SPIRIT 2013: new guidance for content of clinical trial protocols. Lancet. 2013;381(9861):91–2. ▶https://doi.org/10.1016/s0140-6736(12)62160-6.

24. Chan AW, Tetzlaff JM, Altman DG, Laupacis A, Gotzsche PC, Krleza-Jeric K, et al. SPIRIT 2013 statement: defining standard protocol items for clinical trials. Ann Intern Med. 2013;158(3):200–7. ▶https://doi.org/10.7326/0003-4819-158-3-201302050-00583.

25. Chan AW, Tetzlaff JM, Gotzsche PC, Altman DG, Mann H, Berlin JA, et al. SPIRIT 2013 explanation and elaboration: guidance for protocols of clinical trials. BMJ. 2013;346:e7586. ▶https://doi.org/10.1136/bmj.e7586.

26. Ahrens W, Pigeot I. Handbook of epidemiology. New York: Springer; 2014.

27. Jadad AR, Enkin MW. Randomized controlled trials. Questions, answers and musings. Malden: Wiley-Blackwell; 2007.

28. Dragt E. How to research trends: move beyond trend watching to kick start innovation. Amsterdam: BIS Publishers; 2017.

29. Elliot P, Cuzick D, English D, Stern R. Geographical and environmental epidemiology. Methods for small-area studies. Oxford: Oxford University Press; 1996.

30. Flick U. An introduction to qualitative research. London: Sage Publications Ltd; 2014.

31. Maxwell JA. Qualitative research design: an interactive approach. Thousands Oaks: Sage Publications Ltd; 2013.

32. Wehling M. Principles of translational science in medicine: from bench to bedside. London: Academic Press; 2015.

33. de Vet HCW, Terwee CB, Mokkink LB, Knol DL. Measurement in medicine. Cambridge: Cambridge University Press; 2011.

34. Gough D, Oliver S, Thomas J. An introduction to systematic reviews. Los Angeles: Sage Publications Ltd; 2017.

35. Cleophas TJ, Zwinderman AH. Modern meta-analysis. Review and update of methodologies. New York: Springer; 2017.

36. Muennig P. Cost-effectiveness analysis in health: a practical approach. 2nd ed. San Fransisco: Jossey-Bass; 2007.

37. Neumann PJ, Ganiats TG, Russel LB, Sanders GD, Siegel JE. Cost-effectiveness in health and medicine. New York: Oxford University Press; 2016.

38. Elashoff JD, Lemeshow S. Sample size determination in epidemiologic studies. In: Ahrens W, Pigeot I, editors. Handbook of epidemiology. New York: Springer; 2014.

39. Siegel JP. Equivalence and noninferiority trials. Am Heart J. 2000;139(4):S166–70. ▶https://doi.org/10.1016/s0002-8703(00)90066-8.

40. Walker E, Nowacki AS. Understanding equivalence and noninferiority testing. J Gen Intern Med. 2011;26(2):192–6. ▶https://doi.org/10.1007/s11606-010-1513-8.

Medical Statistics – the Basics

Abstract

Statistics is classified in two main fields: descriptive statistics and inferential statistics. Descriptive statistics summarize and visualize important features of the collected data, whereas inferential statistics generalize the results from the study population to the research population. In this chapter, we introduce important, basic statistical terminology as well as concepts that form the basis of the statistical analyses that are described in detail in the next chapters.

© Bohn Stafleu van Loghum is een imprint van Springer Media B.V., onderdeel van Springer Nature 2019
M. M. ter Wee and B. I. Lissenberg-Witte, *A Quick Guide on How to Conduct Medical Research*,
https://doi.org/10.1007/978-90-368-2248-0_2

2.1   Different Types of Variables

The choice of all statistical analyses is always based on the type of variables stated in the research question. The type of outcome variable as well as the type of the determinant are important. The determinant is a variable which affects the nature or outcome of interest. In medical research, this can, for example, be the received medical treatment such as in the COmbinatie Behandeling Reumatoïde Artritis (COBRA)-light trial [1]. Patients characteristics are also determinants, such as being anticyclic citrullinated peptide (aCCP) positive or having a first degree relative (FDR) with rheumatoid arthritis (RA) [2]. Other terms for the determinant are also used in medical research: the independent variable, the explanatory variable, the covariate, the risk factor or the exposure.

The outcome variable, also referred to as the dependent variable, is the variable that is influenced by the determinant. Examples are the disease activity score of 44 joints (DAS44) or the development of RA within 2 years. SPSS always uses the term dependent variable for the outcome variable, and, depending on the statistical analyses, independent variable, covariate or factor for the determinant. However we will use the terms determinant and outcome variable.

The determinant and the outcome variable can be measured at different levels, classified as categorical or continuous. These different levels are called the measurement level of the variable. Categorical variables consist of several mutually exclusive categories. These categories can be ordered or unordered. A categorical variable with unordered categories is called a nominal variable, for example marital status. A categorical variable with ordered categories is called an ordinal variable, such as underweight, healthy weight, overweight and obese. These levels are usually ranked 1, 2, 3, etc. for analyzing purposes, but these ranks are not interpretable. For example, having a healthy weight is not twice as much as having underweight. A categorical variable with only two categories is called a dichotomous variable, for instance being a smoker or non-smoker.

Continuous variables are values measured on a continuous scale and are divided in interval and ratio variables. An interval variable is a variable in which the distance between values is equally spaced and has a meaning. For example, the difference between a body mass index (BMI) of 20 kilograms per square meter (kg/m^2) and of 25 kg/m^2 is the same as the difference in BMI of 15 kg/m^2 and 20 kg/m^2. On the other hand, a BMI of 40 kg/m^2 is not twice as high as a BMI of 20 kg/m^2. A ratio variable is similar to an interval variable, but has an absolute zero that is meaningful. This allows for a relative comparison of values. Weight is an example of a ratio variable, after all 20 kg is twice the weight of 10 kg. The number of swollen joints is another example of a ratio variable.

Note that there is a hierarchy in the levels of measurement. A continuous variable has the highest level of accuracy or precision. If possible, always use a continuous outcome variable. An ordinal variable could be created from a ratio or interval variable, but a ratio or interval variable cannot be derived from an ordinal variable. Data from a continuous variable take on infinitely many values. After categorizing a continuous variable, a patient with an original value close to the lower bound of the category as well as a patient with an original value close to the upper bound of the category, will have the same categorical value and are therefore presumed to be the same. In other words, data is lost in case of categorizing a continuous variable.

A time to event variable, such as the time to development of RA, is a special case of a continuous variable. It measures the time it takes until a certain event occurs. However, the event may not occur during the study period, and analyzing only the patients with an event introduces bias in the results. Therefore, a time to event variable actually consists of two variables: a time variable and a status variable, i.e., indicating whether or not the event of interest occurred.

2.2 Descriptive Statistics

Regardless of the study design, the first step in all statistical analyses, is to become familiar with the data that was collected. With descriptive statistics, all measured variables of interest are summarized and/or visualized. Different descriptive measures are available for the different measurement levels. Categorical variables are generally described by frequencies (e.g., how many men and women) and percentages (e.g., the percentage of men and women).

2.2.1 Continuous Variables

Continuous variables are summarized with two measures: one measure to describe the central tendency of the data (the effect size), and one measure to describe the spread (or variation) of the data. Measures for the central tendency are:
- the mean, which is the sum of all values divided by the total number of values in the study population (or group);
- the median, which is the 'middle' value of all values in the study population (or the mean of the two middle values in case of an even sized study population);
- the mode, which is the value that occurs most often in the study population.

Measures for the spread are:
- the standard deviation (SD), which is calculated by $\sqrt{\frac{1}{n-1}\sum_{i=1}^{n}(x_i - \text{mean})^2}$ where n is the total number of patients in the study population, and x_i is the value of the variable of patient i;
- the range, which is the difference between the highest and the lowest value in the study population;
- the interquartile range (IQR), which is the difference between the 75th percentile and the 25th percentile in the study population.

A measure related to the SD is the variance and is equal to $(\text{SD})^2$. Note that the range and IQR as defined above are single values, representing a difference between two numbers. However, this difference does not provide any information on the observed values in the dataset itself. For example, a range of 10 could correspond to values between -5 and $+5$ or to values between $+25$ and $+35$. The range in combination with the mean or median becomes more evident. However, with a median of zero, a range of 10 could still indicate that the values lie between -8 and $+2$ or between -2 and $+8$. It is important to distinguish these differences, therefore we suggest to report both the range and the IQR when the median is reported.

Example 2.1

Calculating descriptive statistics

In an example database with 15 patients (i.e., $n = 15$), the observed values of a continuous outcome variable are: 2, 4, 4, 9, 2, 9, 8, 2, 1, 8, 1, 1, 2, 4, and 2.

The study population mean is equal to

$$\frac{2+4+4+9+2+9+8+2+1+8+1+1+2+4+2}{15} = \frac{59}{15} = 3.9.$$

The observed values ranked from smallest to largest are 1, 1, 1, 2, 2, 2, 2, 2, 4, 4, 4, 8, 8, 9, and 9. The middle number is the median, in this case 2.

The values one and four are observed three times, the value two five times, and the values eighth and nine are observed twice. The value two is observed the most frequent, hence the mode is 2.

The study population SD is equal to

$$\sqrt{\frac{(2 - 3.9)^2 + (4 - 3.9)^2 + (4 - 3.9)^2 + \ldots + (4 - 3.9)^2 + (2 - 3.9)^2}{15 - 1}} = \sqrt{\frac{129.0}{14}} = 3.04.$$

The range is equal to $9 - 1 = 8$ which we reported as 1–9.

The 25th percentile is equal to 2 (the 4th number of the ordered outcome values) and the 75th percentile is equal to 8 (the 12th number of the ordered outcome values), so the IQR is equal to $8 - 2 = 6$ which we report as [2–8].

2.2.2 Distribution of Continuous Variables

Which descriptive statistics for a continuous variable are reported, depends on the distribution of the continuous variable. The distribution of a continuous outcome variable determines which statistical method needs to be used (► Chap. 3). Although a continuous variable could be distributed in several ways, we only distinguish between normally distributed and non-normally distributed continuous variables. Whether a continuous variable is normally distributed or not could be assessed through different methods, of which we will describe four.

The first option to check normality of a continuous variable is by visual inspection of a histogram. In a histogram, the (relative) frequency of observations falling in each bar is plotted on the y-axis. The histogram of a normally distributed variable is symmetric and follows the bell shape distribution, also known as the Gaussian distribution. □Figure 2.1a shows

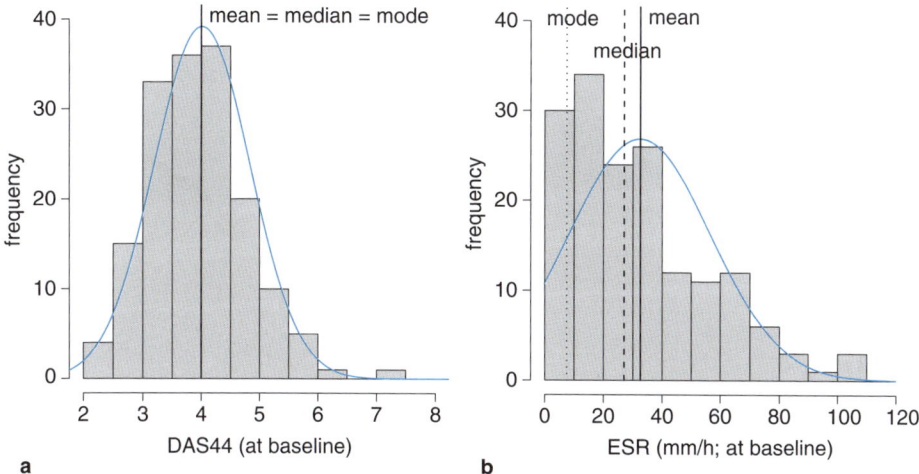

■ **Fig. 2.1** Histogram of a normally distributed variable (**a**) and a non-normally distributed variable (**b**). The curve is the reference curve of the normal distribution

the histogram of the DAS44 and ■Fig. 2.1b shows the histogram of the erythrocyte sedimentation rate (ESR), both measured at baseline in the COBRA-light trial. The histogram in ■Fig. 2.1a follows the Gaussian distribution (the reference line) so we conclude that the DAS44 at baseline is fairly normally distributed, while the ESR at baseline is clearly not.

The histogram of a non-normally distributed continuous variable can have many different shapes, for example, with more than one mode, or long 'tails'. Variables with long 'tails', such as ■Fig. 2.1b, are said to have a skewed distribution, either skewed to the left or to the right. Skewed to the right means that the 'tail' of the distribution is on the right side of the histogram, skewed to the left means that the tail is on the left side of the histogram.

A second option to visually check the distribution of the outcome variable is with a quantile-quantile plot (QQ-plot; ■Fig. 2.2). The QQ-plot plots the quantiles of the observed data against the quantiles of the expected value under the assumption of a normal distribution. If the points of the QQ-plot lie on the reference line, the variable is assumed to be normally distributed. The points with the lowest and highest value always deviate slightly from the reference line, but as long as the majority of the points lie on the reference line, normality could be assumed. Based on the QQ-plots, we again conclude that DAS44 at baseline is normally distributed (■Fig. 2.2a), as most of the dots lie on the reference line, while ESR (■Fig. 2.2b) is not.

The third option is a non-visual check using descriptive measures. For normally distributed variables, the mean, the median and the mode are almost the same (as is seen in ■Fig. 2.1a). Approximately half of the patients have a value smaller than the mean while the other half has a value larger than the mean. Moreover, values close to the mean are observed most frequently. Furthermore, for a non-negative continuous variable, the mean and the SD could be checked. In the case of a normal distribution, approximately 95 % of the patients should have a value between mean $-2 \times$ SD and mean $+2 \times$ SD. Thus, if mean $-2 \times$ SD is negative, the variable cannot be normally distributed.

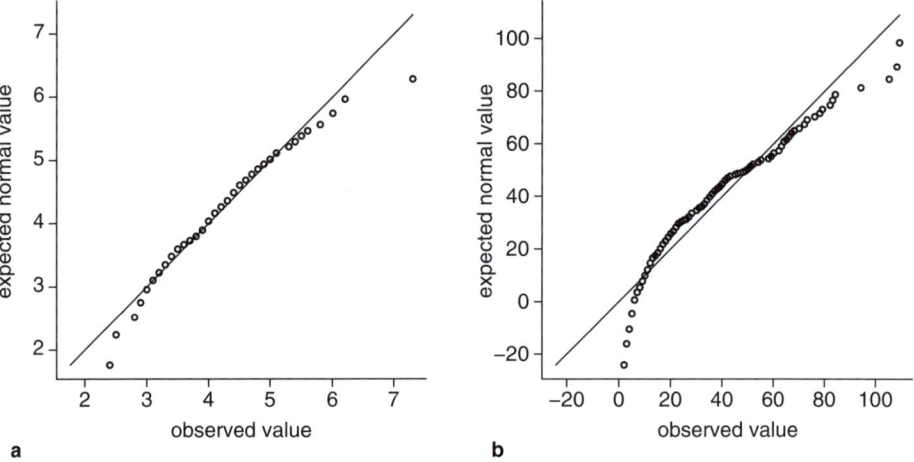

◼ Fig. 2.2   QQ-plot for DAS44 (**a**) and ESR (**b**) at baseline, in the COBRA-light trial

Finally, normality of the continuous variable could be assessed with statistical tests, for example, the Kolmogorov-Smirnov test or the Shapiro-Wilk test. However, these tests are not robust in large study populations: even for a very small deviation from normality, these tests almost always conclude that the variable is not normally distributed. On the other hand, detecting non-normality in small study populations is fairly impossible. We advise to check the distribution of the continuous outcome through the first three mentioned options, and not to solely rely on such statistical tests for normality. It should be noted that many descriptive measures and statistical methods are quite robust against small to moderate deviations from normality. Therefore, unless the data are clearly skewed, one should not worry about normality too much.

2.2.3   Time to Event Variables

When describing time to event variables, it is not sufficient to report the number of patients experiencing the event during the total study period, or the median time to event. This is because occurrence of the event might be censored in some patients. Censoring of the event refers to the phenomenon that not all patients may have experienced the event of interest at the end of a prospective study, or at the date of chart review in a retrospective study, and patients may be lost to follow-up. In many studies, the event of interest is death, and patients are then censored if they did not die before the end of the study or when they are lost to follow-up during the study. The event of interest could also be relapse or progression of a disease, or development of a disease in a high-risk population such as in the RA-cohort [2]. In case the event of interest is not death, patients are censored when they die, are lost to follow-up, or did not develop the disease at the end of the study. It is unknown when the patients would have had the event in case of censoring. Therefore, censoring cannot be ignored in the statistical analyses of a time to event variable.

Two appropriate descriptive measures that combine the time period and the number of experienced events, are the incidence rate and the cumulative incidence. The incidence rate is the number of experienced events (or new cases) divided by the total time during which all patients were at risk. The cumulative incidence at a specific time point t is the number of experienced events before time t divided by the size of the study population initially at risk.

Example 2.2

Incidence rate and cumulative incidence for the development of RA

In a (fictive) prospective cohort study on the development of RA amongst 100 high-risk patients with arthralgia, 10 patients developed RA after 1 year, 8 after 2 years, and 12 after 3 years. The remaining 70 patients did not develop RA within the total follow-up period of 5 years.

The total time at risk for the first 10 patients was $10 \times 1 = 10$ person-years, for the 8 who developed RA after two years this was $2 \times 8 = 16$ person-years, and for the 12 after three years this was $3 \times 12 = 36$ person-years. For the remaining 70 patients, their total time at risk was $70 \times 5 = 350$ person-years. The total person-years for the whole study population of 100 patients is equal to $10 + 16 + 36 + 350 = 412$ person-years. Since 30 patients developed RA during the total follow-up of 412 person-years, the incidence rate is equal to $30/412 = 0.073$. Or equivalently, 7.3 events per 100 person-years or 7.3 events per 100 patients per year.

The cumulative incidence of RA at 1 year is equal to $10/100 = 0.1$ (or 10 %), the cumulative incidence at 5 years is equal to $(10 + 8 + 12)/100 = 0.30$.

If patients are censored before the end of the study, for example due to death or drop-out, the cumulative incidence has to be estimated from the Kaplan-Meier curve. The Kaplan-Meier curve is an estimator for the probability that the event does not occur before a certain time point t, for all values of t up to the last observed follow-up time (◖Fig. 2.3a). This probability function of time is called survival function, and is usually denoted by $S(t)$. The probability that the event occurs before time t is calculated by one minus the probability that it does not occur before time t. The cumulative incidence curve (or one minus survival curve) at time t is estimated by one minus the Kaplan-Meier estimate at time t (◖Fig. 2.3b). The (one minus) Kaplan-Meier curve is the best graphical representation of a time to event outcome variable. At each time t, it provides the probability that the event has not occurred yet (or it has already occurred for the estimated cumulative incidence). In general, Kaplan-Meier curves are used for death related events, such as death itself (called overall survival) or disease specific death, while one minus Kaplan-Meier curves are used for other event types, such as development of RA.

The exact values of the Kaplan-Meier curve at each time t, is standard output in most of the statistical software packages. ◖Table 2.1 shows part of the SPSS output of the survival table of the RA-cohort. The first patient (first row "1") developed RA (under "Status", is equal to 'arthritis') within 0.23 months (under "Time"), and the probability

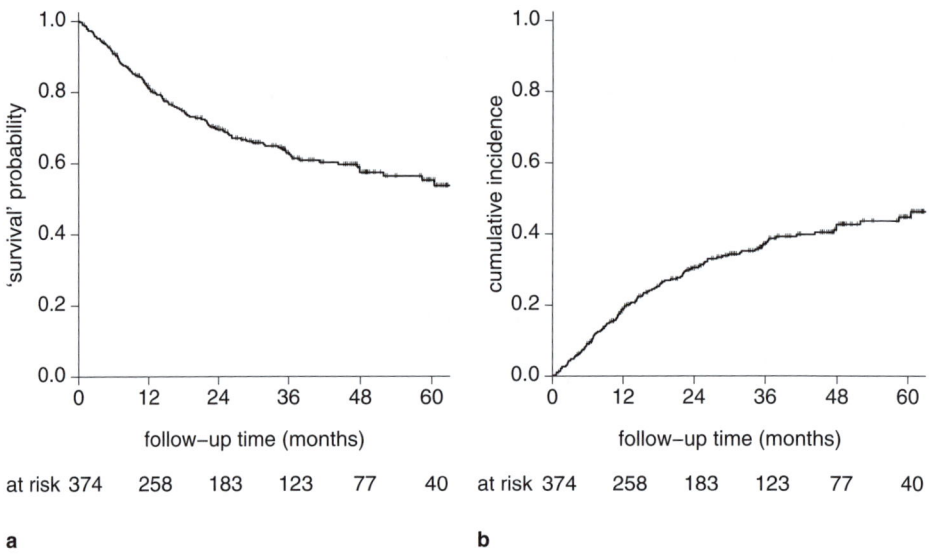

■ **Fig. 2.3**   The Kaplan-Meier curve (**a**) and one minus Kaplan-Meier curve (**b**) for the time to development of RA, in the RA-cohort

■ **Table 2.1**   Part of the SPSS output of the survival table for the probability of developing RA within a time period of 2 years

Survival Table

	Time	Status	Cumulative Proportion Surviving at the Time		N of Cumulative Events	N of Remaining Cases
			Estimate	Std. Error		
1	.230	arthritis	.997	.003	1	373
2	.624	arthritis	.995	.004	2	372
3	.657	arthritis	.992	.005	3	371
4	.690	arthritis	.989	.005	4	370
5	.986	no arthritis	.	.	4	369
6	1.051	arthritis	.987	.006	5	368
110	11.729	arthritis	.812	.021	67	264
111	11.729	no arthritis	.	.	67	263
120	11.959	no arthritis	.	.	67	254
121	12.025	arthritis	.809	.021	68	253
122	12.025	no arthritis	.	.	68	252
123	12.025	no arthritis	.	.	68	251
124	12.189	arthritis	.	.	69	250
125	12.189	arthritis	.803	.021	70	249
189	23.688	arthritis	.695	.026	101	185

◻ **Table 2.2** SPSS output of the estimated mean and median time to development of RA

Means and Medians for Survival Time							
Mean[a]				Median			
Estimate	Std. Error	95 % Confidence Interval		Estimate	Std. Error	95 % Confidence Interval	
		Lower Bound	Upper Bound			Lower Bound	Upper Bound
53.516	2.141	49.319	57.713	72.444	9.210	54.392	90.496

[a]Estimation is limited to the largest survival time if it is censored

of not developing RA before this time was 0.997 (under "Estimate"). Estimated values always have some uncertainty, which we explain in ▶ Sect. 2.3.3, and is reported under "Std. Error". Up to this time point, evidently, only one event occurred (under "N of Cumulative Events"), and 373 patients were still at risk of developing RA (under "N of Remaining Cases"). The second patient developed RA within 0.62 months, and the third within 0.66 months. Furthermore, censoring of a patient occurred for the first time after 0.99 months (the fifth patient in line). The "Cumulative Proportion Surviving at the Time" is not given, because this is equal to the cumulative proportion surviving at the previous time point. Also, the number of cumulative events does not change between the fourth and fifth patient (both equal to 4). However, the number of remaining cases decreased by one (from 370 to 369). The survival table is also used to present the number of patients at risk below the Kaplan-Meier curve.

From the Kaplan-Meier curve, the median time to event is estimated. This is the time point where the Kaplan-Meier curve is below 0.5 (or 50 %). In most statistical software, the median time to event is reported, also in SPSS (by default). SPSS also reports the estimated mean time to event, although this is never reported. After all, time to event outcome variables are never normally distributed, and for non-normally distributed outcome variables, the median is reported instead of the mean. ◻Table 2.2 shows the SPSS output with the estimated mean (under "Mean") and median (under "Median") time to develop RA. Both estimated values are reported under "Estimate". The uncertainty of both estimates are reported under "Std. Error" and are used to calculate the values under "95 % Confidence Interval" (see also ▶ Sect. 2.3.3). From this table, we see that the median time to event of the RA-cohort was 72.4 months. So the Kaplan-Meier curve for the RA-cohort was below 0.5 after 72.4 months. In other words, if all patients were followed until all developed RA, 50 % of the patients would have developed RA within 72.4 months.

2.2.4 Association Between Two Variables

Descriptive statistics can also be used to summarize the association between the determinant and the outcome variable.

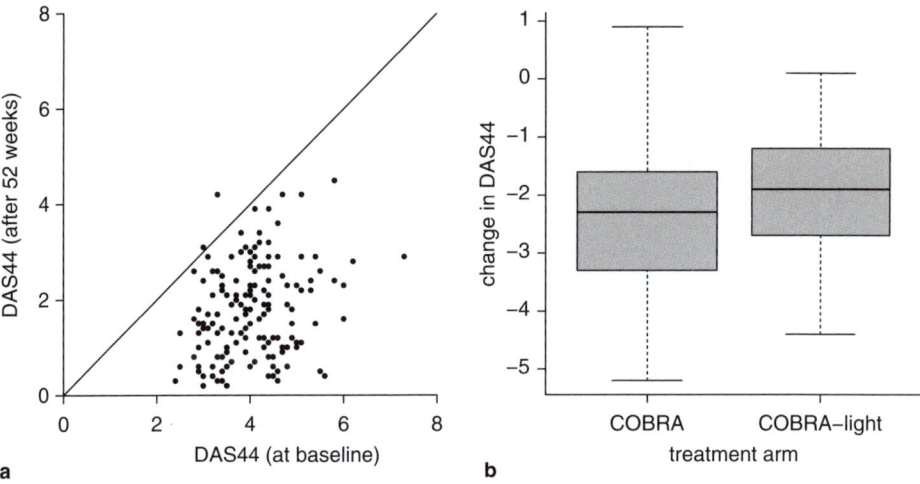

■ **Fig. 2.4**   Scatterplot for the association between the DAS44 at baseline and the DAS44 after 52 weeks in the COBRA-light trial (**a**), and a boxplot of the change in DAS44 after 52 weeks of treatment for the COBRA and the COBRA-light treatment separately (**b**)

The scatterplot is used to visualize the association between two continuous variables (■Fig. 2.4a). Each point in the scatterplot corresponds to a patient: his/her values of the determinant and the outcome variable are plotted on the x- and y-axis, respectively. An increasing pattern in the data points (going from left to right on the x-axis) indicates a positive association between the outcome variable and the determinant. A decreasing pattern indicates a negative association. Absence of an increasing or decreasing pattern indicates that there is no association between the outcome variable and the determinant. The closer the dots lie on an imaginary straight line, the stronger the association between the two variables.

The box-and-whisker plot (or just boxplot) is used to visualize the association between a continuous outcome variable and a categorical determinant (■Fig. 2.4b). The lower and upper part of the box represent the 25th and 75th percentile of the outcome variable within each group, the line in the middle of the box represents the median within each group. The end of the lines (called the whiskers) represent different values, depending on the statistical software used. In SPSS, they are the smallest observed value within $1.5 \times$ IQR above the 25th percentile (lower whisker), and the largest observed value within $1.5 \times$ IQR below the 75th percentile (upper whisker). The values outside the whiskers are considered outliers and are plotted as a separate dot ($\bigcirc$). SPSS distinguishes between outliers between 1.5 and 3 times the IQR and more than 3 times the IQR, the latter ones plotted as asterisks (*).

A $k \times 2$ contingency table (or crosstab, pivot table or multi-dimensional table) is used to summarize the association between a dichotomous outcome variable and categorical determinant with k groups. The two possible outcomes, of which one is the outcome of interest, are listed in the two columns of the table. The different groups of the determinant are listed in the k different rows of the table. ■Table 2.3 shows the general

◼ **Table 2.3** General form of a 2 × 2 crosstab

		Outcome		Total
		Event	No event	
Group	1	a	b	$n_1 = a + b$
	2	c	d	$n_2 = c + d$
Total		$a + c$	$b + d$	$n = n_1 + n_2$

form of a 2 × 2 crosstab, for a dichotomous determinant. The outcome of interest is denoted by event. Usually the number of patients in each cell of the table as well as the percentage per group are reported.

Kaplan-Meier curves are also used to visualize the association between a time to event outcome variable and a categorical determinant. For each group, the Kaplan-Meier curve (or one minus Kaplan-Meier curve) is plotted.

2.2.5 Reporting Descriptive Statistics

It is common practice to describe which descriptive statistics are reported in the statistical analyses section of a scientific paper. The descriptive statistics of the most important variables collected in the study are then summarized in the first table of the scientific paper. Such a table is sometimes referred to as the "Table 1" or "Demographics table". How the descriptive statistics are presented, depends on the design of the study. For example in a randomized controlled trial (RCT), descriptive statistics are reported for each of the arms separately, whereas in a prospective cohort study descriptive statistics are often reported for the whole study population. ◼Tables 2.4 and 2.5 are examples of (parts of) the demographics table of the COBRA-light trial and the RA-cohort. The total number of patients (for each arm in the case of an RCT, or in each group in a case-control study) is reported in the column headings. Information on missing data and the measures of central tendency and spread are printed in footnotes below the table. Moreover, the abbreviations used in the table are explained below the table. For normally distributed variables, the mean and SD are reported and for non-normally distributed variables, the median and (interquartile) range.

2.3 Inferential Statistics

Descriptive statistics provide information on the study population. To answer the research question, inferential statistics is needed. With inferential statistics, results and conclusions from the study population are generalized to the research population. Inferential statistics is divided in three topics: (i) estimating the difference between groups, or an association between the determinant and outcome variable, which we refer to as the effect size, (ii) quantifying the uncertainty of these estimates, and (iii) testing hypotheses.

◻ Table 2.4   Parts of the demographics table of the COBRA-light trial ($n = 162$) [1]. © BMJ & EULAR 2018

	COBRA ($n = 81$)	COBRA–light ($n = 81$)
Female	54 (67 %)	56 (69 %)
Age (years)	53.0 (13.0)	51.0 (12.8)
Disease duration (weeks)	15.5 [9.0–27.5]	16.5 [8.3–35.0]
IgM-RF positive[a]	47 (58 %)	46 (57 %)
aCCP positive[b]	50 (62 %)	53 (65 %)
DAS44	4.1 (0.74)	4.0 (0.90)
DAS28	5.5 (1.1)	5.3 (1.2)
Tender joints	15.0 [10.5–20.0]	14.0 [9.0–18.5]
Swollen joints	13.0 [10.0–17.0]	11.0 [8.5–14.5]
ESR (mm/h)	27.0 [14.5–44.5]	27.0 [12.0–49.0]
CRP (mg/L)	13.0 [4.5–27.0]	13.0 [4.0–31.0]
Patient assessment of global health (VAS; mm)	60.1 (22.9)	57.9 (25.5)

[a]missing for two patients in the COBRA-light arm
[b]missing for one patient in the COBRA-light arm
Continuous variables are described by mean (SD) or median [IQR], depending on its distribution
aCCP anticyclic citrullinated peptide, *CRPC* reactive protein, *DAS28* disease activity score of 28 joints, *DAS44* disease activity score of 44 joints, *ESR* erythrocyte sedimentation rate, *IgM-RF* rheumatoid factors type immunoglobulin M, *mg/L* milligrams per liter, *mm/h* millimeters per hour, *VAS* visual analogue scale

Below, we describe several effect sizes for a continuous and a dichotomous outcome variable. Effect sizes can also be calculated for time to event outcome variables, but this requires some more advanced statistics. We introduce the effect size for a time to event outcome variable in ▶Chap. 5.

2.3.1 Effect Size for a Continuous Outcome Variable

The effect size for the difference in a normally distributed continuous outcome variable between two groups, is the mean difference between the groups. Sometimes, this difference in mean between the groups is divided by the pooled SD of both groups. The pooled SD is equal to

$$\sqrt{\frac{(n_1 - 1) \times SD_1^2 + (n_2 - 1) \times SD_2^2}{n_1 + n_2 - 2}}. \tag{E2.1}$$

In this equation, n_1 and n_2 are the size of the study population of the two groups, and SD_1 and SD_2 are the SDs of the two groups. The standardized differences is called the Cohen's *d* effect size [3]. A Cohen's *d* around 0.2 is considered to indicate a small effect (or a

◘ **Table 2.5** The demographics table of the RA-cohort ($n = 374$)

	n (%)
Age (years)	48.8 (11.5)
FDR with RA	86 (23 %)
Current smoker[a]	113 (30 %)
No alcohol[b]	132 (37 %)
NSAID use	101 (27 %)
Duration of symptoms < 12 months[c]	118 (32 %)
Intermittent symptoms present[d]	128 (36 %)
Symmetric arthralgia[e]	272 (74 %)
Arthralgia in upper and lower extrimities[f]	186 (51 %)
Arthralgia in small joints[c]	256 (70 %)
VAS pain ≥ 50	128 (34 %)
Morning stiffness ≥ 1 h	68 (18 %)
Swollen joint(s) reported	126 (34 %)
Tender joint count	0 [0–3]
CRP positive[f]	35 (10 %)
Antibody status	
IgM-RF positive but aCCP negative	120 (32 %)
IgM-RF negative but aCCP low positive	65 (17 %)
IgM-RF negative but aCCP high positive	78 (21 %)
IgM-RF and aCCP positive	111 (30 %)

[a]missing for 2 patients
[b]missing for 13 patients
[c]missing for 6 patients
[d]missing for 14 patients
[e]missing for 5 patients
[f]missing for 7 patients
Continuous variables are described by mean (SD) or median [IQR], depending on its distribution
aCCP anticyclic citrullinated peptide, *CRP* C reactive protein, *FDR* first degree relative, *h* hour,
IgM-RF rheumatoid factors type immunoglobulin M, *NSAID* non-steroid anti-inflammatory drugs,
RA rheumatoid arthritis, *VAS* visual analogue scale

small difference between the two groups), around 0.5 a moderate, and around 0.8 a large effect (or a large difference between the two groups) [3].

Example 2.3

Effect size in the COBRA-light trial
The mean DAS44 after 52 weeks of treatment in the control arm (COBRA) was 1.70 (SD 0.97, $n = 77$) and in the intervention arm (COBRA-light) 1.88 (SD 0.99, $n = 77$). The effect size (i.e., the difference in mean between both arms) after 52 weeks of

treatment is then equal to $1.88 - 1.70 = 0.18$. That is, the intervention arm had on average a 0.18 points higher DAS44 after 52 weeks of treatment than the control arm. The pooled SD is equal to

$$\sqrt{\frac{(77-1) \times 0.97^2 + (77-1) \times 0.99^2}{77+77-2}} = 0.98.$$

The Cohen's d after 52 weeks is equal to $0.18/0.98 = 0.18$, indicating a small difference between COBRA-light and COBRA treatment.

In case the determinant is categorical, with more than two groups, no single effect size is calculated. Instead, one group is set as the reference group, and for each group separately the difference in mean between that group and the reference group is calculated. For non-normally distributed outcome variables, there is no effect size defined. Instead, the median and (interquartile) range in each group separately is reported. This holds for dichotomous and categorical determinants.

The effect size of the association between a continuous outcome variable and a continuous determinant is the correlation coefficient (or simply correlation). Correlation coefficients are usually denoted by ρ (rho), and lies between -1 and $+1$. A value of zero implies no correlation between the two variables, but that does not automatically imply that there is no association between the two variables. A value of $+1$ implies a perfect positive correlation, and a value of -1 implies a negative correlation. For two normally distributed variables, the Pearson's correlation coefficient is calculated. When at least one of the two variables is not normally distributed, the Spearman's rank correlation is calculated. The Pearson's correlation coefficient is the covariance between the two variables divided by the product of their SDs. The actual mathematical formula can be found in many mathematical statistics books. We refer to the further readings (▶Sect. 2.4) for references to those statistical books. The Spearman's rank correlation is actually the same as the Pearson's correlation coefficient, but it is computed on the ranks of the values instead of the values themselves. The rank of a value is its position in the ordered data (from lowest to highest). In a study population of size n, the lowest observed value is assigned rank 1, the second lowest rank 2, the second highest rank $n - 1$ and the highest rank n. Because both variables are standardized, the interpretation of the correlation coefficient is not straight forward as an effect size. In Chapter 3 we illustrate an effect size that has a clinical interpretation when analyzing the association between a continuous outcome variable and a continuous determinant.

2.3.2 Effect Size for a Dichotomous Outcome Variable

For a dichotomous outcome variable, one outcome is usually considered as 'success' and the other as 'failure'. Two measures are of interest in a dichotomous outcome variable. The first measure is the probability of 'success', parametrized by p, also called risk. The other measure is the odds for 'success', which is equal to the probability of 'success' divided by the probability of a 'failure': $p/(1-p)$. Success and failure are written between quotation marks, because while a successful outcome does not necessarily imply to be the favorable one, the 'success' outcome is defined as the outcome of interest, for example developing RA during follow-up. Based on a 2×2 crosstab ($\blacksquare$Table 2.3), three effect sizes could be calculated for the association between a dichotomous outcome variable and a dichotomous determinant:

- the risk difference (RD), which is equal to $p_1 - p_2$, or $\frac{a}{n_1} - \frac{c}{n_2}$;

- the relative risk (RR), which is equal to $\frac{p_1}{p_2}$, or $\frac{a}{n_1} / \frac{c}{n_2} = \frac{a \times n_2}{n_1 \times c}$; or

- the odds ratio (OR), which is equal to $\frac{p_1/(1-p_1)}{p_2/(1-p_2)}$, or $\frac{a \times d}{b \times c}$.

Here, p_1 and p_2 are the estimated risks in the two groups. One group is set as the reference group, in this case group 2. A negative RD implies that group 1 has a lower risk than the reference group. An RR below one or an OR below one indicates that group 1 has a lower risk or odds compared to the reference group.

Example 2.4

Effect sizes in the RA-cohort

In the RA-cohort, a total of 374 patients were included. The different effect sizes for the association between development of RA within the follow-up period, and having an FDR with RA are estimated from the 2×2 crosstab.

		development of RA		total
		yes	no	
group	FDR with RA	38	48	86
	no FDR with RA	93	195	228
total		131	243	374

For patients with an FDR with RA, the risk to develop RA within the follow-up period is equal to $38/86 = 0.44$ and for patients without an FDR with RA $93/228 = 0.32$.
We set the group 'no FDR with RA' as reference.
Then the RD is equal to $0.44 - 0.32 = 0.12$, i.e., patients with an FDR with RA have 0.12 higher risk of developing RA within the follow-up period than patients without an FRD with RA.
The RR is equal to $0.44/0.32 = 1.38$, i.e., the risk of developing RA is 1.38 times higher in patients with an FDR with RA than in patients without an FDR with RA.
The OR is equal to $\frac{0.44/0.56}{0.32/0.68} = \frac{38 \times 195}{48 \times 93} = 1.66$ i.e., the odds to develop RA is 1.66 times higher in patients with an FDR with RA than in patients without an FDR with RA.

The OR is more difficult to interpret than the RD and RR. However, the actual risk is only computed in prospective cohort studies and not in, for example, case-control studies. ORs are also easier to adjust for influencing factors ($\blacktriangleright$Chap. 6). Finally, the OR is reported as the effect size for the association between a continuous determinant and a dichotomous outcome variable. For rare outcomes (i.e., with a risk or prevalence of the disease/outcome below 1 %), the OR is approximately equal to the RR.

In case of a categorical determinant, as before, no single effect size is available. Instead, one group is set as reference group and the effect sizes of the remaining groups are computed compared to the reference group.

2.3.3 Confidence Interval

To generalize the estimated effect sizes from the study population to the research popula-tion, uncertainty needs to be quantified. The uncertainty of an estimate is measured by the standard error (SE). The smaller the SE, the more certain one is that the effect in the study population is a good estimate of the true effect in the research population. The SE depends on the size of the study population: the larger the study population, the smaller the SE and vice versa. The SE can be computed with several equations (▶Sects. 3.2 and 4.2), depending on the effect size, but they are also generally provided by any statistical software package.

With the SE a confidence interval (CI) is constructed. The CI has a certain precision, which is denoted by α and usually set to 0.05. The general form of a $(1 - \alpha)$ 100 % CI (i.e., 95 % CI) is equal to

$$\left[\text{effect size} - z_{\alpha/2} \times \text{SE}; \text{effect size} + z_{\alpha/2} \times \text{SE}\right]. \tag{E2.2}$$

The precision α determines the value of $z_{\alpha/2}$, which is called the critical value. The criti-cal value can be found in tables provided in many statistical text books [4–7]. Statisti-cal software packages automatically compute the critical value. The most common used critical values are $z_{\alpha/2} = 1.96$ for $\alpha = 0.05$, $z_{\alpha/2} = 1.64$ for $\alpha = 0.1$, and $z_{\alpha/2} = 2.59$ for $\alpha = 0.01$. Consequently, the smaller the α, the wider the CI.

> **Example 2.5**
>
> **95 % CI for the effect size in the COBRA-light trial**
> The SE for the mean difference in DAS44 after 52 weeks treatment is equal to 0.15, so the 95 % CI for the mean difference is equal to
>
> $[0.18 - 1.96 \times 0.15; 0.18 + 1.96 \times 0.15] = [-0.11; 0.47].$

Note that this general form holds for most effect sizes, for large study populations as well as for the natural logarithm (ln) of the RR or the OR. However, it does not hold in case of a very small study population (i.e., groups below 20–50), or for the RR and OR. After computing the 95 % CI for the ln(RR) or ln(OR), the 95 % CI for the RR or the OR are obtained by taking the exponential (exp) of the bounds for ln(RR) or ln(OR).

> **Example 2.6**
>
> **95 % CI for the effect size in RA-cohort**
> The SE for the ln(OR) comparing patients with an FDR with RA to patients without an FDR with RA is equal to 0.25, so the 95 % CI for the ln(OR) is equal to

$$\left[\ln(1.70) - 1.96 \times 0.25; \ln(1.70) - 1.96 \times 0.25\right] = [0.041; 1.02].$$

The 95 % CI for the OR is then equal to

$$\left[\exp(0.041); \exp(1.02)\right] = [1.04; 2.77].$$

The $(1 - \alpha)$ 100 % CI varies between study populations, while the (unknown) population effect is fixed. A common mistake in the interpretation of the CI is that the probability of the population effect lies within the CI, equals $(1 - \alpha)$ 100 %. The correct interpretation of the CI is that the probability that the interval contains the true population effect is equal to $(1 - \alpha)$ 100 %. It is a subtle difference, but if we would repeatedly estimate an effect size in the study population from independent random samples of the same research population and calculate the 95 % CI for each of these samples, on average 19 of every 20 CIs would contain the true population effect size, and one of every 20 would not.

2.3.4 Testing Hypotheses

The CI provides some information on the 'true' population effect, but the estimated study effect or association could also have arisen by chance. As described in ▶ Chap. 1, a null and alternative hypothesis are formulated based on the research question. In inferential statistics, the null hypothesis is the hypothesis that is provisionally assumed to hold (and sometimes called the working hypothesis). The collected data should provide enough evidence to reject it, in favor of the alternative hypothesis. The null hypothesis is tested by computing a test statistic, which follows a certain distribution under the null hypothesis. Many distributions exist, we have already introduced the normal distribution. Other distributions commonly encountered in hypotheses testing are the (Student's) t-distribution, the chi-square (or χ^2-) distribution and the F-distribution. The test statistics and their distributions are described in more detail in ▶ Chaps. 3–5. All these distributions have degrees of freedom. This is the number of values to compute the value of the test statistic freely, to obtain the test statistic.

Example 2.7

Degrees of freedom in study population mean
After 52 weeks of COBRA-light treatment, the mean DAS44 score of $n = 77$ patients was equal to 1.88. To get a mean of 1.88, the DAS44 score of 76 patients 'can vary freely' while only one is fixed. The degrees of freedom are, in this case, 76 (i.e., $n - 1$).

The degrees of freedom are needed to determine the probability of finding the observed value of the test statistic or even more extreme values (favoring the alternative hypothesis). This probability is called the p-value. Many statistical tables exist which list the different p-values for different distributions of the test statistic with corresponding degrees

◻ Table 2.6   All four possible decisions that could be made in hypothesis testing

	H0 is true	H1 is true
H0 is not rejected	Correct decision	Wrong decision (type II error)
H0 is rejected	Wrong decision (type I error, α)	Correct decision (β)

of freedom. These tables can also be found in statistical textbooks [4–7]. From these tables, one usually only concludes whether the p-value is smaller than 0.1, 0.05, 0.01 or 0.001. Of course, statistical software packages provide the exact p-value.

What does the p-value tell us? Well, the smaller the p-value, the stronger the evidence against the null hypothesis. If the p-value is smaller than a predefined significance level, usually also set to 0.05 and denoted by α, the null hypothesis is rejected in favor of the alternative hypothesis. If the p-value is larger than the significance level, the null hypothesis cannot be rejected. This does not mean that the null hypothesis is true, but just that the data does not provide enough evidence against it [8]. As for the SE, the p-value is also influenced by the size of the study population. The larger the study population, the smaller the p-values.

Sometimes, a p-value between 0.1 and 0.05 is interpreted as a trend towards statistical significance. However, the cut-off of 0.05 to indicate statistical significance, is just a rule of thumb [9]. Therefore, some epidemiological journals, such as Epidemiology, the International Journal of Epidemiology and the American Journal of Epidemiology, prohibit the use of the term statistical significance (or significant). They advise to report the effect sizes, with corresponding 95 % CIs and the exact p-values (not just whether it was smaller than the significance level α). Depending on the research field and the journal, the value of the test statistic and the degrees of freedom are also reported.

Different types of outcome variables require different types of effect sizes as well as different statistical tests. How to report results of inferential statistics will be explained in the following chapters. Throughout the following chapters, we do not interpret a p-value between 0.05 and 0.1 as a statistical trend and also do not report the values of the test statistic and the degrees of freedom.

Without dwelling on too many details, we want to provide a bit more information on the meaning of the significance level. Based on the p-value of the statistical test, the null hypothesis is rejected or not. If H0 is not rejected it does not mean that H0 is actually accepted! As either H0 or H1 is really true, two correct and two wrong decisions could be made based on the p-value. ◻Table 2.6 summarizes all possible decisions. Ideally, both the type I error (falsely rejecting a true null hypothesis) and the type II error (falsely accepting a wrong null hypothesis) are zero. This is impossible. By setting the significance level α at a certain level, chosen before the hypothesis test is performed (and stated in the research proposal), one accepts that the probability of the type I error is at most α.

Put differently, for an α of 0.05, one accepts that for every 20 true null hypotheses, one (i.e., 5 %) is falsely rejected. Generally, a larger probability of the type II error is accepted. One minus the probability of the type II error is called the power of a test, denoted by β and usually set at 0.8 or 0.9.

Depending on the sign or direction of the alternative hypothesis, the hypothesis test is either one-sided or two-sided. If the direction of the comparison in the alternative hypothesis is specified, the test is called one-sided; if the direction is unspecified, the test is two-sided. The alternative hypothesis in ▶Example 1.2 is two-sided. A one-sided alternative hypothesis would be, for example, that the decrease in DAS44 is larger in the COBRA-light strategy compared to the COBRA strategy. The direction of the effect is specified in this example.

The significance level and the precision of the CI for the effect size, are based on the same *arbitrary* chosen threshold α of 0.05 and hence are related. If the 95 % CI does not contain the effect under the null hypothesis (called the null value), the *p*-value will be smaller than 0.05, and vice versa, if the *p*-value is smaller than 0.05, the 95 % CI will not contain the null value. For effect sizes that are defined as differences, the null value is usually zero, corresponding to the null hypothesis of no difference. For ratio effect sizes, such as the RR and OR, the null value is equal to one, corresponding to equality of the risks or odds. Although this relation exists, the exact *p*-value as well as the 95 % CI are both reported in scientific papers, as advised by the Epidemiological journals.

Both the *p*-value and the CI are influenced by the size of the study population. A large study population is more likely to provide strong evidence against a null hypothesis in the form of a small *p*-value and a narrow CI. However, small *p*-values and narrow CIs do not provide any clinical relevance of the observed effect. Thus, a significant effect might not be a clinical relevant effect, and the absence of a significant *p*-value does not imply the result is not clinically relevant.

Non-Inferiority or Equivalence Study

In non-inferiority and equivalence studies, a non-inferiority or equivalence margin is defined. This margin, usually denoted by D, has to be set in the research proposal and study protocol before start of the study.

Testing hypotheses in a non-inferiority or an equivalence study, is solely based on CIs, and not on *p*-values. After all, the alternative hypothesis of a non-inferiority study states that the difference between two groups is larger than value $-D$ (or is smaller than $+D$, depending on which direction is more favorable). And the alternative hypothesis of an equivalence study states that the difference between two groups falls completely between the values $-D$ and $+D$. In a non-inferiority study, the null hypothesis is rejected at a significance level α of 0.025, if the lower limit of the 95 % CI is larger than $-D$ (or the upper limit is smaller than $+D$). To test the null hypothesis at a significance level α of 0.05, a 90 % CI needs to be computed. In an equivalence study, the null hypothesis is rejected at a significance level α of 0.05, if the 95 % CI lies completely within the interval $[-D; +D]$.

2.4   Further Readings

There are many books in the field of medical statistics and epidemiology. All of them provide at least two full chapters on the different ways to summarize data, as well as on the fundamentals of statistical methods. They all focus on non-mathematical readers (i.e., medical researchers), but they also provide, to different extents, the statistical theory with mathematical equations. We refer readers who would like to learn more about the statistical theory behind inferential statistics to the books written by, for example, Altman, Riffenburgh, Rothman et al., Armitage et al. and Kirkwood & Sterne [4–7, 10].

References

1. ter Wee MM, den Uyl D, Boers M, Kerstens P, Nurmohamed M, van Schaardenburg D, et al. Intensive combination treatment regimens, including prednisolone, are effective in treating patients with early rheumatoid arthritis regardless of additional etanercept: 1-year results of the COBRA-light open-label, randomised, non-inferiority trial. Ann Rheum Dis. 2015;74(6):1233–40. ▶https://doi.org/10.1136/annrheumdis-2013-205143.
2. van de Stadt LA, Witte BI, Bos WH, van Schaardenburg D. A prediction rule for the development of arthritis in seropositive arthralgia patients. Ann Rheum Dis. 2013;72(12):1920–6. ▶https://doi.org/10.1136/annrheumdis-2012-202127.
3. Cohen J. Statistical power analysis for the behavioral sciences. 2nd ed. Hilllsdale: Erlbaum Associated; 1988.
4. Altman DG. Practical statistics for medical research. London: Chapman & Hall; 1991.
5. Riffenburgh RH. Statistics in medicine. San Diego: Academic Press; 1999.
6. Armitage P, Berry G, Matthews JNS. Statistical methods in medical research. Oxford: Blackwell Science Ltd; 2002.
7. Kirkwood BR, Sterne JAC. Essential medical statistics. 2nd ed. Oxford: Blackwell Science Ltd; 2003.
8. Greenland S, Senn SJ, Rothman KJ, Carlin JB, Poole C, Goodman SN, et al. Statistical tests, P values, confidence intervals, and power: a guide to misinterpretations. Eur J Epidemiol. 2016;31(4):337–50. ▶https://doi.org/10.1007/s10654-016-0149-3.
9. Sterne JAC, Smith GD. Sifting the evidence—what's wrong with significance tests? Phys Ther. 2001;81(8):1464–9. ▶https://doi.org/10.1093/ptj/81.8.1464.
10. Rothman KJ, Lash TL, Greenland S. Modern epidemiology. 3rd ed. Philadelphia: Lippincott-Raven; 2012.

Analyzing Continuous Outcome Variables

Abstract

The association between a continuous outcome variable and a dichotomous, a categorical, or a continuous determinant, is analyzed with different statistical methods. In this chapter, we explain these methods. Furthermore, we explain how to compare two measurements of the same (continuous) outcome variable within a patient. We do this for both normally distributed as well as non-normally distributed continuous outcome variables.

© Bohn Stafleu van Loghum is een imprint van Springer Media B.V., onderdeel van Springer Nature 2019
M. M. ter Wee and B. I. Lissenberg-Witte, *A Quick Guide on How to Conduct Medical Research*,
https://doi.org/10.1007/978-90-368-2248-0_3

3.1   Transformations of a Continuous Outcome Variable

When the outcome variable is continuous, the first step, in general, is to check its ditribution. As described in ▶ Chap. 2, we distinguish between a normally and a non-normally distributed continuous outcome variable. If the outcome variable does not seem to be normally distributed, e.g., investigated by a histogram or QQ-plot, a good solution would be to transform the outcome variable. The transformed outcome variable might be normally distributed. If so, the analyses are performed on the transformed outcome variable. Widely used transformations are:

- the natural logarithmic (ln) transformation, where an outcome variable Y is transformed to $\ln(Y)$;
- the reciprocal transformation, where an outcome variable Y is transformed to $1/Y$;
- the square root or cube root transformation, where an outcome variable Y is transformed to $\sqrt{Y}$ or $\sqrt[3]{Y}$, respectively;
- the square transformation, where an outcome variable Y is transformed to Y^2.

It is important to note that the effect size of the transformed outcome variable has a different interpretation than the effect size of the original (untransformed) outcome variable, because the scale of the variable has changed. Therefore, the obtained effect size needs to be transformed back to the original scale by taking the inverse of the transformation. The inverse of, for example, the natural logarithm is the exponential: e^x or $\exp(x)$. As long as it is explained in the scientific paper what has been done in the case of a non-normal distributed outcome variable, it does not matter which transformation method is chosen.

If transforming the outcome variable does not result in a normally distributed outcome variable, a non-parametric test is required. A non-parametric test is not based on the observed values, but on the ranks of these values. The smallest observed value in the study population is assigned rank 1, the second smallest is assigned rank 2, up the to the largest observed value which is assigned rank n (the total size of the study population). By ranking the observations, any clinical information on the values themselves is lost and, hence, non-parametric tests only provide a p-value and no effect size or confidence interval (CI). Non-parametric tests are also not suitable to correct for potential influencing variables (▶ Chap. 6). Moreover, a non-parametric test will never produce a low p-value in extremely small sized study populations. For example in two groups of three patients each, the p-value will never reach the significance level. Most statistical tests are also rather robust against normality, therefore, we advise to use non-parametric tests only if the size of the study population is small, with 10 to 25 patients per group. We illustrate both solutions to non-normality for comparing two or more groups and for comparing two measurements within the same patient in the following sections.

Normally distributed variables are sometimes transformed too, e.g., to allow for easy comparison between different research populations. These transformations are called centralization and standardization. The centralized variable is obtained by subtracting the study population mean of the variable to each patient's individual value. The standardized variable (or z-score) is obtained by dividing the centralized variable by the standard deviation (SD) of the study population. Consequently, the mean of a centralized or standardized variable is equal to zero and the SD of a standardized variable is equal to one. In ▶Example 3.1 we explain how to calculate the centralized and standardized variables.

Example 3.1

Calculating centralized and standardized variables

In an example dataset ($n = 5$), the observed values of a continuous outcome variable are 0.50, 4.2, 0.60, 2.7, 3.0. The study population mean is equal to 2.18; the study population SD is equal to 1.60.

The centralized values are then equal to: (a) $0.50 - 2.18 = -1.68$; (b) $4.2 - 2.18 = 2.02$; (c) $0.60 - 2.18 = -1.58$; (d) $2.6 - 2.18 = 0.42$; and (e) $3.0 - 2.18 = 0.82$.

The standardized values are then equal to: (a) $-1.68/1.60 = -1.05$; (b) $2.02/1.60 = 1.26$; (c) $-1.58/1.60 = -0.99$; (d) $0.42/1.60 = 0.26$; and (e) $0.82/1.60 = 0.51$.

3.2   In Case of a Dichotomous Determinant

In a randomized controlled trial (RCT), such as the COmbinatie Behandeling Reumatoïde Artritis (COBRA)-light trial [1, 2], an important research question is whether a continuous outcome variable differs between the groups at the end of the follow-up period.

3.2.1 Independent Samples *T*-Test

Differences between two groups (i.e., a dichotomous determinant) are assessed with the independent samples t-test. The null and alternative hypothesis of the independent samples t-test are usually

H0: the mean of the outcome variable is equal in both groups;
H1: the mean of the outcome variable is unequal in both groups.

Put differently, H0 states that the mean difference between both groups is equal to zero, while H1 states the mean difference is unequal to zero. Therefore, the effect size of the independent samples t-test is the mean difference of the outcome variable. The standard error (SE) of the mean difference between the groups is equal to

$$SE_{diff} = \sqrt{\frac{(n_1 - 1) \times SD_1^2 + (n_2 - 1) \times SD_2^2}{n_1 + n_2 - 2}} \sqrt{\frac{1}{n_1} + \frac{1}{n_2}}. \tag{E3.1}$$

Here, n_1 and n_2 are the study population sizes of both groups, and SD_1 and SD_2 are the SDs of the two groups. Note that the first square root equals the pooled SD of both groups (▶Eq. E2.1, ▶Sect. 2.3.1). The 95 % CI for the mean difference is computed with ▶Eq. E2.2 (▶Sect. 2.3.3), which translates to

$$[\text{mean diff} - 1.96 \times SE_{diff}; \text{mean diff} + 1.96 \times SE_{diff}]. \qquad (\text{E3.2})$$

The SE of the mean difference and the corresponding 95 % CI are default output of the independent samples t-test in most statistical software packages. The test statistic of the independent samples t-test, denoted by t, is equal to the mean difference divided by its SE

$$t = \frac{\text{mean diff}}{SE_{diff}}. \qquad (\text{E3.3})$$

The test statistic t has a t-distribution with $n_1 + n_2 - 2$ degrees of freedom. Higher values of the absolute value of t are evidence against the null hypothesis and in favour of the alternative hypothesis.

Let us consider the research question given in ▶Example 1.1 (▶Sect. 1.4)

> ❓ Is there a difference in decrease of the disease activity score of 44 joints (DAS44) between the COBRA-light strategy and the COBRA strategy in patients with early rheumatoid arthritis (RA) after 52 weeks of treatment?

And let us assume that we want to test the null and alternative hypothesis given in ▶Example 1.2 (▶Sect. 1.4)

H0: there is no difference in decrease in the DAS44 between the COBRA-light and the COBRA strategy;

H1: there is a difference in decrease in the DAS44 between the COBRA-light and the COBRA strategy.

The outcome variable of this research question is the change in DAS44 within a patient. To clearly distinguish differences *within* a patient from differences *between* groups of patients, we refer to the differences within a patient as change. The change within a patient is often referred to as the delta-score (or Δ-score) and the variable itself as the delta-variable (or Δ-variable). In an RCT, it is assumed that both groups start at approximately the same level, but in other research designs (such as a cohort study) this might not be the case. When baseline differences exist between groups, we advise to test for differences in changes within a patient between groups rather than test for differences at the end of a time period.

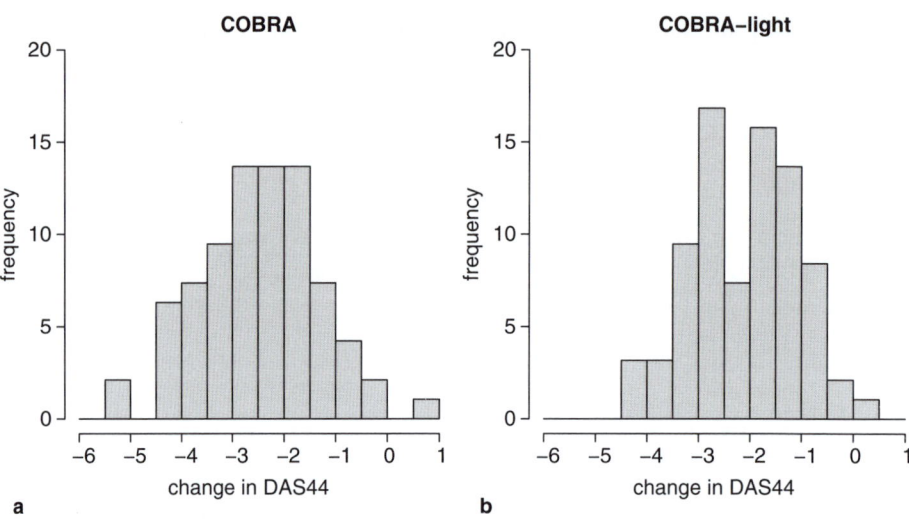

◘ **Fig. 3.1**   Histogram of change in DAS44 after 52 weeks of treatment according to the COBRA strategy (**a**) or COBRA-light strategy (**b**)

Example 3.2

Difference in change in the DAS44 in the COBRA-light trial

In the COBRA-light arm, the mean change in DAS44 was -2.06 (SD 1.03, $n = 77$), and in the COBRA arm -2.41 (SD 1.17, $n = 77$). The effect size, i.e., the mean difference in decrease, is then equal to $-2.41 - (-2.06) = -0.35$.

The SE of the mean difference is equal to

$$\sqrt{\frac{(77-1) \times 0.97^2 + (77-1) \times 0.99^2}{77+77-2}} \times \sqrt{\frac{1}{77} + \frac{1}{77}} \approx 0.98 \times 0.16 = 0.15,$$

and, consequently, the 95 % CI for the mean difference is equal to

$$[-0.35 - 1.96 \times 0.15; -0.35 + 1.96 \times 0.15] = [-0.64; -0.056].$$

Normally Distributed Outcome Variable

The independent samples t-test can only be used when the outcome variable is normally distributed, in each of the two groups separately. ◘Figure 3.1 shows the histograms of the change in DAS44 after 52 weeks of treatment for the COBRA (coded as zero in the database) and the COBRA-light strategy (coded as one in the database) separately. From this figure, we conclude that the DAS44 is normally distributed in both groups: we can use the independent samples t-test.

◘Table 3.1 shows the SPSS output of the independent samples t-test. The SPSS output consists of several rows and columns. The first row is labeled "Equal variances assumed", the second is labeled "Equal variances not assumed". This refers to the assumption of the independent samples t-test: the variances (i.e., the squared SD) of both groups need to be equal. If this assumption does not hold, the degrees of freedom (under "df") of the test

□ Table 3.1 SPSS output of the independent samples t-test, comparing the change in DAS44 after 52 weeks between the COBRA and COBRA-light treatment

Independent Sample Test

| | | Levene's Test for Equality of Variances | | t-test for Equality of Means | | | | | 95 % Confidence Interval of the Difference | |
		F	Sig.	t	df	Sig. (2-tailed)	Mean Difference	Std. Error Difference	Lower	Upper
change in DAS44	Equal variances assumed	.803	.372	−1.932	152	.055	−.343	.177	−.694	.008
	Equal variances not assumed			−1.932	149.413	.055	−.343	.177	−.694	.008

need to be adjusted. The results in the first two columns, under "Levene's Test for Equality of the Variances", correspond to the test of this assumption. The Levene's test tests the following null and alternative hypothesis

H0: the variance in both groups are equal;
H1: the variance in both groups are unequal.

In this example, the *p*-value of the Levene's test (under "Sig.") is larger than the significance level α of 0.05, so we cannot reject the null hypothesis. Put differently, we can assume equal variances, therefore we need to use the results in the row labeled "Equal variances assumed". The test statistic of the Levene's test is also reported (under "F"). The *p*-value (under "Sig. (2-tailed)") for the comparison of the mean change in DAS44 is therefore read from the first row. The mean difference between the two groups (under "Mean Difference"), the SE of the mean difference (under "Std. Error Difference") and the corresponding 95 % CI (under "95 % Confidence Interval of the Difference") are also reported. Furthermore, the value of the test statistic (under "t") and the degrees of freedom (under "df") are reported in SPSS by default. From this table, we conclude that there is not enough evidence to prove that the decrease in DAS44 after 52 weeks of treatment differs between the COBRA and the COBRA-light strategies. In a scientific paper, this is usually reported as follows: there is no evidence for a difference in change in DAS44 after 52 weeks of treatment between the COBRA and COBRA-light strategy (mean difference -0.35, 95 % CI $[-0.69; 0.008]$, $p = 0.055$).

A statistical significant difference between two groups could also be investigated by looking at the 95 % CI for the mean outcome in each group separately. Non-overlapping 95 % CIs of both groups imply a statistical significant difference between the groups, at the significance level α of 0.05. The other way around is not necessarily true: overlapping CIs do not always imply a non-significant difference. If the mean outcome of one group lies in the 95 % CI of the other group (and/or vice versa), the difference between the groups is not significant. However, if this is not the case and the CIs overlap, the difference could be either significant or not [3].

Example 3.3

Difference between two groups based on the 95 % CIs
The mean change in DAS44 in the COBRA-light arm was -2.06 (SD 1.03, $n = 77$, 95 % CI $[-2.29, -1.83]$) and -2.41 (SD 1.17, $n = 77$, 95 % CI $[-2.67, -2.14]$) in the COBRA arm. The 95 % CIs overlap, but the mean in the COBRA-light arm (i.e., -2.06) does not lie within the 95 % CI of the COBRA arm (i.e., $[-2.67, -2.14]$). Also, the mean of the COBRA arm (i.e., -2.41) does not lie within the 95 % CI of the COBRA-light arm. Therefore, in this example, we cannot rule out or confirm a statistically significant difference between the strategies just by looking at the 95 % CIs.

Non-Normally Distributed Outcome Variable

If the continuous outcome variable is not normally distributed in both groups separately, and the size of the study populations in both groups is large enough (e.g., both groups have at least 25 patients), the outcome variable could be transformed. Assume, for example, the primary outcome variable of the COBRA-light trial was not decrease in DAS44 but in the erythrocyte sedimentation rate (ESR) after 52 weeks of treatment. The research question would be

> ❓ Is there a difference in ESR after 52 weeks of treatment between the COBRA-light strategy and the COBRA strategy in patients with early RA?

The null and alternative hypothesis of this new research question are

H0: there is no difference in ESR between the COBRA-light and the COBRA strategy;
H1: there is a difference in ESR between both strategies.

In ▶Chap. 2 we already concluded that ESR at baseline, for the whole study population, is not normally distributed (◻Fig. 2.1, ▶Sect. 2.2.2). ◻Figure 3.2a and b show that ESR after 52 weeks of treatment is also not normally distributed in the COBRA and the COBRA-light arm separately. However, ln(ESR) after 52 weeks seems more normally distributed (◻Fig. 3.2c and d). Because the size of the study population is large enough in both arms, we ignore the small deviation from normality and use the independent samples t-test to test the difference between both groups on the ln-transformed outcome variable.

　◻Table 3.2 shows the SPSS output of this independent samples t-test. From the Levene's test it follows that we can assume equal variances ($p = 0.37$). According to SPSS the p-value is actually 0.368, but we round p-values larger than 0.1 to two decimals and only use three decimals for p-values smaller than 0.1 for the same precision. Furthermore, there is not enough evidence to prove a difference in ln(ESR) after 52 weeks of treatment in the COBRA or COBRA-light strategy (mean difference -0.29, 95 % CI $[-0.58; 0.004]$, $p = 0.053$). Since the independent samples t-test was performed on the ln-transformed outcome variable, the mean difference reported in the output is on the ln-scale and not on the ESR scale. To obtain an effect size on the original scale, the mean difference has to be transformed back with the inverse function of the natural logarithm: the exponential. First, recall that the difference between two natural logarithms is equal to the natural logarithm of the ratio, i.e.,

$$-0.29 = \ln\left(ESR_{52weeks;COBRA-light}\right) - \ln\left(ESR_{52weeks;COBRA}\right)$$
$$= \ln\left(ESR_{52weeks;COBRA-light}/ESR_{52weeks;COBRA}\right).$$

From this it follows that

$$\exp\left(ESR_{52weeks;COBRA-light}/ESR_{52weeks;COBRA}\right) = \exp(-0.29) = 0.75.$$

In other words, the ESR after 52 weeks of COBRA-light treatment is on average (though not significant) 0.75 times higher than the ESR after 52 weeks of COBRA treatment, or is $1 - 0.75 = 0.25$ times lower. To calculate the 95 % CI for this relative difference, the same inverse transformation has to be applied to the values of the 95 % CI for the difference at the ln-scale: $\exp(-0.58) = 0.56$ and $\exp(0.004) = 1.004$. The final conclusion with respect to the difference in ESR after 52 weeks of treatment between the COBRA and

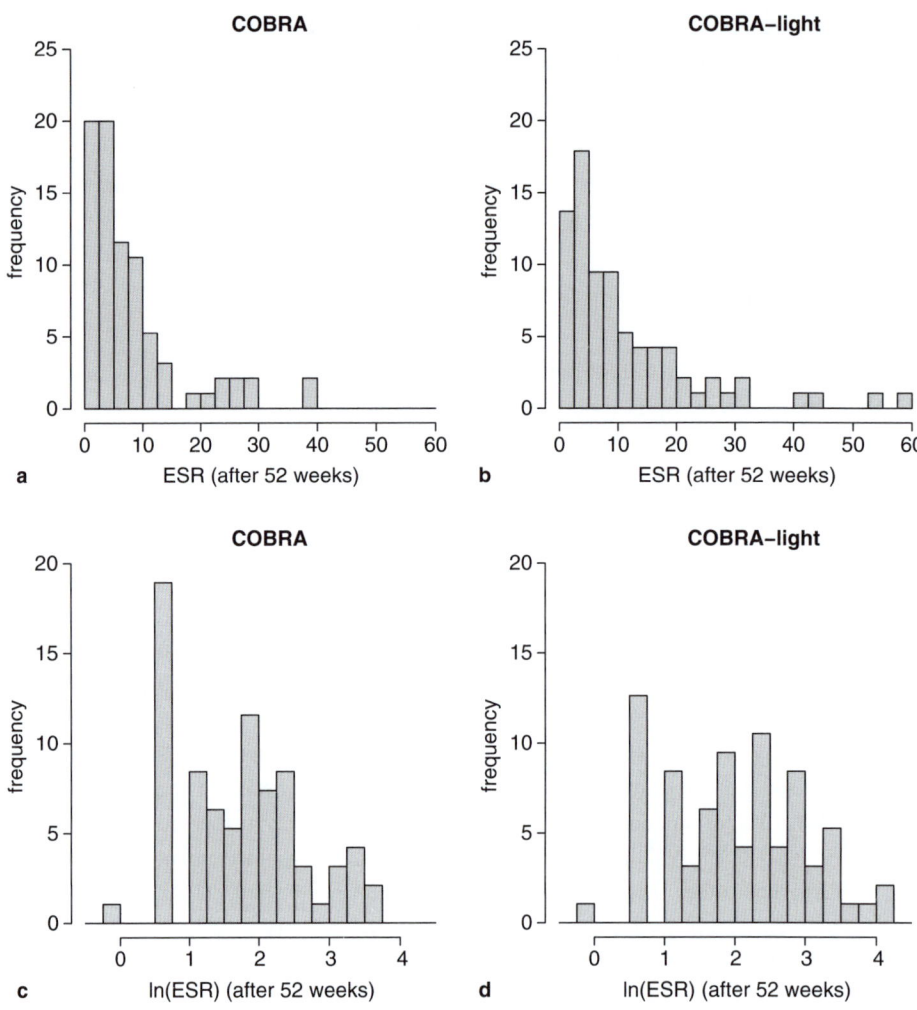

◼ Fig. 3.2 Histograms of ESR (**a, b**) and ln(ESR) (**c, d**) after 52 weeks treatment according to the COBRA strategy (**a, c**) or COBRA-light strategy (**b, d**)

COBRA-light arm, is that there is not enough evidence to prove that ESR after 52 weeks of COBRA-light treatment is different than after 52 weeks of COBRA treatment (relative difference 0.75, 95 % CI [0.25; 1.004], $p = 0.053$).

3.2.2 Mann-Whitney *U* Test

As mentioned in ▶ Sect. 3.1, if the size of the study population is large enough, most tests are quite robust against small deviations from normality. If, for example, only two times 20 patients ($n = 40$) instead of two times 81 patients ($n = 162$) were included in the COBRA-light trial, the difference in ESR after 52 weeks treatment could not be

■ Table 3.2 SPSS output of the independent samples t-test, comparing ln-transformed ESR after 52 weeks of COBRA treatment with COBRA-light treatment

Independent Samples Test

		Levene's Test for Equality of Variances		t-test for Equality of Means					95 % Confidence Interval of the Difference	
		F	Sig.	t	df	Sig. (2-tailed)	Mean Difference	Std. Error Difference	Lower	Upper
ln(ESR) after 52 weeks	Equal variances assumed	.816	.368	−1.949	152	.053	−.289	.148	−.582	.004
	Equal variances not assumed			−1.949	145.791	.053	−.289	.148	−.582	.004

▣ **Table 3.3**   SPSS output of the Mann-Whitney U test, comparing ESR after 52 weeks of COBRA treatment with 52 weeks of COBRA-light treatment

Test Statistics[a]

	ESR after 52 weeks
Mann-Whitney U	155.500
Wilcoxon W	326.500
Z	−.719
Asymp. Sig. (2-tailed)	.472
Exact Sig. [2*(1-tailed Sig.)]	.478[b]

[a]Grouping Variable: treatment arm
[b]Not corrected for ties

investigated with the independent samples t-test on the ln-transformed outcome variable. A non-parametric test should rather be used. The non-parametric version of the independent samples t-test is the Mann-Whitney U test. This test tests the following null and alternative hypothesis

H0: the distribution of ESR is equal in both groups;
H1: the distribution of ESR is unequal in both groups.

Non-parametric tests are based on the ranks of all observed outcome values. The Mann-Whitney U test compares the mean of the ranks in two groups. If the distribution of the outcome variable is (approximately) equal in both groups, the mean ranks of both groups are expected to be similar. Equivalently, large differences in the mean ranks of both groups are in favor of the alternative hypothesis.

▣Table 3.3 shows the SPSS output of the Mann-Whitney U test comparing ESR after 52 weeks of COBRA treatment with 52 weeks of COBRA-light treatment. The mean rank in each group is also reported by SPSS, in a separate table, which we do not illustrate, as they do not contribute to the interpretation of the Mann Whitney U test. In the COBRA arm, the mean rank (of 18 patients, two had incomplete follow-up) was 18.1, while in the COBRA-light arm the mean rank (of 20 patients) was 20.7. This is quite similar to each other, reflected by the p-value which is larger than the significance level α of 0.05. For very small sized study populations, SPSS reports an exact p-value ("Exact Sig. [2*(1-tailed Sig.)]") and an asymptotical p-value ("Asymp. Sig. (2-tailed)"). For larger sized study populations, only the asymptotical one is reported. If possible, report the exact p-value. The test statistic of the Mann-Whitney U test is too complex to provide in this quick guide and is not necessary to know to be able to interpret the results, but the value of the test statistic is reported in the row "Mann-Whitney U", from which a z-score is computed ("Z"). The asymptotical p-value is computed with this z-score. The value in the row "Wilcoxon W" is equal to the sum of the ranks in the COBRA arm.

Since non-parametric tests rank the observations, no effect size with corresponding 95 % CI is available. When using a non-parametric test, it is common practice to report the median and the range or interquartile range (IQR) of both groups. From the Mann-Whitney U test we conclude that there is not enough evidence to prove that ESR after 52 weeks of COBRA-light treatment (median 9 mm/h, IQR [2.3–16.3]) is different than after 52 weeks of COBRA treatment (median 5.5 mm/h, IQR [3.8–9.5]; $p = 0.48$).

3.2.3 Non-Inferiority and Equivalence

The COBRA-light trial was officially designed as a non-inferiority trial, with the primary aim to determine whether the COBRA-light strategy was non-inferior to the COBRA strategy in the decrease of the DAS44 at 26 weeks of follow-up [1]. In other words, the decrease in DAS44 in the COBRA-light arm (the intervention arm of the RCT), is not much worse (or even better) than in the COBRA arm (the control arm of the RCT). This 'not much worse' is quantified by the pre-set non-inferiority margin D. Let us consider the actual research question of the trial (▶Example 1.3, ▶Sect. 1.4):

> ❓ Is the COBRA-light strategy non-inferior compared to the COBRA strategy in change in the DAS44 in patients with early RA after 26 weeks of treatment?

The non-inferiority margin D of the trial was set to 0.50, so the null and alternative hypothesis were equal to

H0: the mean difference in change in DAS44 is smaller than −0.50 (with the COBRA strategy set as the reference group);
H1: the mean difference in change in DAS44 is larger than −0.50.

To test whether the null hypothesis in a non-inferiority study can be rejected, we focus on the 95 % CI for the mean difference in change in DAS44 between the two groups. The null hypothesis will be rejected, at the significance level α of 0.025, if the lower limit of the 95 % CI is larger than $-D$. The 95 % CI can be computed manually, using ▶Eq. E3.2 (▶Sect. 3.2.1). However, the 95 % CI of the mean difference between the groups is also part of the default SPSS output of the independent samples t-test. The mean decrease in the COBRA arm was −2.48 (SD 1.17) and −2.18 (SD 1.14) in the COBRA-light arm. The 95 % CI for the mean difference in decrease of the DAS44 (i.e., −0.30) is [−0.66; 0.059] (◻Table 3.4). Because the lower limit of the 95 % CI is smaller than −0.50, there is not enough evidence to reject the null hypothesis. In other words, there seems to be a difference in the decrease of DAS44 between COBRA and COBRA-light treatment. However, for a 95 % CI, the significance level α of the test is equal to 0.025, instead of the usual 0.05. To test at the significance level of 0.05, a 90 % CI for the mean difference has to be computed. The 90 % CI is equal to [−0.60; 0.00], hence at the 0.05 significance level, there is not enough evidence to reject the null hypothesis either. Summarizing, in a non-inferiority study with a significance level α, the $(1-2\alpha)100$ % CI has to be calculated.

3

■ Table 3.4   SPSS output of the independent samples t-test, comparing the change in DAS44 after 26 weeks between COBRA and COBRA-light treatment

Independent Samples Test

		Levene's Test for Equality of Variances		t-test for Equality of Means					95 % Confidence Interval of the Difference	
		F	Sig.	t	df	Sig. (2-tailed)	Mean Difference	Std. Error Difference	Lower	Upper
change in DAS44	Equal variances assumed	.013	.910	−1.653	159	.100	−.301	.182	−.660	.059
	Equal variances not assumed			−1.653	158.753	.100	−.301	.182	−.661	.059

The researchers of the COBRA-light trial could also have decided to perform an equivalence study. In that case, the research question would have been

> ? Is the COBRA-light strategy equivalent to the COBRA strategy in change in DAS44 in patients with early RA after 26 weeks of treatment?

For an equivalence margin D, the null and alternative hypothesis are:

H0: the mean difference in change in DAS44 is smaller than $-D$ or larger than $+D$ (with the COBRA strategy set as reference);
H1: the mean difference in change in DAS44 lies between $-D$ and $+D$.

The null hypothesis is rejected, at a significance level α of 0.05, if the 95 % CI lies completely between $-D$ and $+D$. For an equivalence margin of 0.50, there is not enough evidence to reject the null hypothesis, since the 95 % CI for the mean difference in change in DAS44 between COBRA and COBRA-light treatment is equal to $[-0.66; 0.059]$ (◘Table 3.4) and contains the value -0.50.

3.3 In Case of a Categorical Determinant

3.3.1 Analysis of Variance

The association between a continuous outcome variable and a categorical determinant (with more than two groups), is analyzed with an analysis of variance (ANOVA). The null and alternative hypothesis of the ANOVA are usually

H0: the mean of the outcome variable is equal in all groups;
H1: the mean of the outcome variable differs between at least two groups.

A common mistake made in formulating the alternative hypothesis for an ANOVA is that the mean of the outcome variable differs between *all* groups. However, since a difference between all groups is much stronger than a difference between at least two groups, the latter is the correct formulation.

The null and alternative hypothesis are written in terms of the mean of the outcome variable. However, the test statistic of the ANOVA is based on two components of the variance (explaining the term analysis of variance): (1) variance within groups, and (2) variance between groups. The variance in the study population is called the total sum of squares and denoted by SS_{tot}. It is equal to the sum of the squared difference between each observed value and the mean of the study population. The SS_{tot} can be decomposed in two separate sums of squares. The first component is the sum of squares between groups (denoted by $SS_{between}$), the second component is the sum of squares within groups (denoted by SS_{within}). The different sum of squares are computed as follows

$$SS_{tot} = \sum_{g=1}^{k} \sum_{i=1}^{n_g} (Y_{i,g} - \bar{Y})^2, \tag{E3.4}$$

$$SS_{between} = \sum_{g=1}^{k} n_g(\bar{Y}_g - \bar{Y})^2, \tag{E3.5}$$

$$SS_{within} = \sum_{g=1}^{k} \sum_{i=1}^{n_g} (Y_{i,g} - \bar{Y}_g)^2. \tag{E3.6}$$

In these equations, $Y_{i,g}$ is the value of the outcome variable for patient i in group g (with k groups in total), $\bar{Y}$ is the mean of the total study population, $\bar{Y}_g$ is the mean in group g, and n_g is the size of group g. The test statistic of the ANOVA is equal to

$$F = \frac{SS_{between}/(k-1)}{SS_{within}/(n-k)}. \tag{E3.7}$$

The larger the value of the test statistic F, the higher the evidence against the null hypothesis. The test statistic F has an F-distribution, with $k-1$ and $n-k$ degrees of freedom.

Example 3.4

Calculating the sum of squares

In an example dataset, three groups with three patients each, are measured. The observed outcome values of the patients in group one are: 5, 4, and 6. The observed outcome values of the patients in group two are: 2, 3, and 4. And in group three: 4, 3, and 5. The study population mean is equal to 4, and the group means are 5 (group 1), 3 (group 2), and 4 (group 3). The total sum of squares is equal to

$$SS_{tot} = (5-4)^2 + (4-4)^2 + (6-4)^2 + (2-4)^2 + (3-4)^2$$
$$+ (4-4)^2 + (4-4)^2 + (3-4)^2 + (5-4)^2 = 12.$$

The sum of squares between groups is equal to

$$SS_{between} = 3 \times (5-4)^2 + 3 \times (3-4)^2 + 3 \times (4-4)^2 = 6.$$

The sum of squares within groups is equal to

$$SS_{within} = (5-5)^2 + (4-5)^2 + (6-5)^2 + (2-3)^2 + (3-3)^2 +$$
$$(4-3)^2 + (4-4)^2 + (3-4)^2 + (5-4)^2 = 6.$$

The sum of squares between groups has 2 (i.e., $k-1 = 3-1$) degrees of freedom, and the sum of squares within groups 6 (i.e., $n-k = 9-3$) degrees of freedom.

Normally Distributed Outcome Variable

To illustrate the ANOVA, we consider the following research question

? Is there a difference between low, moderate and high ESR-level at baseline in decrease in DAS44 in patients with early RA after 52 weeks of treatment?

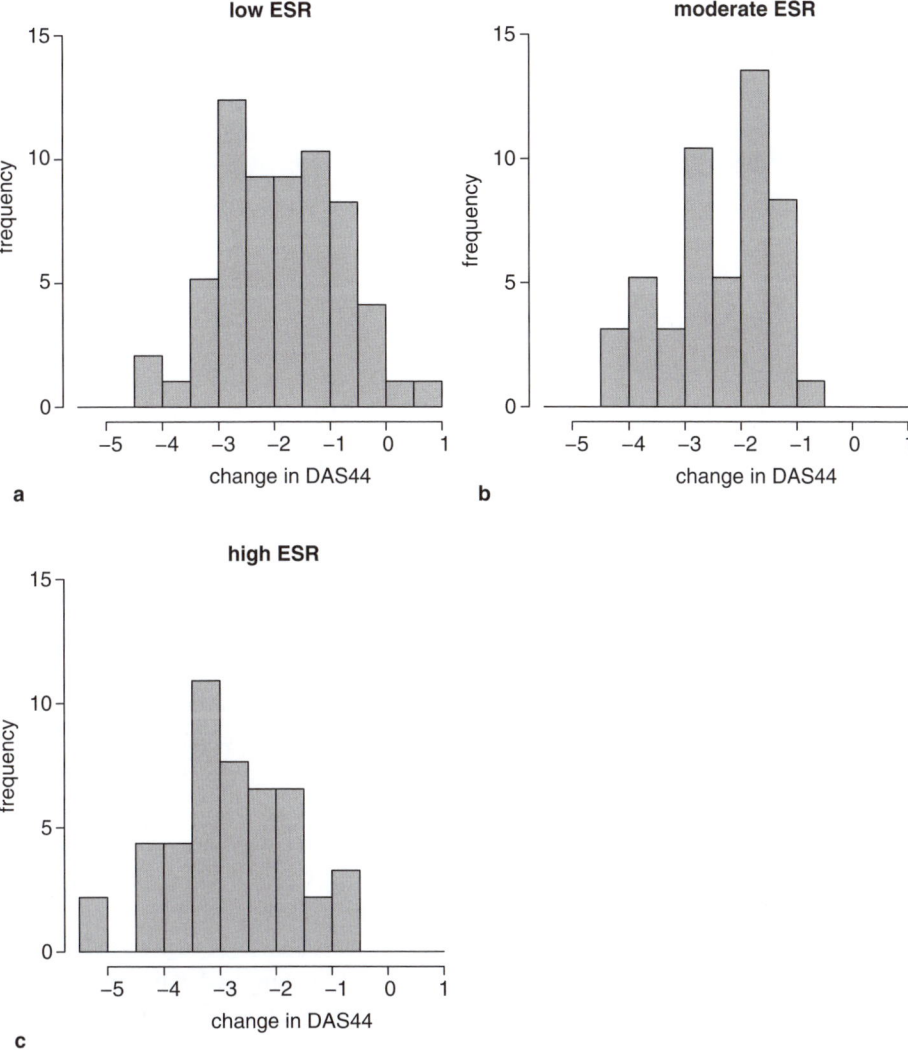

● **Fig. 3.3**   Histogram of the change in DAS44 after 52 weeks of treatment stratified by ESR at baseline: low ESR (**a**), moderate ESR (**b**), and high ESR (**c**)

As the outcome variable is continuous, its distribution needs to be checked in each group separately. ●Figure 3.3 shows the histograms of the change in DAS44 after 52 weeks of COBRA or COBRA-light treatment, stratified by ESR-level at baseline. In all groups, the outcome variable seems fairly normally distributed: therefore we apply the ANOVA on the original DAS44 outcome variable.

In patients with a low ESR at baseline ($n = 62$), the mean decrease in DAS44 is 1.8 millimeters per hour (mm/h) (SD 1.1), for patients with a moderate ESR at baseline ($n = 48$) −2.3 mm/h (SD 0.95), and in patients with a high ESR at baseline ($n = 44$) − 2.8 mm/h (SD 1.1). Since we now are comparing three groups, we cannot report one single effect size summarizing the overall difference between the three groups. Therefore, we

Table 3.5   SPSS output of an ANOVA, comparing the change in DAS44 between patients with low, moderate and high ESR at baseline

ANOVA

Change in DAS44

	Sum of Squares	df	Mean Square	F	Sig.
Between Groups	24.967	2	12.484	11.501	.000
Within Groups	163.897	151	1.085		
Total	188.864	153			

first test whether we can reject the null hypothesis, with the ANOVA. If the null hypothesis is rejected, we need to further investigate which groups differ from each other in a post hoc analysis. ◻Table 3.5 shows the SPSS output of the ANOVA. The different sum of squares ("under Sum of Squares") are provided in the different rows: SS_{tot} in row "Total", $SS_{between}$ in row "Between Groups", and SS_{within} in row "Within Groups". The degrees of freedom for each sum of squares are reported under "df". The sums of squares within and between groups divided by their respective degrees of freedom are reported under "Mean Square". The value of the test statistic is given under "F" and the p-value under "Sig.". From this output we conclude that the null hypothesis is rejected. According to SPSS, the p-value is equal to 0.000. SPSS rounds p-value to three decimals and, since it can never be exactly equal to zero, a p-value of 0.000 means that the p-value is smaller than 0.0005. We report this as $p < 0.001$.

Because the null hypothesis is rejected, a post hoc analysis needs to be performed. In the post hoc analysis, we test whether the difference in change in DAS44 between the groups is significant for each of the three pairs of comparisons. This could be done with three separate independent samples t-tests comparing two groups with each other in every analysis separately. However, the post hoc procedure is also part of the ANOVA analysis in SPSS. It is important to note that in the post hoc analysis, each group is compared to the other groups, and hence multiple null hypotheses are tested. For each combination of two groups, we test

H0: the mean of the outcome variable is equal in both groups;
H1: the mean of the outcome variable differs between both groups.

This means that multiple hypotheses are tested and, consequently, the probability to falsely reject a true null hypothesis increases. For testing one hypothesis, this probability is equal to the significance level of the test (i.e., the value of α). Thus, in a post hoc analysis, we have to correct for multiple testing, either by changing the significance level (i.e., lower the value of α) or adjusting the p-value.

There are many ways to adjust the p-value to account for multiple testing, of which we only illustrate the most conservative method: the Bonferroni correction. With the Bonferroni correction, the p-value of each of the post hoc tests is multiplied by m in case of m post hoc tests. In our example m is equal to three as we compared the change in DAS44 between low and moderate, low and high, and moderate and high ESR

☐ **Table 3.6** SPSS output of post hoc analyses after an ANOVA, comparing the change in DAS44 between patients with low, moderate and high ESR-level at baseline

Multiple Comparisons

Dependent Variable: change in DAS44

Bonferroni

(I) ESR at baseline	(J) ESR at baseline	Mean Difference (I–J)	Std. Error	Sig.	95 % Confidence Interval	
					Lower Bound	Upper Bound
low	moderate	.465	.200	.065	−.020	.950
	high	.983[a]	.205	.000	.486	1.480
moderate	low	−.465	.200	.065	−.950	.020
	high	.518	.217	.055	−.008	1.044
high	low	−.982[a]	.205	.000	−1.480	−.486
	moderate	−.518	.217	.055	−1.044	.008

[a]The mean difference is significant at the 0.05 level

level at baseline. In general, if k groups are compared, $k(k−1)/2$ post hoc tests are performed. For other frequently used correction methods we refer to the further readings (▶ Sect. 3.7). ☐Table 3.6 shows the SPSS output of the post hoc analyses, using the Bonferroni correction to account for multiple testing. Each group (under "(I) ESR at baseline") is compared to any of the other groups (under "(J) ESR at baseline"). The mean difference between each of these pairwise comparisons are reported under "Mean Difference (I–J)". Mean differences that differ significantly between the groups are marked with a footnote; these are corrected for multiple testing. The SE of this difference is reported under "Std. Error" and the p-value corrected for multiple testing under "Sig." The used correction method is stated below "Dependent Variable: change in DAS44", in our case it is "Bonferroni". The 95 % CIs for each pairwise comparison is provided under "95 % Confidence Interval". It is important to note that the 95 % CIs for the mean difference in the post hoc comparison of two groups are based on a different SE than in the independent samples t-test. Instead of using only the two groups that are compared, all other groups (in our example just one) are used as well. If possible, use the post hoc procedure of the statistical test to obtain effect sizes and corresponding 95 % CIs instead of comparing each pair of groups manually. In SPSS, however, not all statistical tests have a post hoc procedure.

Before we finalize the conclusion with respect to our current exemplary research question, we need to check one more assumption of the ANOVA. Just like the independent samples t-test, the ANOVA also assumes that the variances in all groups are equal. Equality of variances across groups is called homogeneity. The test for homogeneity is not a default

Table 3.7   SPSS output of test of homogeneity of variances in an ANOVA

Test of Homogeneity of Variances

Change in DAS44

Levene Statistic	df1	df2	Sig.
.476	2	151	.622

Table 3.8   SPSS output of the ANOVA, comparing the change in DAS44 between patients treated with the COBRA and COBRA-light strategy

ANOVA

Change in DAS44

	Sum of Squares	df	Mean Square	F	Sig.
Between Groups	4.526	1	4.526	3.732	.055
Within Groups	184.339	152	1.213		
Total	188.864	153			

test in SPSS, but can be opted for as additional output. When the test of homogeneity is not statistically significant, the assumption of equal variances is met and the ANOVA test can be used. When the homogeneity assumption does not hold (which is called heterogeneity), other statistical tests need to be used such as the Welch's ANOVA or the Brown-Forsythe ANOVA [4] which are two (optional) methods in SPSS (Apendix A.4.2). ◻Table 3.7 shows the SPSS output of the test of homogeneity. The value of the test statistic, which we do not explain as it is beyond the scope of this quick guide, is reported under "Levene statistic", the p-value under "Sig." and the degrees of freedom under "df1" and "df2". Since the test of homogeneity is not significant ($p = 0.62$), we can assume equal variances in the three groups.

The final conclusion regarding the research question is that the change in DAS44 differs between patients with low, moderate and high ESR at baseline ($p < 0.001$). Post hoc analyses with Bonferroni correction revealed a significantly larger decrease in DAS44 for patients with high ESR at baseline compared to patients with low ESR at baseline (mean differences 0.98 mm/h, 95 % CI [0.49; 1.5], $p < 0.001$ after Bonferroni correction). There was no evidence that patients with moderate ESR at baseline had a different decrease in DAS44, either when compared to patients with low ESR at baseline or to patients with high ESR at baseline.

The ANOVA could also be used to compare a continuous outcome variable between two groups, i.e., in case of a dichotomous determinant. The p-value of the ANOVA is then equal to the p-value of the independent samples t-test, under equal variances assumed (◻Table 3.1, ▶Sect. 3.2.1). ◻Table 3.8 shows the SPSS output of the ANOVA to compare the change in DAS44 after 52 weeks of COBRA treatment with COBRA-light treatment, in which we see the same p-value as in ◻Table 3.1.

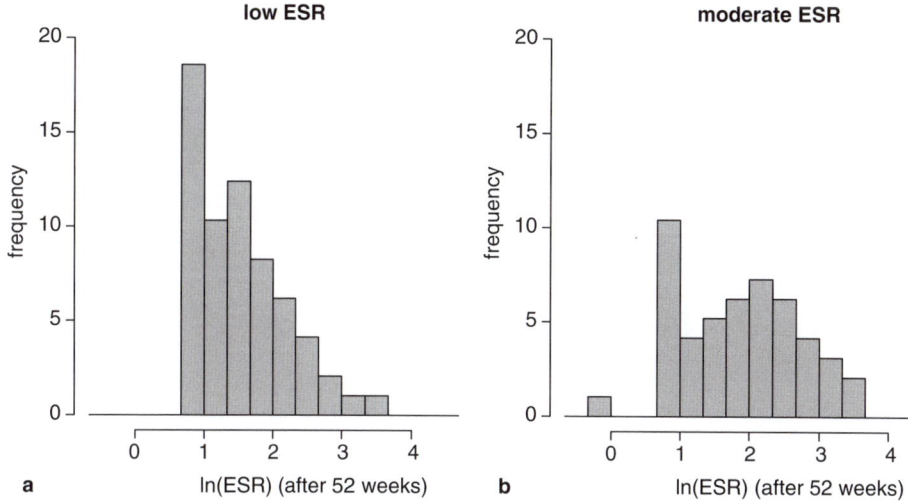

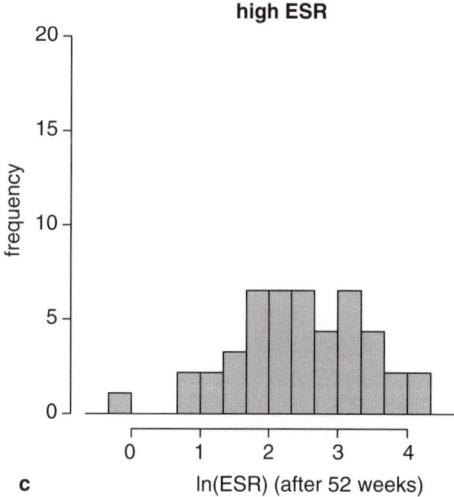

□ **Fig. 3.4**   Histogram of ln-transformed ESR after 52 weeks treatment stratified by ESR at baseline: low ESR (**a**), moderate ESR (**b**), and high ESR (**c**)

Non-Normally Distributed Outcome Variable

Similarly to when comparing two groups, the association between a non-normally distributed continuous outcome variable and a categorical determinant, could be tested by transforming the non-normally outcome variable. We illustrate this with the following research question

❓ Is there a difference in ESR after 52 weeks of treatment between patients with early RA with a low, moderate and high ESR-level at baseline?

We have already seen that ESR is not normally distributed in the whole study population (□Fig. 2.1, ▶Sect. 2.2.2) or within the treatment arm (□Fig. 3.2, ▶Sect. 3.2.1).

◘ **Table 3.9** SPSS output of the test of homogeneity of variances in an ANOVA

Test of Homogeneity of Variances			
ln(ESR) after 52 weeks			
Levene Statistic	df1	df2	Sig.
1.746	2	151	.178

◘ **Table 3.10** SPSS output of ANOVA, comparing the ln-transformed ESR after 52 weeks of treatment between patients with low, moderate and high ESR-level at baseline

ANOVA					
ln(ESR) after 52 weeks					
	Sum of Squares	df	Mean Square	F	Sig.
Between Groups	23.174	2	11.587	16.083	.000
Within Groups	108.789	151	.720		
Total	131.963	153			

Therefore, it is unlikely that ESR after 52 weeks of treatment is normally distributed within the three groups stated in this research question. Although this assumption might hold, we do always check the distribution of the outcome variable in each group. ◘Figure 3.4 shows the histograms of the ln-transformed ESR after 52 weeks of COBRA or COBRA-light treatment, stratified by ESR-level at baseline. In the first group, with low ESR at baseline, the normality assumption of ln(ESR) seems not to be met (◘Fig. 3.4a), while it does in the second and third group with moderate and high ESR at baseline (◘Fig. 3.4b and c, respectively). The ANOVA is quite robust against deviations from normality. Therefore, we use the ANOVA to answer this research question.

The test of homogeneity does not reject the null hypothesis of equal variances across the groups ($p = 0.18$, ◘Table 3.9). Therefore we use the regular ANOVA. The ln-transformed ESR after 52 weeks of treatment differs significantly ($p < 0.001$, ◘Table 3.10), indicating a significant difference between at least two groups. Post hoc analyses, with Bonferroni correction, reveal a significant difference between patients with a high ESR at baseline and patients with a low or moderate ESR at baseline (◘Table 3.11). Remember that, in the output, the mean differences with corresponding 95 % CIs are mean differences on the ln-transformed scale. The differences on the original ESR-scale are obtained by transforming these differences back (with the exponential function). This implies that

$$ESR_{52weeks;\ low}/ESR_{52weeks;\ high} = \exp(-0.95) = 0.39,$$
$$ESR_{52weeks;moderate}/ESR_{52weeks;high} = \exp(-0.59) = 0.55,$$

◻ **Table 3.11** SPSS output of post hoc analyses after an ANOVA, comparing the ln-transformed ESR after 52 weeks of treatment between patients with low, moderate and high ESR-level at baseline

Multiple Comparisons

Dependent Variable: ln(ESR) after 52 weeks

Bonferroni

(I) ESR at baseline	(J) ESR at baseline	Mean Difference (I–J)	Std. Error	Sig.	95 % Confidence Interval	
					Lower Bound	Upper Bound
low	moderate	−.355	.163	.094	−.750	.040
	high	−.948[a]	.167	.000	−1.353	−.543
moderate	low	.355	.163	.094	−.040	.750
	high	−.593[a]	.177	.003	−1.022	−.164
high	low	.948[a]	.167	.000	.543	1.353
	moderate	.593[a]	.177	.003	.164	1.022

[a]The mean difference is significant at the 0.05 level

or, equivalently, that the relative difference in ESR after 52 weeks of treatment between patients with low and high ESR at baseline is 0.39 (95 % CI [0.26; 0.58], $p < 0.001$) and between patients with moderate and high ESR at baseline 0.55 (95 % CI [0.36; 0.85], $p = 0.003$). This is also written as follows: the mean ESR after 52 weeks treatment in patients with high ESR at baseline is $1/0.39 = 2.6$ times higher (95 % CI [1.7; 3.8]) than in patients with low ESR at baseline, and $1/0.55 = 1.8$ times higher (95 % CI [1.2, 2.8]) than patients with moderate ESR at baseline.

3.3.2 Kruskall-Wallis Test

The ANOVA cannot be used to test the association between ESR after 52 weeks of treatment between patients with low, moderate and high ESR at baseline in a much smaller sized study population than the original study population. For example, assume that only 59 patients were included in the study of which 24 had a low ESR at baseline, 15 had a moderate ESR at baseline, and 20 had a high ESR at baseline. In such a case, a non-parametric test had to be used instead of the ANOVA: the Kruskal-Wallis test. The null and alternative hypothesis of this test are

H0: the distribution of ESR is equal in all groups;
H1: the distribution of ESR differs between at least two groups.

◻ Table 3.12   SPSS output of the Kruskal-Wallis test, comparing ESR after 52 weeks of treatment between patients with low, moderate and high ESR at baseline

Test Statistics[a,b]

	ESR after 52 weeks
Chi-Square	10.938
df	2
Asymp. Sig.	.004

[a]Kruskal Wallis Test
[b]Grouping Variable: ESR (mm/h) at baseline

◻ Table 3.13   Combined SPSS outputs for the post hoc pairwise comparisons with the Mann-Whitney *U* test

Test Statistics[a]

	Low vs moderate	Low vs high	Moderate vs high
Mann-Whitney U	155.000	99.500	63.500
Wilcoxon W	275.000	352.500	183.500
Z	−.319	−2.881	−2.754
Asymp. Sig. (2-tailed)	.750	.004	.006
Exact Sig. [2*(1-tailed Sig.)]	.772[b]	.[c]	.005[b]

[a]Grouping Variable: ESR at baseline
[b]Not corrected for ties
[c]Not reported by SPSS

The Kruskal-Wallis test is similar to the Mann-Whitney U test, but it computes and compares the mean rank of the three groups. Mean ranks that are similar in all groups are in favor of the null hypothesis, while differences between mean ranks are in favor of the alternative hypothesis.

◻Table 3.12 shows the SPSS output of the Kruskal-Wallis test. The value of the test statistic of the Krusal-Wallis test is reported in the first row ("Chi-Square"), the degrees of freedom of this test statistic in the second row ("df") and the p-value in the last row ("Asymp. Sig."). Again, the definition for the test statistic ("Z") is skipped; it is beyond the scope of this quick guide, and the definition is not necessary to interpret the results. From this table, we conclude that also in this small sized study population, ESR after 52 weeks of treatment differs between patients with low, moderate and high ESR at baseline ($p = 0.004$). In case of an overall difference between the groups, post hoc analyses reveal which groups differ significantly from each other. This is done with the Mann-Whitney U test because there is no post hoc procedure in the Kruskal-Wallis test in SPSS. ◻Table 3.13 shows the results of the post hoc analyses, in which three Mann-Whitney U tests were run for the pairwise comparisons. After applying the Bonferroni correction manually (i.e., multiply the p-value with the total number of comparisons), we conclude that patients with high ESR at baseline have a higher ESR after 52 weeks of treatment (median 11 mm/h, IQR [6−25]) than patients with low ESR at baseline (median 4 mm/h, IQR [2–9], $p = 0.012$) and moderate ESR at baseline (median 3, IQR [2–8], $p = 0.018$). In a scientific paper, we would report the median and IQR in each group, since no effect size is computed with non-parametric tests.

3.4   In Case of a Continuous Determinant

In a longitudinal study, the value of the outcome variable at the end of the follow-up period could be related to the value of the outcome variable at the beginning of the study. For example, patients with a lower DAS44 at baseline might also have a lower DAS44 or a smaller decrease in DAS44 after 52 weeks of COBRA-light treatment. In this case, both the determinant and the outcome variable are continuous. To illustrate how an association between a continuous outcome variable and a determinant is tested, we consider the following research question

> ❓ Is decrease in DAS44 after 52 weeks of COBRA-light treatment associated with the DAS44 at the start of study in patients with early RA?

The null and alternative hypothesis for this research question are:

H0: the decrease in DAS44 is not associated with the DAS44 at baseline;
H1: the decrease in DAS44 is associated with the DAS44 at baseline.

The association between two continuous variables is best visualized with a scatterplot (▶ Sect. 2.2.4), and tested with a correlation coefficient. For two normally distributed variables, the Pearson's correlation coefficient is used, so we first have to assess normality of the determinant (DAS44 at baseline) as well as the outcome variable (change in DAS44). Normality of the change in DAS44 was already shown in ◻Fig. 3.1 (▶ Sect. 3.2.1); normality of the DAS44 at baseline is concluded from the histogram in ◻Fig. 3.5.

   In terms of the correlation coefficient, the null and alternative hypothesis of our research question are

H0: there is no correlation between decrease in DAS44 and the DAS44 at baseline
   (i.e., $\rho = 0$);
H1: there is a correlation between decrease in DAS44 and the DAS44 at baseline
   (i.e., $\rho \neq 0$).

◻Table 3.14 shows the SPSS output of the Pearson's correlation coefficient between the decrease in change in DAS44 (named dDAS44) and the DAS44 at baseline. SPSS calculates the correlations between the two different variables in the cells "DAS44" and "dDAS44" as well as the correlation of both variables with themselves, in the cells "DAS44" and

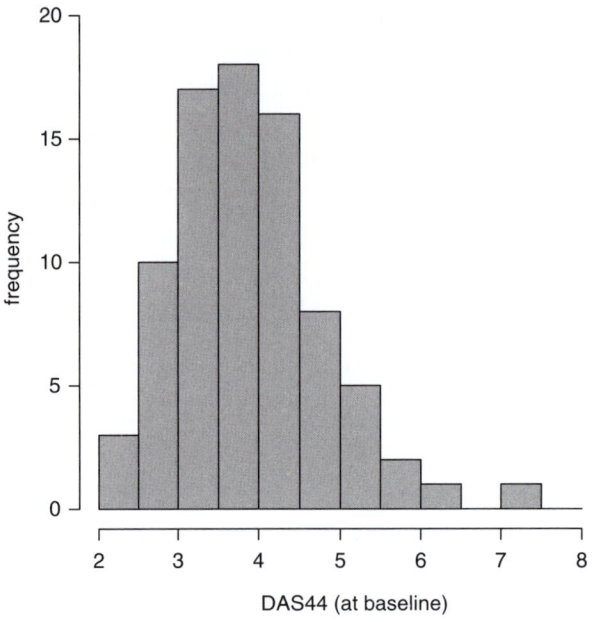

☐ Fig. 3.5   Histogram of the DAS44 at baseline for the COBRA-light treatment arm

☐ Table 3.14   SPSS output of the Pearson's correlation coefficient between decrease in DAS44 ('dDAS44') and the DAS44 at baseline in patients treated with the COBRA-light strategy

Correlations		DAS44	dDAS44
DAS44	Pearson Correlation	1	−.493[a]
	Sig. (2-tailed)		.000
	N	81	77
dDAS44	Pearson Correlation	−.493[a]	1
	Sig. (2-tailed)	.000	
	N	77	77

[a]Correlation is significant at the 0.01 level (2-tailed)

"DAS44" or "dDAS44" and "dDAS44". By default, the later ones are always equal to one. The correlation between any two variables is reported in the row "Pearson Correlation", the p-value in the row "Sig. (2-tailed)" and the number of patients with a non-missing value for both variables in the row "N". For example, among the 81 patients with a baseline assessment, a delta-score could be computed for only 77 of them. From this output, we conclude that there is a significant correlation between the two variables ($\rho = -0.49$, $p < 0.001$).

3.4.1 Linear Regression Model

The interpretation of the correlation coefficient is not as straight forward as an effect size: the correlation coefficient does not have a dimension, since both variables are standardized. A better effect size to measure the effect of the determinant on the continuous outcome variable, is a statistic that directly relates differences in the outcome variable to differences in the determinant. Such a relation between the differences is obtained by a linear regression model. In the linear regression model, the outcome variable is modeled by a linear function of the determinant. The model in our example is

$$\text{mean dDAS44} = b_0 + b_1 \times \text{DAS44\_wk0}, \tag{M3.1}$$

where the coefficients b_0 and b_1 are called regression coefficients. The coefficients are estimated by the least squares estimation method. This method minimizes the squared difference between the observed values of the outcome variable (generally denoted by $Y_1, Y_2, \ldots, Y_n$ for a study population of size n) and a linear (straight) line with intercept b_0 and slope b_1. The interpretation of the regression coefficients are derived from the linear function:

- b_0 is the mean change in DAS44 for a patient with a DAS44 of zero at baseline [the intercept of the line];
- b_1 is the mean difference in change in DAS44 between two patients who differ by one point in their DAS44 at baseline [the slope of the line].

Note that the value of the intercept b_0 is not always clinically meaningful, after all, patients with a DAS44 of zero at baseline would probably not have been included in the trial. In that case, the determinant (i.e., DAS44 at baseline) could be centralized so that b_0 is the mean outcome at the mean value of the determinant. The null and alternative hypothesis regarding the association between the change in DAS44 and the DAS44 at baseline can be translated to a null and alternative hypothesis involving the regression coefficient b_1

H0: $b_1 = 0$;
H1: $b_1 \neq 0$;

◻Table 3.15 shows the SPSS output of the linear regression model, relating a decrease in the change in DAS44 to an increase of the DAS44 at baseline. The table consists of two rows, one labeled "(Constant)", the other labeled "DAS44 (at baseline)". The first row reports the estimated regression coefficient b_0 (under "B"), with its SE (under "Std Error"), the corresponding 95 % CI (under "95 % Confidence Interval for B"), the p-value (under "Sig"), and the test-statistic (under "t"). These values are, however, not important, because b_0 is only the intercept and not the result of interest. The second row reports the estimated regression coefficient for the slope b_1, its SE with corresponding 95 % CI, the p-value and the test-statistic. The value of the standardized coefficient (under "Beta"), is equal to the Pearson's correlation coefficient. At this stage, we do not look at

◻ Table 3.15   SPSS output of a linear regression analysis, relating the change in DAS44 to the DAS44 at baseline

Coefficients[a]

Model		Unstandardized Coefficients		Standardized Coefficients	t	Sig.	95 % Confidence Interval for B	
		B	Std. Error	Beta			Lower Bound	Upper Bound
1	(Constant)	.101	.453		.223	.824	−.801	1.003
	DAS44 (at baseline)	−.548	.112	−.493	−4.905	.000	−.771	−.326

[a]Dependent Variable: change in DAS44

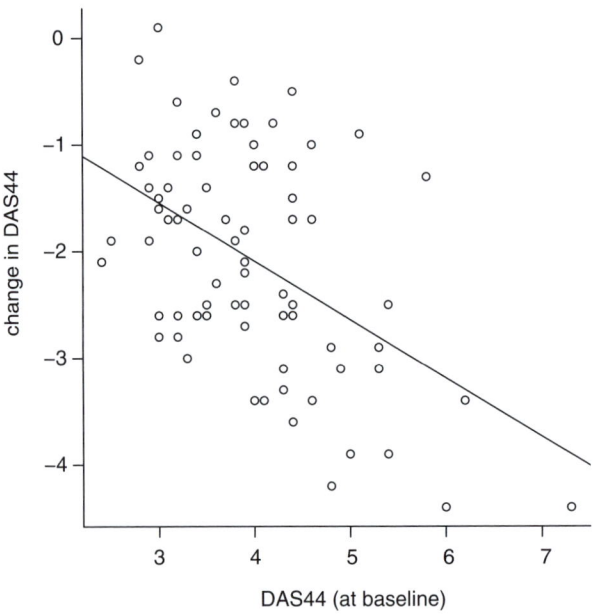

◻ Fig. 3.6   Scatterplot of the association between the change in DAS44 and the DAS44 at baseline after 52 weeks of COBRA-light treatment. The reference line represents the estimated regression line

the standardized coefficients any further, but we will discuss them again when discussing multivariable regressions models (including multiple determinants) in ▶ Chap. 6. The final conclusion with regard to our research question is as follows: the change in DAS44 after 52 weeks of COBRA-light treatment is associated with the DAS44 at baseline ($p < 0.001$). A higher score at baseline implies a stronger decrease in DAS44 after 52 weeks of treatment: 0.55 points per difference of 1 point at baseline (95 % CI [0.33; 0.77]). Beside reporting the results of the linear regression model in a table, a scatterplot with the regression function provides a nice visual summary of the data and the model (◻Fig. 3.6).

3.4.2 Assumptions of the Linear Regression Model

As we have seen up until now, assumptions need to be checked for all analyses, to see if the statistical test can indeed be used. Contrary to the independent samples t-test and the ANOVA, the assumptions of the linear regression model can only be checked after estimating the model. The assumptions and how to test them, need to be explained with the help of a mathematical equation. The general linear regression model relating the outcome variable Y to the determinant x has the form

$$\text{mean } Y = b_0 + b_1 \times x. \tag{M3.2}$$

Since some unobserved variation between patients is always present which is caused by factors not included in the regression model, the linear regression model is also written as

$$Y = b_0 + b_1 \times x + \varepsilon. \tag{M3.3}$$

This unobserved variation is captured in the variable ε (epsilon; also referred to as the error-variable). The linear regression models assumes that
1. ε is normally distributed with mean equal to zero (normality);
2. the variance of ε does not depend on the determinant x (which is called homoscedasticity); and
3. the relation between Y and x is linear (which is referred to as linearity).

To test assumptions 1. and 2., the error-variable has to be estimated because it is unobserved. To do so, we use the linear regression equation with the estimated regression coefficients to 'predict' the value of the outcome variable for every subject i with determinant value x_i by $\hat{Y}_i = b_0 + b_1 x_i$. The difference between the predicted value $\hat{Y}_i$ and the observed value Y_i is called the residual (for subject i) and is considered an estimate of the error-variable. Assumptions 1. and 2. are investigated by checking whether the residuals are normally distributed with mean equal to zero and whether their variances do not depend on the determinant x.

In SPSS, the residuals can be saved in a linear regression analysis query (Supplementary Information A.4.3), which are then added to the database as a new variable. Normality of the residuals is then investigated with a histogram (◻Fig. 3.7a). From this figure, we conclude that the residuals seem fairly normally distributed. Homoscedasticity can be investigated with a residual-versus-predictor plot. On the x-axis of this plot, the value of the determinant (or predictor) for each patient is plotted, and on the y-axis the corresponding residual is plotted. If the residuals form a 'horizontal band' around the reference line at zero, homoscedasticity is assumed. In ◻Fig. 3.7b, we see this band lies between the lines -2 and $+2$, so homoscedasticity seems a valid assumption. The opposite of homoscedasticity is heteroscedasticity, which means that the variance of the error-variable ε depends on the determinant x and the residuals do not form a horizontal band around the reference line at zero. In ▶ Sect. 3.4.5, we explain how to deal with heteroscedasticity The third assumption, linearity, is explained in ▶ Sect. 3.4.4 because we first have to explain how to interpret a linear regression model with a categorical determinant.

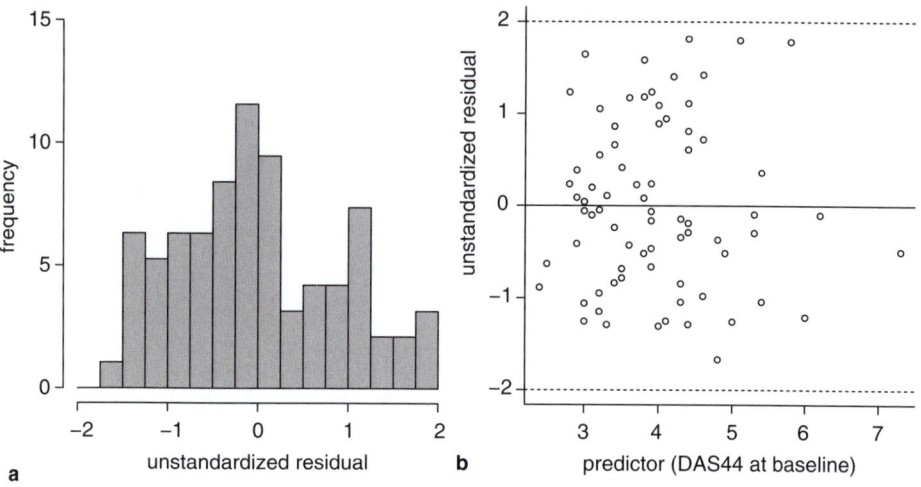

◻ Fig. 3.7 Histogram of the residuals of the linear regression model relating the change in DAS44 after 52 weeks of COBRA-light treatment to the DAS44 at baseline (**a**), and the residual-versus-predictor plot for the same linear regression model (**b**)

3.4.3 Linear Regression Model with a Dichotomous or Categorical Determinant

Linear regression also works for analyzing the association between a continuous out-come and a categorical determinant. To illustrate this, let us consider the research question of ▶Example 1.1 (▶Sect. 1.4) again: the mean differences in decrease of DAS44 between COBRA and COBRA-light treatment after 52 weeks of treatment. The linear regression model with treatment arm as determinant is equal to

$$\text{mean dDAS44} = b_0 + b_1 \times \text{treatment.} \tag{M3.4}$$

From ▶Model M3.4 it follows that the mean change in DAS44 in patients treated with the COBRA strategy is equal to $b_0 + b_1 \times 0 = b_0$ and with the COBRA-light strategy to $b_0 + b_1 \times 1 = b_0 + b_1$. So, b_1 is the mean difference in change in DAS44 between 52 weeks of COBRA and COBRA-light treatment, and b_0 is the mean change in DAS44 after 52 weeks of COBRA treatment (as the COBRA arm was set as reference group). ◻Table 3.16 shows the results of the linear regression model. The unstandardized coeffi-cient is equal to the mean difference between the arms as obtained with the independent samples t-test (◻Table 3.1, ▶Sect. 3.2.1), except for the minus sign. This is because in the linear regression model the COBRA strategy is set as reference category, whereas in the independent samples t-test the COBRA-light strategy is set as the reference category.

Assumptions 1. and 2. of the linear regression model need to be checked for a cat-egorical determinant too. This is similar to what is done for a continuous determinant, with a histogram (◻Fig. 3.8a) and a residual-versus-predictor-plot (◻Fig. 3.8b). Homo-scedasticity (assumption 2.) can also be formally tested with the Levene's test for equality of variances, through the independent samples t-test on the residuals (◻Table 3.17).

■ **Table 3.16** SPSS output of a linear regression model, comparing the change in DAS44 after 52 weeks of COBRA treatment with COBRA-light treatment

Coefficients[a]

Model		Unstandardized Coefficients		Standardized Coefficients	t	Sig.	95 % Confidence Interval for B	
		B	Std. Error	Beta			Lower Bound	Upper Bound
1	(Constant)	−2.405	.125		−19.165	.000	−2.653	−2.157
	treatment	.343	.177	.155	1.932	.055	−.008	.694

[a]Dependent Variable: change in DAS44

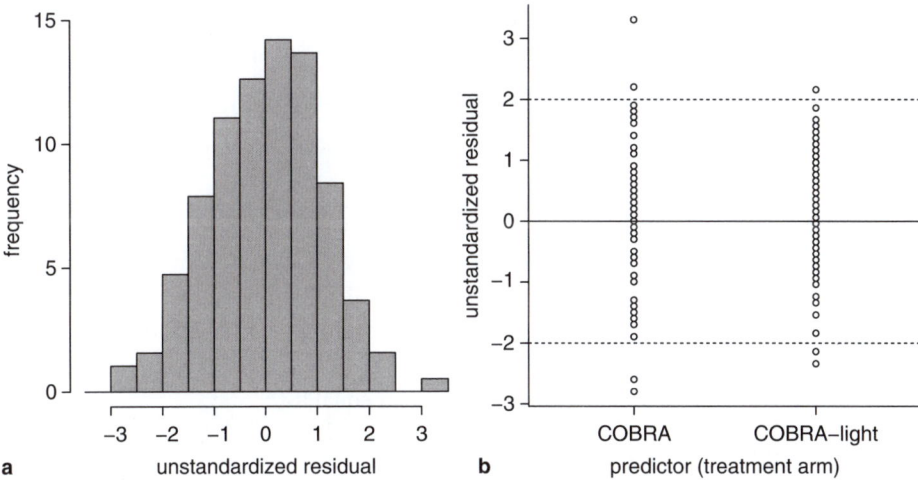

a   b

■ **Fig. 3.8** Histogram of residuals in linear regression model relating the change in DAS44 after 52 weeks to treatment arm (**a**), and the residual-versus-predictor plot for the same linear regression model (**b**)

Since the p-value of the Levene's test is larger than the significance level α of 0.05, we cannot reject the null hypothesis, and we assume that the variance of the residuals is equal in the COBRA and the COBRA-light arm.

For a categorical determinant with more than two groups, dummy variables need to be created for the linear regression model. Otherwise, the regression coefficient b_1 is interpreted as the mean difference between any pair of consecutive groups. Apart from the linearity assumption in case of a continuous determinant, this is usually not assumed when comparing multiple groups. Dummy variables are dichotomous indicator variables, and are created such that the regression coefficient is interpreted as the mean difference between two groups. For a categorical determinant with k groups, $k-1$ dummy variables are created and one category is set as the reference group. The value of the dummy variable for this group is set to zero for all dummies, while the values of the remaining dummy variables are set to one for each of the other groups separately.

Table 3.17   SPSS output of the Levene's test to check homoscedasticity of the residuals of a linear regression model with a dichotomous determinant, as part of the independent samples t-test

Independent Samples Test

		Levene's Test for Equality of Variances	
		F	Sig.
Unstandardized Residual	Equal variances assumed	.803	.372
	Equal variances not assumed		

Table 3.18   Categorical dummy coding for a linear regression model with ESR at baseline in three groups

ESR at baseline	d_1	d_2
Low	0	0
Moderate	1	0
High	0	1

Consider the research question of ▶Sect. 3.3.1 again in which we investigated the change in DAS44 between patients with low, moderate and high ESR at baseline. Let us set low ESR at baseline as the reference group. Dummy d_1 is equal to one only for patients with moderate ESR at baseline and zero otherwise, and dummy d_2 is equal to one only for patients with high ESR at baseline (▪Table 3.18).

The linear regression model for these dummies is equal to

$$\text{mean dDAS44} = b_0 + b_1 \times d_1 + b_2 \times d_2. \tag{M3.5}$$

From ▶Model M3.5 it follows that the mean change in DAS44 for patients with low ESR at baseline is equal to $b_0 + b_1 \times 0 + b_2 \times 0 = b_0$, for patients with moderate ESR at baseline to $b_0 + b_1 \times 1 + b_2 \times 0 = b_0 + b_1$, and for patient with high ESR at baseline to $b_0 + b_1 \times 0 + b_2 \times 1 = b_0 + b_2$.

In other words, b_0 is the mean change in DAS44 in patients with low ESR at baseline, b_1 is the mean difference (in change) between patients with moderate and low ESR at baseline, and b_2 between patients with high and low ESR at baseline. The difference between patients with high and moderate ESR at baseline could also be derived from the regression coefficients b_1 and b_2 and is equal to $b_2 - b_1$. ▪Table 3.19 shows the SPSS output of this linear regression model. From this output we conclude that the mean difference in change in DAS44 between patients with moderate ESR at baseline and low ESR at baseline is −0.47. In other words, the change in DAS44 is 0.47 points lower in patients with moderate ESR than the change in DAS44 in patients with low ESR. The difference in mean change in DAS44 between high ESR and low ESR is −0.98.

The differences between patients with moderate or high ESR at baseline, and patients with low ESR at baseline are equal to what we found in the post hoc analyses

◘ **Table 3.19** SPSS output of a linear regression model comparing the change in DAS44 between patients with low, moderate and high ESR at baseline

Coefficients[a]

Model		Unstandardized Coefficients		Standardized Coefficients	t	Sig.	95 % Confidence Interval for B	
		B	Std. Error	Beta			Lower Bound	Upper Bound
1	(Constant)	−1.808	.132		−13.665	.000	−2.069	−1.547
	d1	−.465	.200	−.194	−2.321	.022	−.861	−.069
	d2	−.983	.205	−.401	−4.786	.000	−1.389	−.577

[a]Dependent Variable: change in DAS44

of the ANOVA, but the 95 % CIs are not. This is due to the fact that the 95 % CIs in the post hoc analyses of the ANOVA were based on a different SE. The p-values comparing patients with moderate or high ESR at baseline with patients with low ESR at baseline ($p = 0.022$ and $p < 0.001$, respectively) in a linear regression analysis are not corrected for multiple testing. In conclusion, a continuous outcome variable could be compared with a linear regression model or an ANOVA. The advantage of ANOVA is that SPSS has an option to correct for multiple testing, which cannot be done with linear regression. However, the advantage of linear regression is that the analyses could be corrected for potential influencing factors (►Chap. 6).

3.4.4 Investigating the Linearity Assumption

We needed the set-up and interpretation of a linear regression model with a categorical determinant to investigate the third assumption, i.e., linearity, in a linear regression model, with a continuous determinant. The third assumption implies that the difference in the outcome variable is constant per unit increase of the determinant. This assumption is checked with the residual-versus-predictor plot. Linearity holds if the residuals 'bounce randomly' around the reference line at zero. That is, there is no increasing (or decreasing) trend visible, or for small and large values the residuals are almost all negative, while they are positive in the middle. Similarly as for the assumption of homoscedasticity, this is based on eye-balling and this procedure will not work for other types of outcome variables.

Another method to investigate linearity between the outcome variable and the determinant is to add a quadratic term to the linear regression model. Let us go back to the research question relating the change in DAS44 after 52 weeks of COBRA-light treatment to the DAS44 at baseline. We add the square of DASS44 at baseline to the linear regression model

$$\text{mean dDAS44} = b_0 + b_1 \times \text{DAS44\_wk0} + b_2 \times \text{DAS44\_wk0}^2. \tag{M3.6}$$

■ **Table 3.20**   SPSS output of the linear regression model for the association between the change in DAS44 and DAS44 at baseline, with a quadratic term for DAS44 at baseline

Coefficients

	Unstandardized Coefficients		Standardized Coefficients	t	Sig.
	B	Std. Error	Beta		
DAS44 (at baseline)	.223	.701	.200	.318	.752
DAS44 (at baseline) ** 2	−.088	.079	−.702	−1.114	.269
(Constant)	−1.497	1.504		−.995	.323

To investigate the linearity assumption, we then test the following null and alternative hypothesis

H0: $b_2 = 0$;
H1: $b_2 \neq 0$;

After all, if the regression coefficient b_2 would be equal to zero, it indicates that the relation between the change in DAS44 and DAS44 at baseline is at least not quadratic. ▶Model M3.6 can be estimated in two ways in SPSS. First of all, a new variable could be computed, with the square of DAS44 at baseline. Secondly, the curve estimation query in SPSS can be used (Supplementary Information A.4.3). This procedure creates the square automatically. ▢Table 3.20 shows the SPSS output of ▶Model M3.6, using the curve esti-mation query. The first row in the SPSS output corresponds to the regression coefficient b_1 for the linear term, the second row to the regression coefficient b_2 for the quadratic term, and the third row to the regression coefficient b_0 for the intercept. The estimated regression coefficients can be found under "B", its SE under "Std. Error", the value of the test-statistic under "t" and the p-value under "Sig.". Again, a standardized coefficient is calculated (under "Beta"), which we ignore for now. In the curve estimation query, SPSS does not provide the 95 % CI for the regression coefficients. If the quadratic term would have been created manually and then added to the model in the linear regression query, the 95% CI would have been provided if selected as additional option (Supplementary Information A.4.3). Because the p-value for b_2 is larger than the significance level α of 0.05 ($p = 0.27$), we cannot reject the null hypothesis, and conclude that the relation is at least not quadratic. However, a cubic relation would be possible, i.e., a model were also DAS44_wk0^3 is included, or even relations in which a higher power of DAS44 at baseline are included. The question is then, when to stop including higher powers of the determi-nant. The same holds, if the null hypothesis would be rejected; is the relation then quad-ratic, or even cubic? Moreover, we cannot interpret the regression coefficients anymore, and only visualize the association between the outcome variable and the determinant with the estimated regression curve.

◫ **Table 3.21** Categorical dummy coding for a linear regression model with four groups

Quartile	n	Range	d_1	d_2	d_3
1	20	2.4–3.2	0	0	0
2	18	3.3–3.8	1	0	0
3	26	3.9–4.4	0	1	0
4	17	4.6–7.3	0	0	1

◫ **Table 3.22** SPSS output of a linear regression model with DAS44 at baseline in four categories (three dummy variables)

Coefficients[a]

Model		Unstandardized Coefficients		Standardized Coefficients	t	Sig.	95 % Confidence Interval for B	
		B	Std. Error	Beta			Lower Bound	Upper Bound
1	(Constant)	−1.600	.206		−7.781	.000	−2.010	−1.190
	d1	−.141	.303	−.057	−.465	.643	−.746	.463
	d2	−.492	.278	−.223	−1.766	.082	−1.047	.063
	d3	−1.338	.308	−.532	−4.336	.000	−1.952	−.723

[a]Dependent Variable: change in DAS44

Therefore we suggest another method to investigate linearity between the outcome variable and the determinant: categorization of the determinant in more than two groups. Assume, for example, that the determinant is categorized in four groups. Then, linearity implies that the mean difference between the first two groups is approximately equal to the difference between the third and second group and also between the last and third group. This can be done by checking the differences between consecutive groups with an ANOVA, but is easier to check with a linear regression model.

Another way to investigate whether the association between the change in DAS44 after 52 weeks of COBRA-light treatment to the DAS44 at baseline is indeed linear, is to divide the DAS44 at baseline in four groups of approximately the same size (called quartiles). We choose groups of approximately the same size in order to prevent a small group being the reference group, which makes the results of the linear regression model less stable. For these four groups, three dummy variables are created (◫Table 3.21).

◫Table 3.22 shows the SPSS output of the linear regression with the three dummy variables. In this output, we see that the difference in change in DAS44 between the first and second group is −0.14, between the third and first group is −0.49, and between the fourth and first group is −1.34. The difference between the third and second group is equal to −0.49 − (−0.14) = −0.35, and the difference between the fourth and third

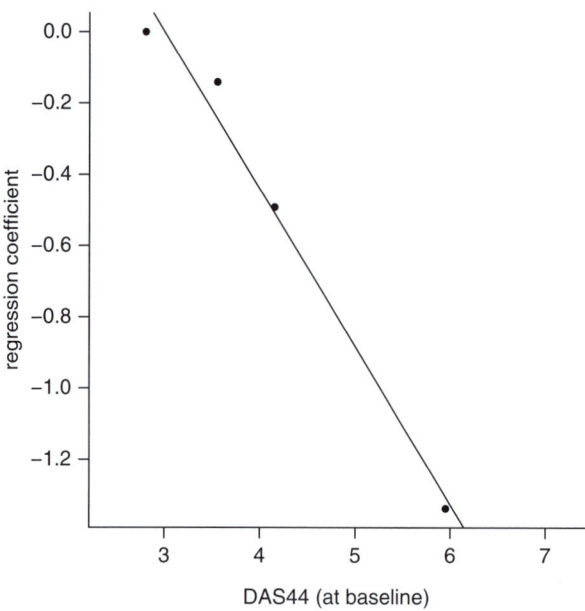

◘ Fig. 3.9   Scatterplot of the midpoints of the four DAS44 at baseline groups and the corresponding regression coefficients for the groups

group is equal to $-1.34 - (-0.49) = -0.85$. Linearity would hold if these differences are approximately equal to the difference between the first and second group. This doesn't seem to be the case. However, the DAS44 at baseline was divided into four groups of approximately the same size, not of approximately the same width. Therefore, we plot the regression coefficients at the mid-point of the groups to find out whether the points lie more or less on a straight line (◘Fig. 3.9). We use the mid-points, because fewer patients had a high DAS44 at baseline, therefore covering a wider range of DAS44 scores. We conclude that the linearity assumption in the association between change in DAS44 and the DAS44 at baseline holds. In conclusion, the change in DAS44 after 52 weeks of COBRA-light treatment is associated with the DAS44 at baseline ($p < 0.001$, ◘Table 3.15). A higher score at baseline implies a stronger decrease in DAS44 after 52 weeks of treatment: 0.55 points per increase of 1 point at baseline (95 % CI [0.33; 0.77]).

3.4.5 Violation of the Assumptions, What to Do?

In all the examples above, all three assumptions for the linear regression model are met. What to do if this was not the case?

1. If normality of the residuals does not hold, try to transform the outcome variable. Note that the assumption of normality is on the error-variable, not on the outcome variable itself. First, estimate the linear regression model and save the residuals. Then make a histogram or QQ-plot of the residuals. Linear regression models are robust

against small deviations from normality. However, if the size of the study population is small and the outcome variable is highly skewed, the Spearman's rank correlation is the only way to test the association between two continuous variables in that case (▶ Sect. 2.3.1).

2. If homoscedasticity does not hold, try to transform the outcome variable and/or continuous determinants. If this does not help, consult a statistician. There are other mathematical models to deal with heteroscedasticity, but they are far beyond the scope of this quick guide. For more advanced readers, we refer to further readings (▶ Sect. 3.7) for references on these advanced models.

3. If linearity does not hold, analyze the association between the outcome variable and the determinant by categorizing the latter one (▶ Sect. 3.4.4). It is then advised to create clinically relevant categories instead of quartiles, while keeping in mind that the reference group should not be too small compared to the other categories.

3.5　In Case of Repeated Measurements

In many prospective studies, variables are repeatedly measured within patients, such as in the COBRA-light trial where patients were measured at study entry (baseline), and after 13, 26, 39 and 52 weeks of treatment. All examples in the previous sections are based on a change between two measurements (i.e., between baseline and after 26 or 52 weeks of treatment). In these sections we illustrated how to test for differences between groups, but the primary or secondary objective of a study could also be to test for a change between two measurements within the same patient. If the outcome variable is measured twice within the same patient, the measurements cannot be considered independent, as was the case in the independent samples t-test. In this section, we illustrate how to test for differences in analyses of repeated measurements of the outcome variable within patients.

3.5.1　Paired Sample *T*-Test

If the outcome variable is normally distributed at both measurements, the paired sample t-test is used. The null and alternative hypothesis of the paired sample t-test usually are

H0: the mean of the outcome variable is equal at both measurements;
H1: the mean of the outcome variable is unequal at both measurements.

This is the same as testing

H0: the mean differences (within each patient) is equal to zero;
H1: the mean difference is unequal to zero.

The effect size of this test is the mean difference and it could be computed in two ways: either by computing the mean outcomes at both measurements and then taking the difference, or by computing the difference (delta-score) between the measurements within each patient separately and then computing the mean of this new outcome variable. The test statistic for the paired sample t-test is equal to

$$t = \frac{\text{mean difference}}{\text{SD}_\Delta / \sqrt{n}}.$$

(E3.8)

Here SD_Δ is the SD of the delta-variable, and n the size of the study population. The test statistic t has a t-distribution with $n-1$ degrees of freedom. Higher values of the absolute value of t are evidence against the null hypothesis and in favor of the alternative hypothesis.

Example 3.5

Effect size after 52 weeks of COBRA-light treatment
Four out of 81 patients (4.9 %) missed a DAS44 measurement after 52 weeks of COBRA-light treatment. The baseline score of the remaining 77 patients was 3.95 (SD 0.92) which decreased to 1.88 (SD 0.99) after 52 weeks. The mean decrease is then equal to $1.88-3.95 = -2.06$.

Normally Distributed Outcome Variable

Assume, for example, that we want to answer the following research question

❓ Does the DAS44 change within 52 weeks of treatment with the COBRA-light strategy in patients with RA (compared to before treatment)?

Note that we formulate this research question only for the patients who received the COBRA-light strategy. Before the paired sample t-test is used, normality of the outcome variables at both measurements has to be checked, or, equivalently, normality of the delta-variable. ◘Figure 3.10 shows the histograms of the DAS44 at baseline and after 52 weeks of COBRA-light treatment. The DAS44 seems normally distributed at baseline, but not after 52 weeks of treatment. Also the delta-variable does not seem to be normally distributed (◘Fig. 3.1b, ▶Sect. 3.2.1). However, since the size of the study population is not so small ($n = 81$), and the deviation from normality is probably only mild, we use the paired sample t-test anyway, to answer the research question.

◘Table 3.23 shows the SPSS output of the paired sample t-test. As with the independent samples t-test, the mean difference is reported (under "Mean"), together with the SE (under "Std. Error Mean"), the 95 % CI (under "95 % Confidence Interval of the Difference") and the p-value (under "Sig. (2-tailed)"). In addition, the test statistic ("t"), the degrees of freedom (under "df") and the SD (under "Std. Deviation") are reported. We conclude that the DAS44 decreases significantly after 52 weeks of COBRA-light treatment. This is reported as follows: the mean DAS44 decreased by 2.1 points (95 % CI [1.8; 2.3], $p < 0.001$) after 52 weeks of COBRA-light treatment.

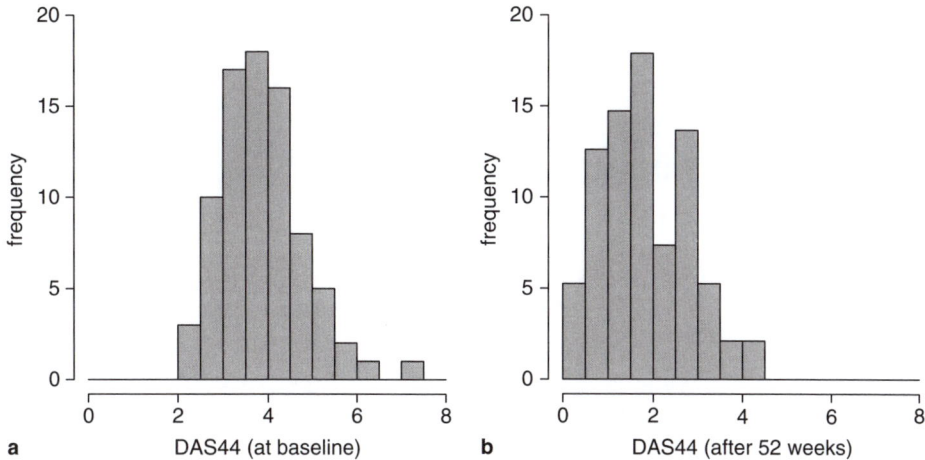

a   DAS44 (at baseline)   b   DAS44 (after 52 weeks)

◻ **Fig. 3.10**   Histograms of the DAS44 at baseline (**a**) and after 52 weeks (**b**) of COBRA-light treatment

◻ **Table 3.23**   SPSS output of the paired sample t-test to investigate the change in DAS44 after 52 weeks COBRA-light treatment

Paired Samples Test

	Paired Differences					t	df	Sig. (2-tailed)
	Mean	Std. Deviation	Std. Error Mean	95 % Confidence Interval of the Difference				
				Lower	Upper			
DAS44 (52 weeks) – DAS44 (baseline)	−2.062	1.026	.117	−2.295	−1.829	−17.634	76	.000

Non-Normally Distributed Outcome Variable

If the effect of 52 weeks of COBRA-light treatment would have been investigated using the ESR instead of the DAS44, the paired sample t-test could not be used directly. In ►Chaps. 2 and 3 we already saw that ESR is not normally distributed at baseline (◻Fig. 2.1, ►Sect. 2.2.2) and after 52 weeks (◻Fig. 3.2, ►Sect. 3.2.2). Consequently, the difference between the measurement after 52 weeks and the measurement at baseline is also not likely to be normally distributed (data not shown). However, the outcome variable can be transformed. The ln-transformation works well in this case: ◻Fig. 3.11 shows the histogram of the change in ln(ESR) between baseline and after 52 weeks, which resembles the normal distribution.

Since the change in ln(ESR) is normally distributed, the paired sample t-test is used to investigate whether ESR changed significantly after 52 weeks COBRA-light treatment. ◻Table 3.24 shows the SPSS output of the paired sample t-test. The mean ln(ESR) decreased by 1.1 (95 % CI [0.90; 1.3], $p < 0.001$). However, this decrease is

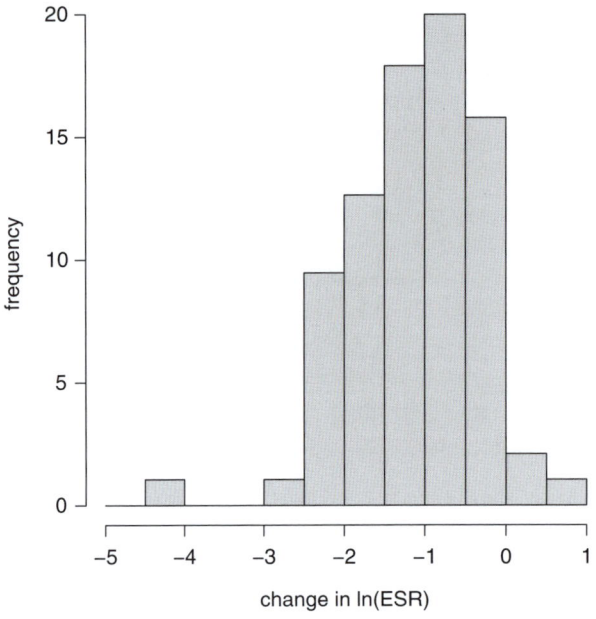

Fig. 3.11 Histogram of the change in ln(ESR) after 52 weeks COBRA-light treatment

Table 3.24 SPSS output of the paired sample *t*-test to investigate the change in ESR after 52 weeks COBRA-light treatment

Paired Samples Test

	Paired Differences					t	df	Sig. (2-tailed)
	Mean	Std. Deviation	Std. Error Mean	95 % CI				
				Lower	Upper			
ln(ESR) (52 weeks) − ln(ESR) (baseline)	−1.092	.827	.094	−1.280	−.904	−11.582	76	.000

measured on the ln-scale and not on the ESR-scale. To get the effect size at the original ESR-scale (i.e., mm/h), the mean difference has to be back-transformed with the exponential function (exp). Since

$$-1.09 = \ln(\text{ESR}_{52\text{weeks}}) - \ln(\text{ESR}_{\text{baseline}}) = \ln(\text{ESR}_{52\text{weeks}}/\text{ESR}_{\text{baseline}}),$$

the relative difference in ESR baseline and after 52 weeks of COBRA-light treatment is

$$\text{ESR}_{52\text{weeks}}/\text{ESR}_{\text{baseline}} = \exp(-1.09) = 0.34.$$

In other words, the ESR after 52 weeks of COBRA-light treatment is 0.34 times higher than the ESR at baseline, or is $1 - 0.34 = 0.66$ times lower than at baseline. To obtain the 95 % CI for this relative difference, the same inverse transformation is applied

$[\exp(-1.28); \exp(-0.90)] = [0.28; 0.41]$.

The final conclusion with respect to the change in ESR after 52 weeks of COBRA-light treatment is as follows: ESR decreases significantly after 52 weeks of COBRA-light treatment (relative difference 0.34, 95 % CI [0.28; 0.41], $p < 0.001$).

Note that the interpretation of the effect size as a relative difference only holds because we first transformed the outcome variable at both measurements and then took the difference. If we first computed delta-scores of ESR, this interpretation would not hold, because

$$\ln(ESR_{52weeks} - ESR_{baseline}) \neq \ln(ESR_{52weeks}) - \ln(ESR_{baseline}).$$

Moreover, the natural logarithm cannot be taken from a negative number. Adding a number to all delta-scored does not help, because it cannot be interpreted as a relative difference for the same reason.

3.5.2 Wilcoxon Signed Rank Test

In the above section, we used the paired sample t-test despite small deviations from normality, because the size of the study population was not too small. In the case of a small sized study population, for example, 20 patients, the paired sample t-test is not advised. Rather, a non-parametric test should be used. The non-parametric version of the paired sample t-test is the Wilcoxon signed rank test. The null and alternative hypothesis of this test are

H0: the distribution of change in the outcome variable is equal at both measurements;
H1: the distribution of change in the outcome variable is not equal at both measurements.

Non-parametric tests are based on ranks, in this case the ranks of the absolute differences in the outcome variable. In addition to the ranks, the Wilcoxon signed rank test also takes into account whether the differences between both measurements are positive or negative. If the null hypothesis is true, i.e., no difference in outcome between the two measurements, the sum of the signed ranks (i.e., minus the rank if the difference is negative and the rank itself if the difference is positive) is close to zero. A large or very small sum of the signed ranks is therefore supportive for the alternative hypothesis.

◻Table 3.25 shows the SPSS output of the Wilcoxon signed rank test, based on the data of only the first 20 patients treated with the COBRA-light strategy. The value of the test-statistic is reported in the first row ("Z"), the p-value in the second ("Asymp. Sig. (2-tailed)"). We conclude that treatment by COBRA-light strategy significantly influences the DAS44 after 52 weeks. Recall that non-parametric tests do not provide effect sizes and CIs, so to gain some insight on the effect, descriptive statistics need to be reported. The final conclusion then is that, within 20 patients, the DAS44 decreased significantly after 52 weeks of COBRA-light treatment, with a median decrease of 2.3 (IQR [1.4–3.0], $p < 0.001$).

◪ **Table 3.25** SPSS output of the Wilcoxon signed ranked test to investigate the change in DAS44 after 52 weeks COBRA-light treatment

Test Statistics[a]

	DAS44 (52 weeks)–DAS44 (baseline)
Z	−3.922[b]
Asymp. Sig. (2-tailed)	.000

[a]Wilcoxon Signed Rank Test
[b]Based on positive ranks

◪ **Table 3.26** Summary of the statistical test with the corresponding effect sizes and assumptions, to investigate associations with a continuous outcome variable

		Normally distributed	Non-normally distributed
Dichotomous determinant	Statistical test	Independent samples t-test	Mann-Whitney U test
	Effect size	Mean difference	None
Categorical determinant	Statistical test	ANOVA	Kruskal-Wallis
	Effect size	Mean difference (one group set as reference)	None
Continuous determinant	Statistical model	Linear regression model	
	Effect size	Regression coefficient (mean difference; per increase of 1 unit)	
	Assumptions	Normality residuals	
		Homoscedasticity	
		Linearity	
Repeated measures	Statistical test	Paired sample t-test	Wilcoxon signed rank test
	Effect size	Mean difference	None

3.6   Summary of Analyses

◪Table 3.26 summarizes the effect sizes and assumptions for all statistical tests described in this chapter.

3.7 Further Readings

All statistical tests, including the independent samples t-test, the paired sample t-test, the ANOVA, and their non-parametric counterparts are described in more details in the classic books on medical statistics and epidemiology [4–7]. Other frequently used methods to correct post hoc analyses of an ANOVA are the Šidák correction, the Holm-Bonferroni correction, and the Tukey's test [8]. We only described the one-way ANOVA, but the ANOVA can also be used to investigate differences in a continuous outcome variable between 2 or more categorical (including dichotomous) determinants. For example, to investigate the change in DAS44 between patients treated with COBRA and COBRA-light treatment and between males and females at the same time, to see if the effect of treatment is different for males than for females. This is called an interaction between two determinants, and is tested with a two-way ANOVA, see for example the books written by Armitage et al. and by Kirkwood & Sterne [4, 7], or with a linear regression model, as will be explained in ▶Chap. 6. A short description of generalized linear models, which are used to deal with heteroscedasticity in a linear regression model, can be found in the book written by Steyerberg [9].

In the exemplary research questions of this chapter, we tested for differences in the change in a continuous outcome variable between two time points, either between groups (▶Sects. 3.2–3.4) or within a patient (▶Sect. 3.5). However, in many examples, patients are measured more than twice during the study period, called a longitudinal study. Investigating differences of a continuous variable between groups or within one group over time, is beyond the scope of this quick guide. Twisk has written a book on the analyses of longitudinal data from an applied point of view [10]. A more in-depth theoretical book on longitudinal analyses, still intended for medical researchers, is the book written by Verbeke & Molenberghs [11]. Repeated measures within the same patients are also used to assess the reliability, repeatability and validity of a measurement instrument. More information on the analyses of such repeated measures can be found in the book by de Vet et al. [12].

References

1. den Uyl D, ter Wee MM, Boers M, Kerstens P, Voskuyl A, Nurmohamed M, et al. A non-inferiority trial of an attenuated combination strategy ('COBRA-light') compared to the original COBRA strategy: clinical results after 26 weeks. Ann Rheum Dis. 2014;73(6):1071–8. ▶https://doi.org/10.1136/annrheumdis-2012-202818.
2. ter Wee MM, den Uyl D, Boers M, Kerstens P, Nurmohamed M, van Schaardenburg D, et al. Intensive combination treatment regimens, including prednisolone, are effective in treating patients with early rheumatoid arthritis regardless of additional etanercept: 1-year results of the COBRA-light open-label, randomised, non-inferiority trial. Ann Rheum Dis. 2015;74(6):1233–40. ▶https://doi.org/10.1136/annrheumdis-2013-205143.
3. Greenland S, Senn SJ, Rothman KJ, Carlin JB, Poole C, Goodman SN, et al. Statistical tests, P values, confidence intervals, and power: a guide to misinterpretations. Eur J Epidemiol. 2016;31(4):337–50. ▶https://doi.org/10.1007/s10654-016-0149-3.
4. Armitage P, Berry G, Matthews JNS. Statistical methods in medical research. Oxford: Blackwell Science Ltd; 2002.
5. Altman DG. Practical statistics for medical research. London: Chapman & Hall; 1991.
6. Rothman KJ, Lash TL, Greenland S. Modern epidemiology. 3rd ed. Philadelphia: Lippincott-Raven; 2012.

7. Kirkwood BR, Sterne JAC. Essential medical statistics. 2nd ed. Oxford: Blackwell Science Ltd; 2003.
8. Miller RG Jr. Simultaneous statistical inference. New York: Springer-Verlag Inc; 1981.
9. Steyerberg EW. Clinical prediction models. New York: Springer; 2009.
10. Twisk JWR. Applied longitudinal data analysis for epidemiology. New York: Cambridge University Press; 2003.
11. Verbeke G, Molenberghs G. Introduction to longitudinal data analysis. New York: Springer-Verlag Inc; 2000.
12. de Vet HCW, Terwee CB, Mokkink LB, Knol DL. Measurement in medicine. Cambridge: Cambridge University Press; 2011.

Analyzing Dichotomous Outcome Variables

Abstract

In this chapter, we illustrate how to test the association between a dichotomous outcome variable and a dichotomous, categorical or a continuous determinant. We also illustrate how to compare repeated measurements of a dichotomous outcome within the same patient. In medical research, dichotomous outcomes generally refer to a disease status (healthy or not). The presence or absence of the disease is diagnosed by means of a diagnostic test. In this chapter, we also elaborate on the accuracy measures of a diagnostic test and how to determine a cut-off value used to classify a patient as having the disease.

© Bohn Stafleu van Loghum is een imprint van Springer Media B.V., onderdeel van Springer Nature 2019
M. M. ter Wee and B. I. Lissenberg-Witte, *A Quick Guide on How to Conduct Medical Research*,
https://doi.org/10.1007/978-90-368-2248-0_4

4.1   Proportions: Probabilities, Risks and Odds

A dichotomous outcome variable can only take two values, such as healthy or sick and alive or diseased. One of the values is the outcome of interest, and considered as the 'success' outcome. The other value refers to the absence of the outcome of interest and is considered the 'failure'. Success and failure are written between quotation marks: a successful outcome does not necessarily refer to a favorable outcome. The probability of 'success' is denoted by p, and also called the risk. A measure related to the risk is the odds: the probability of a 'success' divided by the probability of a 'failure', i.e., $p/(1 - p)$. The risk is a chance, a number between zero and one (or between 0 % and 100 %), while the odds is a ratio of two probabilities and can take any value larger than zero. A risk of 10 % to develop Rheumatoid Artritis (RA) within 2 years means that one out of every 10 patients will develop RA within 2 years. The odds corresponding to a risk of 10 % is equal to $0.1/(1 - 0.1) = 0.1/0.9 = 1/9$. This means that for every patient that develops RA within 2 years, nine patients will not develop RA within 2 years.

Another disease-related measure commonly reported in epidemiological cross-sectional or cohort studies, is the prevalence of the disease. This is the proportion of patients who have the disease, in a cohort study usually measured at baseline. Comparing the prevalence of a disease between two or more groups, is similar to comparing risks between groups. Almost all exemplary research questions in this chapter are formulated for a prospective cohort study, where the prevalence of the disease is 0 % at the start of the study. The methods described can be translated directly to a research question involving the prevalence.

4.2   In Case of a Dichotomous Determinant

The first step in analyzing the association between a dichotomous outcome and a dichotomous determinant is to create a 2×2 contingency table (or crosstab). In a crosstab, the results of each group are summarized. ◻Table 4.1 shows the general lay-out of a 2×2 crosstab. The two possible outcomes are put in two different columns, for now labeled as 'event' and 'no event', i.e., 'success' and 'failure'. The two different groups are put in the rows. The letters a, b, c, and d correspond to the number of patients in each group with an event (a and c) and without an event (b and d). From a general 2×2 crosstab, the risk and the odds in each group can be calculated:

- the risk in group 1, denoted by p_1, is equal to a/n_1 and the odds in group 1 are equal to $\frac{a/n_1}{1 - a/n_1} = \frac{a/n_1}{b/n_1} = a/b$;
- the risk in group 2, denoted by p_2, is equal to c/n_2 and the odds in group 2 are equal to c/d.

■ **Table 4.1** General lay-out of a 2 × 2 crosstab

		Outcome		total
		Event	No event	
Group	1	a	b	n_1
	2	c	d	n_2
Total		a + c	b + d	n

4.2.1 Different Effect Sizes

To compare a dichotomous outcome variable between two groups, several effect sizes could be reported (see also ▶ Sect. 2.3.2), either based on the risks or on the odds for the outcome of interest:

- risk difference (RD) = $p_1 - p_2$;
- relative risk (RR) = p_1/p_2; or
- odds ratio (OR) = $\frac{p_1/(1-p_1)}{p_2/(1-p_2)} = \frac{c/d}{a/b} = \frac{a \times d}{b \times c}$.

Here, p_1 and p_2 are the risks in both groups. One group is set as the reference group, in this case group 2. A negative RD implies that group 1 has a lower risk compared to group 2 (the reference group). An RR or OR below one indicates that group 1 has a lower chance or odds for a favorable outcome compared to group 2. The effect size of a case-control study can only be the OR, whilst the RR can be the effect size of both a case-control study as well as of a cohort study. However, an OR is easy to adjust for influencing factors (▶ Chap. 6), and is the only effect size for the association between a dichotomous outcome variable and a continuous determinant. In the case of a rare outcome (e.g. with a risk or prevalence below 1 %), the OR is approximately equal to the RR. Otherwise, the OR is an over- or underestimation of the RR.

The 95 % confidence interval (CI) for the RD is calculated with the standard form of the 95 % CI (▶ Eq. E2.2, ▶ Sect. 2.3.3), where the standard error (SE) of the RD is equal to

$$\text{SE}_{\text{RD}} = \sqrt{\frac{p_1 \times (1 - p_1)}{n_1} + \frac{p_2 \times (1 - p_2)}{n_2}}, \tag{E4.1}$$

The standard form of the 95 % CI cannot be used for the RR and OR, because these effect sizes are ratios and consequently do not follow a normal distribution. The 95 % CIs of the RR and OR are not symmetrically distributed around the effect size. Instead, their natural logarithms (ln) are normally distributed, and the 95 % CIs of the ln-transformed effects sizes can be computed with the standard equations for CIs:

$$[\ln(\text{RR}) - 1.96 \times \text{SE}_{\ln(\text{RR})}; \ln(\text{RR}) + 1.96 \times \text{SE}_{\ln(\text{RR})}], \text{and} \tag{E4.2}$$

$$[\ln(\text{OR}) - 1.96 \times \text{SE}_{\ln(\text{OR})}; \ln(\text{OR}) + 1.96 \times \text{SE}_{\ln(\text{OR})}] \tag{E4.3}$$

The SE for the ln-transformed effect sizes are equal to

$$SE_{\ln(RR)} = \sqrt{\frac{1}{a} + \frac{1}{c} - \frac{1}{n_1} - \frac{1}{n_2}}, \tag{E4.4}$$

$$SE_{\ln(OR)} = \sqrt{\frac{1}{a} + \frac{1}{b} + \frac{1}{c} + \frac{1}{d}}. \tag{E4.5}$$

In these two equations, a, b, c and d are taken from ◻Table 4.1. To calculate the 95 % CI for the RR or the OR, the 95 % CI of $\ln(RR)$ or $\ln(OR)$ has to be back-transformed by taking the exponential (exp) of the upper and lower bound. These equations for the SEs are only valid for large enough sized study populations, i.e., with at least 25 patients in each group. SPSS provides the estimates of the OR and RR (with corresponding 95 % CIs) as additional options in the crosstable query (Supplementary Information A.5.1), but not for the RD.

4.2.2 Chi-Square Test

Differences in the risks or odds for a dichotomous outcome variable between groups are assessed with the Pearson chi-square test (or just chi-square test or χ^2-test). To illustrate this test with the different effect sizes, we study the following research question, using data of the RA-cohort [1]

? Is there a difference in risk to develop RA within 2 years between seropositive arthralgia patients with and without a first-degree relative (FDR) with RA?

Another commonly used paraphrasing of the research question is to assess whether there is an association between the development of RA within 2 years and having an FDR with RA. Then the research question is as follows

? Is there an association between the development of RA within 2 years and having an FDR with RA?

The null and alternative hypothesis for such a research question are

H0: there is no difference in risk to develop RA within 2 years between patients with an FDR with RA and without an FDR with RA (or no association between the two);
H1: there is a difference in risk to develop RA within 2 years between patients with an FDR with RA and without an FDR with RA (or an association between the two).

A total of 374 patients were included in the RA-cohort. However, some patients had less than 2 years of follow-up and did not develop RA within their follow-up period ($n = 91$). These patients were excluded from the analyses. ◻Table 4.2 shows the SPSS output of the crosstab summarizing the results of the remaining 283 patients with at least 2 years follow-up. Of the 214 patients without an FDR with RA (under "Total" in the

◻ Table 4.2 SPSS output of the crosstab for the association between development of RA within 2 years and having an FDR with RA

FDR * arthritis within 2 years Crosstabulation

| | | | arthritis within 2 years | | Total |
			no	yes	
FDR	no RA	Count	139	75	214
		% within FDR	65.0 %	35.0 %	100.0 %
	RA	Count	43	26	69
		% within FDR	62.3 %	37.7 %	100.0 %
Total		Count	182	101	283
		% within FDR	64.3 %	35.7 %	100.0 %

◻ Table 4.3 SPSS output of the estimated OR and RR, comparing development of RA within 2 years in patients with and without an FDR with RA

Risk Estimate

| | Value | 95 % Confidence Interval | |
		Lower	Upper
Odds Ratio for FDR with RA (no RA/RA)	1.121	.639	1.966
For cohort arthritis within 2 years = no	1.042	.846	1.284
For cohort arthritis within 2 years = yes	.930	.653	1.325
N of Valid Cases	283		

row "no RA"), 75 (35 %) developed RA within 2 years (under "yes" in the row "no RA") and of the 69 patients with an FDR with RA (under "Total" in the row "RA"), 26 (38 %) developed RA within 2 years (under "yes" in the row "RA").

The RR to develop RA within 2 years of patients with an FDR with RA compared to patients without an FDR with RA is equal to $0.38/0.35 \approx 1.1$. That is, patients with an FDR with RA have a slightly higher risk (RD 3 %, or RR 1.1) to develop RA within 2 years than patients without an FDR with RA. Also the OR is slightly larger than one: OR $= (26 \times 139)/(43 \times 75) \approx 1.1$. ◻Table 4.3 shows the optional SPSS output of the estimated OR and RR, with corresponding 95 % CI. Important to note is that SPSS computes the RR to develop RA within 2 years by dividing the risk in patients without an FDR with RA by the risk in patients with an FDR with RA (in the row "For cohort RA within 2 years = yes") while we computed it the other way around. That is, we set the group without an FDR with RA as the reference group, whereas SPSS sets the group with an FDR with RA as the reference group. The 95 % CI of the RR is calculated by hand and is equal to $[1/1.325; 1/0.653] \approx [0.75; 1.5]$ for not developing RA within 2 years, of patients without an FDR with RA compared to patients with an FDR with RA (in the row "For cohort arthritis within 2 years = no"). For the calculation of the OR, SPSS sets the group with an FDR with RA as the reference group, this is specified in the row "Odds Ratio for FDR with RA (no RA/RA)", hence the 95 % CI for the OR is equal to [0.64; 2.0] (under "95 % Confidence Interval"). The total number of patients included in the calculation of the OR and RR are reported in the last row ("N of Valid Cases").

In terms of the RR or OR, the null and alternative hypothesis are equal to

H0: $RR = 1$, or $OR = 1$;
H1: $RR \neq 1$, or $OR \neq 1$.

So, since the null value (i.e., 1) is contained in the 95 % CI for the RR as well as for the OR, we could already conclude that there is not enough evidence (at the significance level α of 0.05) to prove a difference in the risk to develop RA within 2 years between patients with and without an FDR with RA.

The null hypothesis is tested statistically with the chi-square test. This test compares the number of observed patients in each of the four cells of the crosstab to the expected number of patients in each of these cells, under the null hypothesis. The test statistic of the chi-square test is equal to

$$X^2 = \sum_{i,j=1}^{2} \frac{(O_{i,j} - E_{i,j})^2}{E_{i,j}},$$

(E4.6)

where $O_{i,j}$ is the observed number of patients in row i and column j of the crosstab, and $E_{i,j}$ the expected number of patients in row i and column j. The larger the difference between the observed and expected number of patients in each cell, the stronger the evidence against the null hypothesis and in favor of the alternative hypothesis. The test statistic X^2 follows a chi-square distribution with 1 degree of freedom.

◻Table 4.4 shows the SPSS output of the chi-square test (in the row "Pearson Chi-Square"). The value of the test statistic is reported under "Value", the degrees of freedom under "df" and finally the p-value under "Asymp. Sig. (2-sided)". However, the chi-square test is only valid when the expected number of patients is at least five in each of the cells of the crosstab. The expected number of patients (referred to as "expected count" by SPSS) in each cell ($E_{i,j}$ in ▶Eq. (E4.6)) can be calculated by hand, but SPSS computes it as well. SPSS reports the number of cells with an expected count less than five in footnote a. In our example, the footnote states that "0 cells (.0 %) have an expected count of less than five. The minimum expected count is 24.63". Consequently, for our example, the chi-square is valid. For small sized study populations, with less than 20–25 patients, as well as for studies with very rare events, the expected count will probably be less than five. In that case the Fisher's exact test needs to be used. The Fisher's exact test is an additional test SPSS always performs on a 2 × 2 crosstab. The p-value of the Fisher's exact test is reported under "Exact Sig. (2-sided)". Another p-value is reported for this test under "Exact Sig. (1-sided)", corresponding to a one-sided hypothesis test. However, usually hypotheses are tested two-sided, hence this column could be ignored. The Fisher's exact

□ **Table 4.4** SPSS output of the chi-square test, comparing development of RA within 2 years in patients with and without an FDR with RA

Chi-Square Tests

	Value	df	Asymp. Sig. (2-sided)	Exact Sig. (2-sided)	Exact Sig. (1-sided)
Pearson Chi-Square	.158[a]	1	.691		
Continuity Correction[b]	.064	1	.800		
Likelihood Ratio	.157	1	.692		
Fisher's Exact Test				.773	.398
Linear-by-Linear Association	.157	1	.692		
N of Valid Cases	283				

[a]0 cells (.0 %) have expected count less than 5. The minimum expected count is 24.63
[b]Computed only for a 2 × 2 table

test is an exact test, which means that it is not based on a test statistic but it uses statistical theory. Therefore de columns "Value", "df" and "Asymp. Sig. (2-sided)" are empty for this test. In both cases (i.e., the chi-square or the Fisher's exact test), however, the effect size for comparison of a dichotomous outcome variable between two groups is always the RR or the OR, with the corresponding 95 % CI.

Besides the results of the chi-square and the Fisher's exact test, SPSS also reports the results of several other tests, as well as the number of patients included in the analysis in the row "N of Valid Cases". The results in the row "Linear-by-linear association" is only of interest when the risk is compared between more than two groups, covered in ▶ Sect. 4.3. For more information on the results in the rows "Continuity Correction" and "Likelihood Ratio", we refer to references on these topics in the further readings (▶ Sect. 4.8). The final conclusion with respect to our research question is that there is no evidence to prove that patients with an FDR with RA have a different risk to develop RA within 2 years than patients without an FDR with RA (OR 1.1, 95 % CI [0.64; 2.0], $p = 0.69$). In other words, the odds to develop RA within 2 years is 1.1 times higher (but not significantly) for patients with an FDR with RA than the odds to develop RA within 2 years for patients without an FDR with RA. Note that the effect size is the OR, while the research question was formulated in terms of the risk. This is because the OR is the effect size for an association between a dichotomous outcome variable and a continuous determinant. Moreover, if the effect of the determinant on the outcome variable is corrected for influencing variables (▶ Chap. 6), the corrected effect size is also an OR and not an RR or RD.

4.2.3 Non-Inferiority and Equivalence

Prospective cohort studies, such as the RA-cohort, are usually not designed to prove non-inferiority or equivalence, in contrast to clinical trials. So to illustrate non-inferiority and equivalence for a dichotomous outcome variable, let us consider the dichotomous outcome variable whether or not the disease activity score in 44 joints (DAS44) after 52 weeks of COBRA or COBRA-light treatment reaches a value below a cut-off of 1.6 in the COmbinatie Behandeling Reumatoïde Artritis (COBRA)-light trial [2]. Proving non-inferiority (or equivalence) in case of a dichotomous outcome variable is done exactly the same as in case of a continuous outcome variable. A priori, a non-inferiority margin is set, either on the RR or on the OR. It could also be set on the RD, but SPSS does not provide a 95 % CI for the RD. So if the non-inferiority margin is set on the RD, the 95 % CI has to be calculated by hand, where the SE of the RD is given in ▶ Eq. E4.1 (▶ Sect. 4.2.1). To illustrate how to prove non-inferiority with a dichotomous outcome variable, let us consider the following research question

> ❓ Is the COBRA-light strategy non-inferior compared to the COBRA strategy in reaching a DAS44 below 1.6 in patients with early RA within 52 weeks?

Assume that the non-inferiority margin for the RR is set at 0.8. That is, the COBRA-light strategy is deemed non-inferior to the COBRA strategy if the RR to reach a DAS44 below 1.6 after 52 weeks of treatment is at least 0.8. After all, an RR below one indicates that the chance that a patient treated with the COBRA-light strategy will reach a DAS44 below 1.6 is lower than the chance to reach a DAS44 below 1.6 in patients treated with the COBRA strategy (i.e., COBRA-light is less effective than COBRA strategy). Hence, the null and alternative hypothesis of the research question (with this non-inferiority margin) are

H0: RR $\leq$ 0.8;
H1: RR $>$ 0.8.

In other words, non-inferiority is proven (at the significance level α of 0.025), if the lower bound of the 95 % CI for the RR is above 0.8.

◻Table 4.5 shows the SPSS output of the crosstab comparing reaching a DAS44 below 1.6 after 52 weeks of treatment between the COBRA and COBRA-light arm. ◻Table 4.6 shows the estimated RR and OR. Remember that SPSS sets the COBRA-light arm as the reference group for the RR. The result of the COBRA-light arm is shown in the row "For cohort DAS44 (after 52 weeks) = < 1.6", so the RR and corresponding 95 % CI are equal to 0.816 (i.e., 1/1.226) and [0.573; 1.163] (i.e., [1/1.746; 1/0.860]). Based on the 95 % CI, we conclude that there is not enough evidence to reject the null hypothesis. In other words, the COBRA-light strategy might be less effective than the COBRA strategy to reach a DAS44 below 1.6 (RR 0.82, 95 % CI [0.57; 1.2]). Note that the p-value of the chi-square test is not reported because the null hypothesis of the chi-square test (in terms of the RR) is equal to

H0: RR $=$ 1.

◻ **Table 4.5**   SPSS output of the crosstab, relating reaching a DAS44 below 1.6 after 52 weeks of treatment, to the treatment arm

treatment arm * DAS44 (after 52 weeks) Crosstabulation

			DAS44 (after 52 weeks)		Total
			>= 1.6	<1.6	
treatment arm	COBRA	Count	39	38	77
		% within treatment arm	50.6 %	49.4 %	100.0 %
	COBRA-light	Count	46	31	77
		% within treatment arm	59.7 %	40.3 %	100.0 %
Total		Count	85	69	154
		% within treatment arm	55.2 %	44.8 %	100.0 %

◻ **Table 4.6**   SPSS output for the risk estimates, relating to reaching a DAS44 below 1.6 after 52 weeks of treatment, to the treatment arm

Risk Estimate

	Value	95 % Confidence Interval	
		Lower	Upper
Odds Ratio for treatment arm (COBRA/COBRA-light)	.692	.365	1.309
For cohort DAS44 (after 52 weeks) = >= 1.6	.848	.636	1.129
For cohort DAS44 (after 52 weeks) = <1.6	1.226	.860	1.746
N of Valid Cases	154		

▶Example 4.1 illustrates how to test non-inferiority of the COBRA-light strategy over the COBRA strategy using the RD.

Example 4.1

Non-inferiority based on RD
Assume the non-inferiority margin for the RD was set at 5 %, i.e., the RD between COBRA-light and COBRA treatment is at most -5 % for the COBRA-light strategy to be non-inferior.
Forty-nine percent of the 77 patients treated with the COBRA strategy reached a DAS44 below 1.6 after 52 weeks of treatment, while 40 % of the 77 patients treated with the COBRA-light strategy reached a DAS44 below 1.6 points. Hence, the RD is equal to $40 - 49 = -9$ % and the SE is equal to

$$SE_{RD} = \sqrt{\frac{0.49 \times (1 - 0.49)}{77} + \frac{0.40 \times (1 - 0.40)}{77}} \approx \sqrt{0.0064} = 0.080.$$

The 95 % CI for the RD is then equal to

$$[-0.09 - 1.96 \times 0.080; -0.09 + 1.96 \times 0.080] \approx [-0.25; 0.067].$$

Because the lower bound of the 95 % CI for the RD (i.e., −25 %) is smaller than the non-inferiority margin −5 %, we cannot conclude that the COBRA-light strategy is non-inferior to the COBRA strategy to reach a DAS44 below 1.6 after 52 weeks of treatment.

Now, let us investigate equivalence between the COBRA-light and the COBRA strategy with respect to reaching a DAS44 below 1.6 after 52 weeks of treatment, with the following research question

Is the COBRA-light strategy equivalent to the COBRA strategy in reaching a DAS44 below 1.6 in patients with early RA within 52 weeks?

Now, two a priori fixed margins need to be set (again, either for the RD, the RR or the OR): the lower and upper bound for equivalence (RD_L and RD_U, or RR_L and RR_U, or OR_L and OR_U, respectively). Since the RR and the OR are a ratio, which is anti-symmetric, these two bounds need to be anti-symmetric as well, i.e., $RR_L = 1/RR_U$ or $OR_L = 1/OR_U$. To keep the lower bound RR_L equal to 0.8, the upper bound RR_U should be equal to $1/0.8 = 1.25$. Then, the alternative hypothesis of the research question is that the true RR lies between RR_L and RR_U whereas the null hypothesis is that the true RR is either 0.8 below or 1.25 or above, i.e.,

H0: RR ≤ 0.8 or RR ≥ 1.25;
H1: 0.8 < RR < 1.25.

If the 95 % CI for the RR lies completely between the lower and upper bound of equivalence, equivalence is proven. Although the upper bound of the 95 % CI in our example (i.e., 1.2) is smaller than RR_U, the null hypothesis cannot be rejected, since the lower bound of the 95 % CI (i.e., 0.57) is smaller than RR_L.

4.3 In Case of a Categorical Determinant

Differences between more than two groups, in case of a categorical determinant, are also assessed with the chi-square test. We illustrate this with the following research question

Is there a difference in risk to develop RA within 2 years for seropositive arthralgia patients with different antibody status at baseline?

□ **Table 4.7** SPSS output of the crosstab for the association between the development of RA within 2 years and antibody status at baseline

antibody * arthritis within 2 years Crosstabulation

			arthritis within 2 years		Total
			no	yes	
antibody	IgM-RF +, aCCP −	Count	72	10	82
		% within antibody	87.8 %	12.2 %	100.0 %
	IgM-RF −, aCCP low +	Count	34	13	47
		% within antibody	72.3 %	27.7 %	100.0 %
	IgM-RF −, aCCP high +	Count	37	26	63
		% within antibody	58.7 %	41.3 %	100.0 %
	IgM-RF +, aCCP +	Count	39	52	91
		% within antibody	42.9 %	57.1 %	100.0 %
Total		Count	182	101	283
		% within antibody	64.3 %	35.7 %	100.0 %

□ **Table 4.8** SPSS output of the chi-square test, comparing development of RA within 2 years between patients with different antibody status at baseline

Chi-Square Tests

	Value	df	Asymp. Sig. (2-sided)
Pearson Chi-Square	40.144[a]	3	.000
Likelihood Ratio	42.872	3	.000
Linear-by-Linear Association	39.979	1	.000
N of Valid Cases	283		

[a]0 cells (.0 %) have expected count less than 5. The minimum expected count is 16.77

Antibody status at baseline is classified as: (i) rheumatoid factor type immunoglobulin M (IgM-RF) positive but anticyclic citrullinated peptide (aCCP) negative, (ii) IgM-RF negative but aCCP low positive, (iii) IgM-RF negative but aCCP high positive, and (iv) both IgM-RF and aCCP positive. The null and alternative hypothesis of this research question are

H0: there is no difference in risk to develop RA within 2 years between patients with different antibody status at baseline;

H1: at least two groups (of patients with different antibody status at baseline) differ in risk to develop RA within 2 years.

As for comparing a continuous outcome variable between more than two groups, the alternative hypothesis only states a difference in risk between at least two groups, not between all groups.

4.3.1 Chi-Square Test

A 4 × 2 crosstab is used to summarize the outcome in each of the groups: four rows for the four different groups, and two columns for the two possible outcomes (◘Table 4.7). Patients who are IgM-RF positive but aCCP negative have the lowest risk to develop RA within 2 years (12 %), and patients who are both IgM-RF and aCCP positive have the highest risk to develop RA within 2 years (57 %).

◘Table 4.8 shows the SPSS output of the chi-square test. From this table, we conclude that there is an overall difference in risk to develop RA within 2 years between patients with different antibody status ($p < 0.001$). The difference in the SPSS output between ◘Tables 4.8 and 4.4, comparing two groups, is the number of the degrees of freedom, which is now 3. In general, when a dichotomous outcome variable is compared between k groups, the degrees of freedom is equal to $k - 1$.

There is also no overall effect size measuring the differences in risk to develop RA within 2 years between the four antibody status groups at once, as was the case in the association between a continuous outcome variable and a categorical determinant. Again, a post hoc analysis (corrected for multiple testing) has to be performed, to investigate which groups differ significantly from each other. SPSS has an option for the post hoc analysis in the case of a dichotomous outcome variable, but only reports which groups differ significantly from each other. The corresponding effect sizes have to be computed by hand. Therefore we do not illustrate this post hoc option, but will analyze each of the pairs separately and apply the Bonferroni correction to account for multiple testing.

For the manual post hoc analysis, we first select only patients from group 1 (IgM-RF positive but aCCP negative) and from group 2 (IgM-RF negative but aCCP low positive), and perform the chi-square test with the option of the risk table. ◘Table 4.9 summarizes the relevant parts of the SPSS output. The corrected p-values (under "Sig. corrected") are computed by multiplying the uncorrected p-value of the Pearson chi-square test (under "Sig. uncorrected") with 6, since there are six pairwise comparisons. Secondly, only patients from group 1 and 3 are selected and used for the chi-square test with the optional output of the risk table output. This procedure is repeated until all groups are compared to each other. The corresponding ORs for the different post hoc comparisons are reported under "Odds Ratio (J vs I)" and the corresponding 95 % CIs under "95 % Confidence Interval".

From these analyses we conclude that patients who are IgM-RF negative but aCCP high positive, as well as patients who are IgM-RF positive and aCCP positive have a higher risk to develop RA within 2 years compared to patients who are IgM-RF positive but aCCP negative (OR 5.1, 95 % CI [2.2; 11.6], $p < 0.001$ and OR 9.6, 95 % CI [4.4; 21.0], $p < 0.001$, respectively). Patients who are IgM-RF positive and aCCP positive also have a higher risk to develop RA within 2 years, compared to patients who are IgM negative but aCCP low positive (OR 3.5, 95 % CI [1.6; 7.5], $p = 0.006$).

4

□ **Table 4.9** Summary of pairwise comparisons in the post hoc analysis, comparing development of RA within 2 years in patients with different antibody status at baseline

(I) antibody status at baseline	(J) antibody status at baseline	Odds Ratio (J vs I)	95 % Confidence Interval		Sig.	
			Lower Bound	Upper Bound	uncorrected	corrected[a]
IgM-RF +, aCCP −	IgM-RF −, aCCP low +	2.753	1.097	6.906	.027	.162
	IgM-RF −, aCCP high +	5.059	2.206	11.604	.000	.000
	IgM-RF +, aCCP +	9.600	4.397	20.962	.000	.000
IgM-RF −, aCCP low +	IgM-RF −, aCCP high +	1.838	.816	4.141	.140	.840
	IgM-RF +, aCCP +	3.487	1.627	7.463	.001	.006
IgM-RF −, aCCP high +	IgM-RF +, aCCP +	1.897	.989	3.639	.053	.318

[a]Bonferroni correction

◪ **Table 4.10** SPSS output of the crosstab for the association between the development of RA within 2 years and antibody status at baseline, in the first 100 patients only

antibody * arthritis within 2 years Crosstabulation

			arthritis within 2 years		Total
			no	yes	
antibody	IgM-RF +, aCCP −	Count	34	2	36
		% within antibody	94.4 %	5.6 %	100.0 %
	IgM-RF −, aCCP low +	Count	13	4	17
		% within antibody	76.5 %	23.5 %	100.0 %
	IgM-RF −, aCCP high +	Count	13	5	18
		% within antibody	72.2 %	27.8 %	100.0 %
	IgM-RF +, aCCP +	Count	13	16	29
		% within antibody	44.8 %	55.2 %	100.0 %
Total		Count	73	27	100
		% within antibody	73.0 %	27.0 %	100.0 %

◪ **Table 4.11** SPSS output of the chi-square test with additional Fisher's exact test, comparing development of RA within 2 years in patients with different antibody status at baseline, in the first 100 patients only

Chi-Square Tests

	Value	df	Asymp. Sig. (2-sided)	Exact Sig. (2-sided)	Exact Sig. (1-sided)	Point Probability
Pearson Chi-Square	20.187[a]	3	.000	.000		
Likelihood Ratio	21.491	3	.000	.000		
Fisher's Exact Test	20.496			.000		
Linear-by-Linear Association	19.101[b]	1	.000	.000	.000	.000
N of Valid Cases	100					

[a]2 cells (25.0 %) have expected count less than 5. The minimum expected count is 4.59
[b]The standardized statistic is 4.370

Two final remarks need to be made with respect to the SPSS output of the chi-square test in ◻Table 4.8. First of all, the chi-square test with a categorical determinant has the same assumption as the chi-square test with a dichotomous determinant: the expected count in all cells should be at least 5. In the 2×2 crosstab, the Fisher's exact test is reported by default. However, this is not the case for a 4×2 crosstab (or more generally, for any $r \times 2$ crosstab). There is an option for the exact p-value in SPSS. ◻Table 4.10 shows the 4×2 crosstab of the first 100 patients, and ◻Table 4.11 shows the corresponding SPSS output with the extra Fisher's exact test for these 100 patients. Based on the results from these 100 patients, using the Fisher's exact test, we also conclude that there is an association between the development of RA within 2 years and antibody status at baseline.

Secondly, when the categorical determinant is an ordinal variable, the result of the linear-by-linear association (in the row "Linear-by-Linear Association") tests whether the ordering in the categorical determinant is also present in the odds for the outcome. This test is also known as the Mantel-Haenszel test for trend and tests the following null and alternative hypothesis:

$$H0: \text{odds}_1 = \text{odds}_2 = \ldots = \text{odds}_k;$$
$$H1: \frac{\text{odds}_2}{\text{odds}_1} = \frac{\text{odds}_3}{\text{odds}_2} = \ldots = \frac{\text{odds}_{k-1}}{\text{odds}_k}.$$

Here odds_i is the odds for the outcome in the group i, with i equal to 1, 2, ..., k. This means that the OR comparing group 3 with groups 1 is twice the OR comparing group 2 with 1 (or half depending on which group has the lowest risk: the first or the last (k-th) group). For ordinal variables, this is however a rather strict assumption which is hardly really tested. Unfortunately, it is a common mistake to interpret the p-value of the linear-by-linear association as a p-value for general trend, that is, testing the above null hypothesis against the following alternative hypothesis

$$H1: \text{odds}_1 < \text{odds}_2 < \ldots < \text{odds}_k.$$

If this is the alternative hypothesis of interest, the Cochran–Armitage test for trend should be used instead. We refer to the further readings (▸ Sect. 4.8) for references with more information on this test.

4.4   In Case of a Continuous Determinant

The association between two continuous variables could be visualized with a scatterplot; the association between a continuous outcome variable and a dichotomous determinant by a boxplot. Neither of these plots are suited to assess the association between a dichotomous outcome variable and a continuous determinant, nor is the independent samples t-test. The only way to assess the association between a dichotomous outcome variable and a continuous determinant is with a regression model, more specifically with a logistic regression model.

◘ **Table 4.12** SPSS output of a logistic regression model relating development of RA within 2 years to the VAS pain score at baseline

Variables in the Equation

		B	SE	Wald	df	Sig.	Exp(B)	95 % C.I. for EXP(B)	
								Lower	Upper
Step 1[a]	VAS	.024	.006	15.684	1	.000	1.024	1.012	1.037
	Constant	−1.719	.321	28.670	1	.000	.179		

[a]Variable(s) entered on step 1: VAS

4.4.1 Logistic Regression Model

A dichotomous outcome variable can only take two values: 'success' (usually coded as one), and 'failure' (usually coded as zero). Instead of modeling the outcome variable directly, the odds for the successful outcome is modeled by the logistic regression model. However, since the odds itself is a ratio (the probability of a 'success' divided by the probability of a 'failure'), and consequently can only take positive values, the natural logarithm of the odds is the outcome of the model. We illustrate this regression model with the following research question

❓ Is the risk to develop RA within 2 years associated with the visual analogue scale (VAS) pain score at baseline?

The null and alternative hypothesis to this research question are

H0: there is no association between the risk to develop RA within 2 years and the VAS pain score at baseline;
H1: there is an association between the risk to develop RA within 2 years and the VAS pain score at baseline.

In the RA-cohort, the VAS pain score was only recorded as a dichotomous variable: below or above 50. For illustrative purposes, we simulated the original VAS pain score ('VAS_pain') for each patient separately, in such a way that the simulated score matched with the official recorded VAS pain score. The logistic regression model to investigate this research question is as follows

$$\ln(\text{odds for RA within 2 years}) = b_0 + b_1 \times \text{VAS\_pain} \tag{M4.1}$$

The regression coefficients have a similar interpretation as in a linear regression model:
- b_0 is the ln(odds) to develop RA within 2 years for a patient with a VAS pain score of zero at baseline;
- b_1 is the difference in ln(odds) to develop RA within 2 years between two patients who differ by 1 point in their VAS pain score at baseline.

Just as in a linear regression model, the value of the intercept b_0 is not always clinically meaningful. In that case, the determinant could be centralized so that b_0 is the ln(odds) at the mean value of the determinant (in our case, the VAS pain score at baseline). However, this would then be a descriptive statistic for the outcome variable, measured at the ln(odds) level. Also the slope b_1 is measured at the ln(odds) level. Therefore, the regression coefficients need to be back transformed with the exponential function. Then, $\exp(b_0)$ is the 'baseline' odds, and $\exp(b_1)$ is the OR between two patients who differ by 1 point in their VAS pain score at baseline. After all, for two patients who differ in the VAS pain score at baseline by 1 point, for example with VAS pain scores 30 and 31 at baseline,

$$b_1 = \ln(\text{odds}_{31}) - \ln(\text{odds}_{30}) = \ln(\text{odds}_{31}/\text{odds}_{30}) = \ln(\text{OR})$$

◘Table 4.12 shows the SPSS output for the logistic regression model for the association between development of RA within 2 years and the VAS pain score at baseline. SPSS produces more tables than just this one, but for now, we only consider the table called "Variables in the Equation". The set-up of the table is similar as to the SPSS output of the linear regression model: two rows, one labeled "VAS" and the other labeled "Constant". The first row reports the estimated regression coefficient b_1 (under "B") with its corresponding SE (under "SE"), the p-value, (under "Sig.") and the exponential of the regression coefficient (the OR, under "Exp(B)") with its corresponding 95 % CI (under "95 % C.I. for EXP(B)"). The 95 % CI is not the default output of SPSS and has to be selected as an additional option in the logistic regression query (Supplementary Information A.5.2). Also the value of the Wald statistics and corresponding degrees of freedom (under "Wald" and "df", respectively) are reported. The p-value of this row tests the null hypothesis of no association (or equivalently H0: $b_1 = 0$) against the alternative hypothesis of an association (i.e., H1: $b_1 \neq 0$). The second column corresponds to the estimated regression coefficient b_0 and is not of interest since it tests whether the baseline ln(odds) is equal to zero. From this table, we conclude that development of RA within 2 years is associated with the VAS pain score at baseline, with an OR of 1.016 per increase of 1 point in the VAS pain score (95 % CI [1.006; 1.026]).

An OR per increase of 1 point in the VAS pain score might not be informative. In ▶Example 4.2 we illustrate how to calculate the OR per increase of 5 or 10 points in the VAS pain score, which might be more informative in clinical practice.

Example 4.2

OR per increase of 5 or 10 points in the VAS pain score at baseline
The OR for an increase of 5 or 10 points in the VAS pain score at baseline is easily derived from the OR per 1 point.
Assume we have two patients, one with a VAS pain score of 30 and one with a VAS pain score of 35 at baseline. The difference in the ln(odds) is equal to

$$b_0 + b_1 \times 35 - (b_0 + b_1 \times 30) = 35 \times b_1 - 30 \times b_1 = 5 \times b_1 = 5 \times 0.024 = 0.12.$$

The ratio of these odds is then equal to $\exp(0.12) \approx 1.13$, which is equal to $1.024^5 \approx 1.13$.

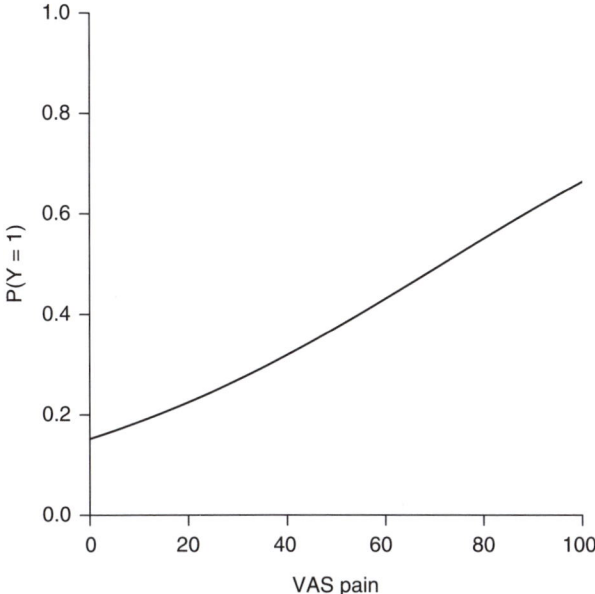

■ **Fig. 4.1**   Estimated probability to develop RA within 2 years as function of the VAS pain score at baseline

The 95 % CI for the OR per increase in 5 points in the VAS pain score at baseline is then equal to $\left[1.012^5; 1.037^5\right] \approx [1.06; 1.20]$.
Similarly, the OR per increase of 10 points in VAS pain score at baseline is equal to $1.024^{10} \approx 1.27$, with corresponding 95 % CI $\left[1.012^{10}; 1.037^{10}\right] \approx [1.13; 1.44]$.

The logistic regression model is formulated in terms of the ln(odds), and can be trans-formed to an OR. The OR, however, does not provide any information on the prob-ability that a patient with a certain VAS pain score at baseline will develop RA within 2 years. Recall that the odds to develop RA within 2 years is equal to the probability that a patients develops RA within 2 years divided by the probability that he/she does not develop RA within 2 years (▶ Sect. 4.1). In mathematics, the probability to develop RA within 2 years would by denoted by $P(Y = 1)$ so that the odds are equal to

$$\text{odds for RA within 2 years} = \frac{P(Y = 1)}{1 - P(Y = 1)}. \qquad (E4.7)$$

Therefore, the probability to develop RA within 2 years can be derived from the logistic regression model

$$P(Y = 1) = \frac{1}{1 + \exp(-(b_0 + b_1 \times \text{VAS\_pain}))}. \qquad (E4.8)$$

This function could be used to visualize the probability to develop RA within 2 years, over the whole range of VAS pain scores at baseline (■Fig. 4.1).

4.4.2 Assumptions of the Logistic Regression Model

Both the linear as well as the logistic regression model assume that the relation between the outcome of the model and the determinant is linear. For the logistic regression model this assumption is investigated in the same way as for the linear regression model. The first option is to add a quadratic/cubic/etc. term to the logistic regression model and test whether the regression coefficients are unequal to zero or not. However, the interpretation of the regression coefficients disappears. The other option is to categorize the continuous determinant, plot the regression coefficients of the groups against the mid-points and check whether these values lie (more or less) on a straight line. The latter option is advised, for the same reasons as in a linear regression model (▶ Sect. 3.4.4).

Contrary to the linear regression model, SPSS creates dummy variables for a categorical determinant automatically, with the 'Categorical' button in the logistic regression query (Supplementary Information A.5.2). By default, SPSS sets the last group (i.e., with the highest value) as the reference group, but the first could also be selected (Supplementary Information A.5.2). The dummy coding of the groups is provided by SPSS, in the table named "Categorical Variables Codings". ◻Table 4.13 shows an example of such a table, for the percentile groups of VAS pain (VAS pain is divided in quartiles, called NVAS by SPSS). The first group is set as the reference, as all three dummies are zero for this group. That is, the first dummy variable (under "(1)") is equal to one for patients in the second percentile group of VAS pain and zero for patients in the other percentile groups. The second dummy (under "(2)") is equal to one for patients in the third percentile group and zero for patients in the other percentile groups and the third dummy (under "(3)") is equal to one for patients in the fourth percentile group and zero for patients in the other percentile groups.

◻Table 4.14 shows the SPSS output of the logistic regression model. From this table we conclude that the linearity assumption does not hold: the ln(odds) increases between the first two quartiles (0.43), then decreases between the second and the third quartile (from 0.43 to 0.12), and then increases again between the third and fourth (from 0.12 to 1.18). This increasing, decreasing and increasing pattern is not linear at all. Therefore, we do not need to plot the regression coefficient any further and conclude that the association between ln(odds) and the VAS pain score at baseline is not linear. Consequently, we need to use the categorized VAS pain score at baseline as categorical determinant in the association between development of RA within 2 years and the VAS pain score at baseline. Note that whenever the difference between two consecutive regression coefficients is positive and two other consecutive regression coefficients is negative, the relation can never be linear.

The association between the development of RA within 2 years and the categorized VAS pain score at baseline is tested either with the chi-square test, providing only an overall p-value but no effect sizes for pairwise comparisons, or with a logistic regression model, providing an overall p-value and ORs for comparisons with the reference group. For illustrative purposes, we divided the VAS pain score at baseline into three groups: below 30, between 30 and 49, or 50 and above. ◻Table 4.15 shows the crosstab of this

◻ **Table 4.13** SPSS categorical variables coding table, indicating the dummies of a categorical variable

Categorical Variables Codings

		Frequency	Parameter coding		
			(1)	(2)	(3)
Percentile Group of VAS	1	67	.000	.000	.000
	2	64	1.000	.000	.000
	3	72	.000	1.000	.000
	4	80	.000	.000	1.000

◻ **Table 4.14** SPSS output of a logistic regression model, relating development of RA within 2 years to the VAS pain score at baseline in quartiles (NVAS)

Variables in the Equation

		B	SE	Wald	df	Sig.	Exp(B)	95 % C.I.for EXP(B)	
								Lower	Upper
Step 1[a]	NVAS			14.473	3	.002			
	NVAS(1)	.432	.385	1.261	1	.261	1.541	.725	3.275
	NVAS(2)	.123	.385	.103	1	.749	1.131	.532	2.405
	NVAS(3)	1.179	.359	10.778	1	.001	3.251	1.608	6.571
	Constant	−1.079	.281	14.765	1	.000	.340		

[a] Variable(s) entered on step 1: NVAS

new variable in relation to the outcome variable. ◻Table 4.16 shows the SPSS output of the corresponding chi-square test. From this table we conclude that the development of RA within 2 years is associated with the VAS pain score at baseline (in three categories, $p = 0.035$).

4.4.3 Logistic Regression Model with a Categorical Determinant

The interpretation of a logistic regression model with a categorical (or dichotomous) determinant is similar as of a linear regression model with a categorical determinant. If we analyze the VAS pain score at baseline in three categories (▶Sect. 4.4.2), setting the VAS pain score below 30 as the reference group and dummy d_1 and d_2 representing a VAS pain score between 30 and 49 and of 50 or above, respectively, the logistic regression model is as follows

$$\ln(\text{odds for RA within 2 years}) = b_0 + b_1 \times d_1 + b_2 \times d_2$$ (M4.2)

◻ **Table 4.15**   SPSS output of the crosstab for the association between development of RA within 2 years and the VAS pain score at baseline, in three groups

VAS3 * arthritis within 2 years Crosstabulation

			arthritis within 2 years		Total
			no	yes	
VAS3	<30	Count	50	17	67
		% within VAS3	74.6 %	25.4 %	100.0 %
	30–49	Count	76	39	115
		% within VAS3	66.1 %	33.9 %	100.0 %
	>=50	Count	56	45	101
		% within VAS3	55.4 %	44.6 %	100.0 %
Total		Count	182	101	283
		% within VAS3	64.3 %	35.7 %	100.0 %

◻ **Table 4.16**   SPSS output of the chi-square test, relating development of RA within 2 years to the VAS pain score at baseline, in three groups

Chi-Square Tests

	Value	df	Asymp. Sig. (2-sided)
Pearson Chi-Square	6.723[a]	2	.035
Likelihood Ratio	6.792	2	.033
Linear-by-Linear Association	6.667	1	.010
N of Valid Cases	283		

[a] 0 cells (.0 %) have expected count less than 5. The minimum expected count is 23.91

Then:
- b_0 is the ln(odds) to develop RA within 2 years in the reference group, i.e., patients with a VAS pain score at baseline below 30, and $\exp(b_0)$ the odds to develop RA within 2 years in this groups;
- b_1 is the difference in ln(odds) between patients with a VAS pain score at baseline between 30 and 49, and patients with a VAS pain score at baseline below 30, and $\exp(b_1)$ the OR between these two groups;
- b_2 is the difference in ln(odds) between patients with a VAS pain score at baseline of 50 or above, and patients with a VAS pain score at baseline below 30, and $\exp(b_2)$ the OR between these two groups.

☐ **Table 4.17** SPSS output of a logistic regression model, relating development of RA within 2 years to the VAS pain score at baseline in three groups (VAS3)

Variables in the Equation

		B	SE	Wald	df	Sig.	Exp(B)	95 % C.I.for EXP(B)	
								Lower	Upper
Step 1[a]	VAS3			6.607	2	.037			
	VAS3(1)	.412	.343	1.441	1	.230	1.509	.771	2.956
	VAS3(2)	.860	.345	6.222	1	.013	2.363	1.202	4.646
	Constant	−1.079	.281	14.765	1	.000	.340		

[a] Variable(s) entered on step 1: VAS3

☐Table 4.17 shows the output of this logistic regression model. The first row of this output corresponds to the overall association, similarly as the chi-square test in ☐Table 4.16, which is significant. Rows two and three report the estimated regression coefficients and ORs comparing patients with a VAS pain score between 30 and 49 or 50 or above to patients with a VAS pain score below 30. The OR to develop RA within 2 years for patients with a VAS pain score between 30 and 49 compared to patients with a VAS pain score below 30 is equal to 1.5 (95 % CI [0.77; 3.0]). The OR for patients with a VAS pain score of 50 or above compared to patients with a VAS pain score below 30 is equal to 2.4 (95 % CI [1.2; 4.6]). The first comparison is insignificant ($p = 0.23$), the second is significant ($p = 0.013$). Note that these p-values are not corrected for multiple testing. The OR of the third comparison could be derived from the first two. After all, the OR for patients with a VAS pain score at baseline of 50 or above compared to patients with a VAS pain score between 30 and 49 is equal to

$$\frac{\text{odds}_{\geq 50}}{\text{odds}_{30-49}} = \frac{\text{odds}_{\geq 50}/\text{odds}_{<30}}{\text{odds}_{30-49}/\text{odds}_{<30}} = \frac{2.363}{1.509} = 1.566.$$

However, whether this is significant or not is difficult to say. To obtain the corresponding 95 % CI and p-value, the group of patients with a VAS pain score of 50 or above needs to be set as reference group in a new logistic regression model. However, in general, only the comparisons with one reference group are reported, not all pairwise comparisons. In summary, the risk to develop RA within 2 years is associated with the VAS pain score at baseline ($p = 0.037$): patients with a VAS pain score of 50 or above have a higher odds to develop RA than those with a VAS pain score below 30 (OR 2.4, 95 % CI [1.2; 4.6]).

☐Table 4.18 shows an exemplary table of how to report all results in ▶Sects. 4.2–4.4 in a scientific paper. The one in the OR-column for the groups 'an FDR with RA: no RA', 'antibody status: IgM-RF + but aCCP −' and 'VAS pain score: < 30' indicate that these groups were set as the reference group. The overall p-value is obtained with the chi-square test, not the logistic regression model. Significance for each of the ORs could also be concluded based on their corresponding 95 % CIs. However, remember that this is not corrected for multiple testing.

□ **Table 4.18**   Example of a results table, relating the risk to develop RA within 2 years to different baseline scores

	OR	95 % CI	p-value
an FDR with RA			0.69
no RA	1		
RA	1.1	0.64; 2.0	
antibody status			<0.001
IgM-RF positive but aCCP negative	1		
IgM-RF negative but aCCP low positive	2.7	1.1; 6.9	
IgM-RF negative but aCCP high positive	5.1	2.2; 11.6	
IgM-RF and aCCP positive	9.6	4.4; 21.0	
VAS pain score			0.035
<30	1		
50–49	1.5	0.77; 3.0	
≥50	2.4	1.2; 4.6	

4.5   In Case of Repeated Measurements

A dichotomous outcome can also be measured repeatedly over time, i.e., longitudinal, within the same patient. In the COBRA-light trial, the primary outcome variable was reaching a DAS44 below 1.6 (yes/no). A possible research question is

? Does the chance to reach a DAS44 below 1.6 change between 26 and 52 weeks of COBRA-light treatment?

The null and alternative hypothesis of this research question are

H0: there is no difference in the chance to reach a DAS44 below 1.6 after 26 and
    52 weeks of COBRA-light treatment;
H1: there is a difference in the chance to reach a DAS44 below 1.6 after 26 and 52 weeks
    of COBRA-light treatment.

4.5.1 McNemar Test

We could just estimate the chance that a patient treated with the COBRA-light strategy has a DAS44 below 1.6 at 26 weeks and 52 weeks, and calculate, for instance, the RD between these two probabilities. However, patients with a DAS44 below 1.6 after 26 weeks of treatment might be more likely to also have a DAS44 below 1.6 after 52 weeks of treatment. And therefore, the repeated measures structure of the data has to be taken into account to answer this research question. Consequently, the McNemar test is used instead of the chi-square test. This test also uses the 2 × 2 crosstab, in which the results after 26 weeks of treatment are reported in the rows, and the results after 52 weeks of treatment in the columns (□Table 4.19).

◻ **Table 4.19** SPSS output of the crosstab comparing reaching a DAS44 below 1.6 after 26 weeks of treatment with 52 weeks of treatment

DAS44 (after 26 weeks) * DAS44 (after 52 weeks) Crosstabulation

Count

		DAS44 (after 52 weeks)		Total
		> = 1.6	<1.6	
DAS44 (after 26 weeks)	> = 1.6	33	11	44
	<1.6	13	20	33
Total		46	31	77

◻ **Table 4.20** SPSS output of the McNemar test comparing reaching a DAS44 below 1.6 after 26 weeks of treatment with 52 weeks of treatment

Chi-Square Tests

	Value	Exact Sig. (2-sided)
McNemar Test		.839[a]
N of Valid Cases	77	

[a]Binomial distribution used

Before we explain the mechanism behind the McNemar test, let us have a closer look at the crosstab in ◻Table 4.19. In total, 77 patients treated with the COBRA-light strategy had a DAS44 score at both week 26 and 52. After 26 weeks of treatment, 33 out of 77 patients (43 %) reached a DAS44 below 1.6. After 52 weeks of treatment, only 31 out of 77 patients (40 %) reached a DAS44 below 1.6, of which 20 patients already had a DAS44 below 1.6 after 26 weeks of treatment. Moreover, of the 33 patients with a DAS44 below 1.6 after 26 weeks, 13 had a score of 1.6 points or higher after 52 weeks of treatment. In total 33 patients did not reach a DAS44 below 1.6 after 26 and 52 weeks of treatment. Patients with the same outcome at both measurements (i.e., after 26 and 52 weeks) are called concordant cases; patients with different outcomes at both measurements are called discordant cases. If the number of discordant cases is much higher at one measurement than at the other, e.g., many more patients had a DAS44 below 1.6 after 52 weeks and a DAS44 of 1.6 points or higher after 26 weeks or vice versa, there is evidence in favor of the alternative hypothesis and against the null hypothesis. Hence, instead of comparing the probabilities to reach a DAS44 below 1.6 points at both times, the McNemar compares the number of discordant cases. ◻Table 4.20 shows the SPSS output of the McNemar test.

This test is an exact test, i.e., it does not use a test statistic such as the chi-square test, so in the first row ("McNemar Test") only the exact p-value is reported (under "Exact Sig. (2-sided)"), and in the second row ("N of Valid Cases") the number of patients included in the analysis is reported (under "Value"). The footnote "a. Binomial distribution used" can be ignored; it provides information on the statistical method used to compute the p-value, which is not required to interpret the results. From this table we conclude that there is not enough evidence to prove that the probability to reach a DAS44 below 1.6 changes between 26 and 52 weeks of COBRA-light treatment. At both time points approximately 40 % of the patients reached a DAS44 below 1.6 (more specifically, 43 %, 95 % CI [32 %; 54 %] after 26 weeks, and 40 %, 95 % CI [26 %; 51 %] after 52 weeks). The 95 % CIs for these probabilities are calculated from the standard form of the 95 % CI (▶Eq. E2.2, ▶Sect. 2.3.3), in which the SE of one proportion is equal to

$$SE_p = \sqrt{\frac{p \times (1 - p)}{n}}.$$

(E4.9)

In this equation, p is the proportion of patients with the 'success' outcome (i.e., reaching a DAS44 below 1.6) and n is the total number of patients in the study population (▶Example 4.3).

Example 4.3

95 % CI for one proportion

Thirty-three of 77 patients reached a DAS44 below 1.6 after 26 weeks of COBRA-light treatment corresponding to a probability of 43 %, hence the SE for this probability is equal to

$$SE_p = \sqrt{\frac{33/77 \times (1 - 33/77)}{77}} \approx \sqrt{0.0032} \approx 0.057.$$

Consequently, the 95 % CI for this probability is equal to

$$[0.43 - 1.96 \times 0.057; 0.43 + 1.96 \times 0.057] \approx [0.32; 0.54].$$

Similarly, for 30 out of 70 patients (40 %) who reached a DAS44 below 1.6 after 52 weeks, the SE and 95 % CI are equal to

$$SE_p = \sqrt{\frac{30/77 \times (1 - 30/77)}{77}} \approx \sqrt{0.0031} \approx 0.056, \text{ and}$$

$$[0.40 - 1.96 \times 0.056; 0.40 + 1.96 \times 0.056] \approx [0.29; 0.51].$$

4.6   In Case of Diagnosing a Disease

A disease is almost always diagnosed by means of a diagnostic test. This diagnostic test usually yields a dichotomous outcome: positive or negative, i.e., presence or absence of the disease. For example, RA is diagnosed by combining several tests, such as a physical examination of each joint for tenderness, swelling, warmth and painful or limited movement, blood tests to detect biomarkers such as the IgM-RF, and aCCP, and inflammation markers such as the erythrocyte sedimentation rate (ESR) and C-reactive protein (CRP).

◻ **Table 4.21** General format for a 2 × 2 crosstab used to estimate the diagnostic accuracy of a diagnostic test

		gold standard test		total
		positive ('cases')	negative ('controls')	
diagnostic test	positive	a	b	m_+
	negative	c	d	m_-
total		n_+	n_-	n

4.6.1 Measures of Diagnostic Accuracy

Diagnostic tests are not perfect: sometimes a subject who has the disease is falsely diagnosed as healthy or a subject who does not have the disease is falsely diagnosed as sick. Subjects with the disease are usually called 'cases' in medical research, and subjects without the disease 'controls'. The diagnostic accuracy of the test provides information on the probabilities of these two types of misdiagnosis and is measured by:

- the sensitivity: the proportion of truly positive cases among all cases;
- the specificity: the proportion of truly negative controls among all controls;
- the positive predictive value (PPV): the proportion of truly positive cases among all subjects with a positive test;
- the negative predictive value (NPV): the proportion of truly negative controls among all subjects with a negative test.

We use the word subject here instead of patients, to make it clear that some subjects do not have the disease and consequently cannot be considered patients. The sensitivity, specificity, PPV and NPV can be determined from a 2 × 2 crosstab as well. The true status of the subject (case or control) is usually assessed with a gold standard test as reference test. ◻Table 4.21 shows the general format of a 2 × 2 crosstab to determine the diagnostic accuracy of a diagnostic test. The true status of the subject is summarized in the columns, and the outcome of the diagnostic test in the rows. The letters a, b, c, and d correspond to the number of subjects in each group with the disease (i.e., cases; a and c) and without the disease (i.e., controls; b and d). From the numbers a, b, c, and d we can obtain the number of subjects with a positive and a negative diagnostic test, m_+ and m_- respectively, as well as the number of cases and controls, n_+ and n_- respectively. Note that b and c are the number of false positive controls and false negative cases, respectively. The diagnostic accuracy measures are then equal to

$$\text{sensitivity} = \frac{a}{n_+},$$ (E4.10)

$$\text{specificity} = \frac{d}{n_-},$$ (E4.11)

$$\text{PPV} = \frac{a}{m_+}, \tag{E4.12}$$

$$\text{NPV} = \frac{d}{m_-}. \tag{E4.13}$$

For each of the diagnostic accuracy measures, the 95 % CI can be calculated from the standard form of the CI (▶Eq. E2.2, ▶Sect. 2.3.3), with the SE for each proportion as provided in ▶Eq. E4.9 (▶Sect. 4.5.1).

4.6.2 Determining the Optimal Cut-off Value

The outcome of the diagnostic test usually classifies a subject as being positive or negative. In general, the output of the test itself is, however, a value measured on a continuous or ordinal scale. A receiver operating characteristics (ROC) curve is used to determine the optimal cut-off value at which the diagnostic test is classified as positive or negative. In an ROC curve, the sensitivity and one minus specificity (i.e., the proportion of false positive controls) for different values of a possible cut-off value are plotted on the y- and x- axis, respectively. To illustrate how to interpret the ROC curve and the different accuracy measures, let us consider the following research question

❓ What is the optimal cut-off value for ESR to diagnose RA, and what are the diagnostic properties of this cut-off value?

To answer this research question, subjects of the COBRA-light trial and subjects of the RA-cohort were pooled. Subjects of the COBRA-light trial were defined as cases since they all were diagnosed with RA, while subjects in the RA-cohort did not have RA yet at the time of inclusion and therefore were defined as controls. Only subjects who did not develop RA within 6 months were eligible as controls; subjects who developed RA within 6 months or had a follow-up shorter than 6 months were excluded. The original database of the RA-cohort did not contain ESR at baseline, and therefore these values were simulated for illustrative purposes.

In total, 162 cases were included and 328 controls. ◘Figure 4.2 shows the ROC of these 490 subjects. The diagonal line, i.e., the line $x = y$ (or sensitivity $= 1 -$ specificity), is called the line of no-discrimination, and reflects the situation where the diagnostic test is nothing but a random guess of the outcome (i.e., a flip of a coin). The point $x = 0$, $y = 1$ corresponds to a perfect classification, after all, this point corresponds to a sensitivity of 100 % and a specificity of 100 % at all relevant cut-off values. In other words, at that point, the test variable (i.e., ESR in our example) perfectly discriminates cases from controls. The closer the ROC curve is to this point, the more discriminating the test variable is. By default, SPSS only produces the ROC curve itself, without the reference line. The reference line is an additional checkbox in the ROC curve query (Supplementary Information A.5.2).

Another option in the ROC curve query in SPSS is a table with all coordinate points of the ROC curve. ◘Table 4.22 shows a part of such a table. SPSS determines all possible cut-off values for the test variable in the following way. The first possible cut-off value

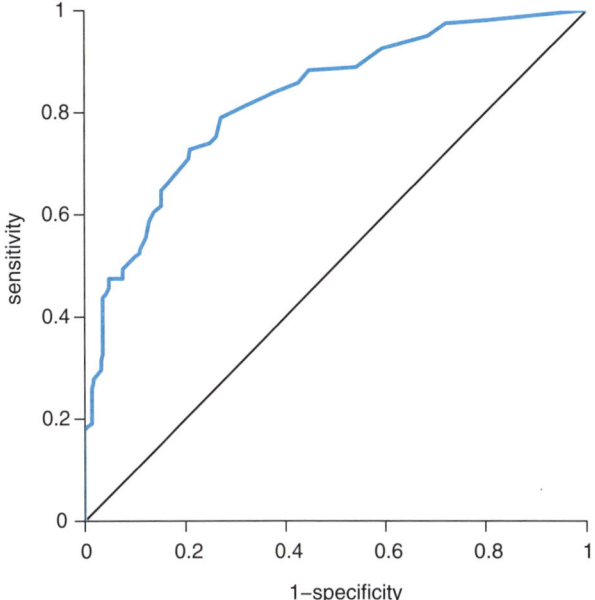

■ **Fig. 4.2**   ROC curve for ESR at baseline to discriminate subjects with RA from subjects without RA

SPSS considers (under "Positive if Greater Than or Equal To"), is the lowest observed value of the test variable minus one, which is 0 mm/h for our exemplary dataset, as can be seen in the first row of the table. This cut-off value of 0 mm/h corresponds to a sensitivity of one (or 100 %; under "Sensitivity") and a specificity of zero (or 0 %), as one minus the specificity is equal to one (under "1-Specificity"). All subsequent cut-off values SPSS considers, lie exactly between two observed values of the test variable. From ■Table 4.22, we furthermore see that for an ESR of 1.5 mm/h or higher, the sensitivity is still one while the specificity increases to 0.012 (i.e., 1 − 0.988). These values of the sensitivity and specificity are also observed if the cut-off value for ESR would be 2 mm/h or higher, because the third row in ■Table 4.22 corresponds to a cut-off value of 2.5 mm/h. That is, for all values between 1.5 mm/h and 2.5 mm/h the sensitivity and specificity do not change. At 2.5 mm/h, the sensitivity slightly decreases to 0.981, but the specificity increases quite a bit to 0.195 (i.e., 1 − 0.805). SPSS continues untill the maximal observed value of the test variable plus one, in ■Table 4.22 110 mm/h. The corresponding sensitivity for this cut-off value is zero while the specificity is one.

Increasing the cut-off of the test variable always increases the specificity, but at the cost of a decrease in the sensitivity. Ideally, the sensitivity and specificity of the diagnostic test are both 100 %, but this is rarely the case. Hence, to determine the optimal cut-off value, a trade-off has to be made between a high sensitivity and a high specificity. There are several possible choices for this trade off. For some diseases a high sensitivity (e.g., above 90 or 95 %) is desirable, because subjects with the disease need to be treated as soon as possible. For other diseases, a high specificity is desirable, because treating healthy subjects is not expedient.

□ **Table 4.22**   Part of the SPSS output of the coordinate points of the ROC curve for different values of the cut-off for ESR to discriminate subjects with RA from subjects without RA

Coordinates of the Curve		
Test Result Variable(s): ESR		
Positive if Greater Than or Equal To[a]	Sensitivity	1–Specificity
.00	1.000	1.000
1.50	1.000	.988
2.50	.981	.805
3.50	.975	.723
4.50	.951	.686
5.50	.926	.595
10.50	.815	.323
11.50	.790	.271
12.50	.753	.262
36.50	.352	.037
37.50	.340	.037
38.50	.327	.037
39.50	.315	.034
56.50	.185	.006
58.50	.179	.000
59.50	.167	.000
110.00	.000	.000

The test result variable(s): ESR has at least one tie between the positive actual state group and the negative actual state group
[a]The smallest cutoff value is the minimum observed test value minus 1, and the largest cutoff value is the maximum observed test value plus 1. All the other cutoff values are the averages of two consecutive ordered observed test values

Another method to determine the best possible cut-off value is with the Youden's *J* statistic. This statistic is equal to the sum of the sensitivity and specificity minus one. The optimal cut-off value is then selected as the cut-off value which has the highest Youden's *J* statistic. The table with coordinates of the ROC curve could be exported to Excel, in which the Youden's *J* statistic is computed for every possible cut-off value. For our dataset, this turned out to be at 11.5 mm/h (data not shown). This value is not observed in clinical practice, hence we set the optimal cut-off value (with the highest Youden's *J* statistic) at 12 mm/h. The sensitivity and specificity corresponding to this cut-off value are 79 % and 73 %, respectively (□Table 4.22). □Table 4.23 shows the 2 × 2 crosstab for this cut-off value. From this table, the PPV and the NPV of this cut-off value can be computed: the PPV is equal to $122/208 \approx 0.59$ (i.e., 59 %) and the NPV is equal to $242/282 \approx 0.86$ (i.e., 86 %).

◻ **Table 4.23** SPSS output of the crosstab corresponding to the optimal cut-off of 12 mm/h for ESR

ESR * group Crosstabulation

Count

		group		Total
		controls	cases	
ESR	< = 11	242	40	282
	> = 12	86	122	208
Total		328	162	490

Example 4.4

Computation of Youden's J statistic

For the first cut-off value for ESR, the sensitivity is equal to 1 and the specificity to 0, hence the Youden's J statistic is equal to $1 + 0 - 1 = 0$.

For the cut-off value of 1.5, the Youden's J statistic is equal to $1 + 0.012 - 1 = 0.012$.

The optimal cut-off value is 11.5, for which the Youden's J statistic is equal to $0.790 + 0.729 - 1 = 0.519$.

In the ROC curve query, SPSS reports by default the area under the curve (AUC). The sensitivity and one minus the specificity are both values between 0 and 1, therefore the maximum value of the AUC is equal to one. This corresponds to a perfect discrimination. The minimum value of the AUC is zero, but in that case probably the direction of the cut-off should be switched, i.e., values smaller than the cut-off value are indicative of the disease while values larger than the cut-off value are indicative for a healthy status. After all, this corresponds to a sensitivity of 0 % and a specificity of 0 % at all relevant cut-off values. Values of the AUC close to 0.5 indicate a very poor test that is unable to discriminate cases from controls, and is no better than flipping a coin. Roughly, an AUC between 0.5 and 0.6 is considered to indicate very poor discrimination, between 0.6 and 0.7 as poor, between 0.7 and 0.8 as fair, between 0.8 and 0.9 as good and between 0.9 and 1 as excellent discrimination [3]. The AUC of the ROC curve is also considered a C-statistic: it measures the concordance between the test variable and the outcome variable. For two randomly chosen subjects, the AUC is the probability that the value of the test variable of a case will be higher than the value of the control. ◻Table 4.24 shows the SPSS output for the AUC of the ROC curve in ◻Fig. 4.2. The 95 % CI for the AUC is an additional option in the ROC curve query (Supplementary Information A.5.2). The p-value in the output (under "Asymptotic Sig.") tests the null hypothesis that the AUC is equal to 0.5 versus the alternative hypothesis that the AUC is unequal to 0.5. The AUC is reported under "Area", the corresponding SE under "Std. Error" and the 95 % CI under "Asymptotic 95 % Confidence Interval". From this table, we conclude that ESR is a good test variable to discriminate subjects with RA from subject without RA (AUC 0.83, 95 % CI [0.79; 0.87]).

□ **Table 4.24**   SPSS output of the AUC of the ROC for ESR to discriminate subjects with RA from subjects without RA

Area Under the Curve

Test Result Variable(s): ESR

Area	Std. Error[a]	Asymptotic Sig.[b]	Asymptotic 95 % Confidence Interval	
			Lower Bound	Upper Bound
.827	.020	.000	.788	.866

The test result variable(s): ESR has at least one tie between the positive actual state group and the negative actual state group. Statistics may be biased
[a]Under the non-parametric assumption
[b]Null hypothesis: true area = 0.5

ROC curves in SPSS can be created for multiple test variables at once. For each test variable, the AUC is reported so that the different test variables can be compared. Statistical tests exists to test which variable is the best discriminator, but not in SPSS (it is possible to obtain in R and Stata). It is important to remember that only subjects with a value for all test variables (i.e., no missing data) are included when ROC curves of multiple test variables are created at once in SPSS.

4.7   Summary of Analyses

□Table 4.25 summarizes the effect sizes and assumptions for all statistical tests described in this chapter.

4.8   Further Readings

All statistical tests, such as the chi-square test (including the continuity correction), the likelihood ratio test, the test for trends and the McNemar test, and the logistic regression model are described in more detail in the classical textbooks on medical statistics and epidemiology [4–7]. The ROC curve is also explained in more detail in these classical textbooks. Dichotomous outcome variables can also be measured repeatedly over time, not just twice. The analyses of such longitudinal data is beyond the scope of this quick guide. Twisk has written a book on the analyses of longitudinal data from an applied point of view [10]. Dichotomous outcome variables are also measured repeatedly to assess agreement between raters, i.e., pathologists or physicians, on the diagnosis. The agreement between raters is measured by the κ (kappa) statistic. More information of the κ statistic can be found in the books written by Armitage et al., Kirkwood & Sterne and de Vet et al. [6, 7, 11]. Crosstabs can also be used to investigate differences in a categorical outcome variable between two or more groups. For more information on analyzing a categorical outcome variables we refer to the book written by Agresti [12].

■ **Table 4.25** Summary of the statistical test with their effect sizes and assumptions, to investigate associations with a dichotomous outcome variable

Dichotomous determinant	Statistical test	Chi-square test
	Effect size	OR/RR/RD
	Assumptions	Expected count $\geq$ 5 in all cells
Categorical determinant	Statistical test	Chi-square test
	Effect size	OR/RR/RD (one group set as reference)
	Assumptions	Expected count $\geq$ 5 in all cells
Continuous determinant	Statistical model	Logistic regression model
	Effect size	Exponential of regression coefficient (OR; per increase of 1 unit)
	Assumptions	Linearity
Repeated measures	Statistical test	McNemar test
	Effect size	Percentage positive outcomes
	Assumptions	None

OR odds ratio, *RD* risk difference, *RR* relative risk

References

1. van de Stadt LA, Witte BI, Bos WH, van Schaardenburg D. A prediction rule for the development of arthritis in seropositive arthralgia patients. Ann Rheum Dis. 2013;72(12):1920–6. ►https://doi.org/10.1136/annrheumdis-2012-202127.
2. ter Wee MM, den Uyl D, Boers M, Kerstens P, Nurmohamed M, van Schaardenburg D, et al. Intensive combination treatment regimens, including prednisolone, are effective in treating patients with early rheumatoid arthritis regardless of additional etanercept: 1-year results of the COBRA-light open-label, randomised, non-inferiority trial. Ann Rheum Dis. 2015;74(6):1233–40. ►https://doi.org/10.1136/annrheumdis-2013-205143.
3. Šimundić A-M. Measures of diagnostic accuracy: basic definitions. EJIFCC. 2009;19(4):203–11.
4. Altman DG. Practical statistics for medical research. London: Chapman & Hall; 1991.
5. Rothman KJ, Lash TL, Greenland S. Modern epidemiology. 3rd ed. Philadelphia: Lippincott-Raven; 2012.
6. Armitage P, Berry G, Matthews JNS. Statistical methods in medical research. Oxford: Blackwell Science Ltd; 2002.
7. Kirkwood BR, Sterne JAC. Essential medical statistics. 2nd ed. Oxford: Blackwell Science Ltd; 2003.
8. Siegel JP. Equivalence and noninferiority trials. Am Heart J. 2000;139(4):S166–70. ►https://doi.org/10.1016/s0002-8703(00)90066-8.
9. Walker E, Nowacki AS. Understanding equivalence and noninferiority testing. J Gen Intern Med. 2011;26(2):192–6. ►https://doi.org/10.1007/s11606-010-1513-8.
10. Twisk JWR. Applied longitudinal data analysis for epidemiology. New York: Cambridge University Press; 2003.
11. de Vet HC, Terwee CB, Mokkink LB, Knol DL. Measurement in medicine. Cambridge: Cambridge University Press; 2011.
12. Agresti A. An introduction to categorical data analysis. 2nd ed. Hoboken: John Wiley & Sons; 2002.

Analyzing Time to Event Outcome Variables

Abstract

Sometimes it is not only interesting to know whether a patient developed a disease, but to also know the time it took to develop the disease. After all, two treatments could, for example, be equally effective in preventing progression within 2 years, but the time until progression occurs might differ. Since not all patients progress during the follow-up, time to progression is a time to event outcome variable; it consists of a time variable and a dichotomous variable indicating whether or not the event occurred (e.g., progression). In this chapter, we explain how to analyze the association between a time to event outcome variable and a dichotomous, a categorical, and a continuous determinant.

© Bohn Stafleu van Loghum is een imprint van Springer Media B.V., onderdeel van Springer Nature 2019
M. M. ter Wee and B. I. Lissenberg-Witte, *A Quick Guide on How to Conduct Medical Research*,
https://doi.org/10.1007/978-90-368-2248-0_5

5.1   What Is a Time to Event Outcome Variable?

In ▶Chap. 4, we analyzed the dichotomous outcome variable development of rheuma-toid arthritis (RA) within 2 years, and only included patients who had at least 2 years of follow-up. However, some patients in the RA-cohort [1] had a follow-up period of less than 2 years and did not develop RA during their follow-up period. Because it was unknown whether these patients would have developed RA within 2 years, these patients were excluded from the analyses in ▶Chap. 4. Moreover, the dichotomous outcome variable development of RA within 2 years does not distinguish between 1 and 2 years, while other patients who do not develop RA within 2 years might develop it during the follow-ing years whilst others do not even within 5 years. A dichotomous outcome variable does not distinguish how fast the outcome occurred, yet this time to event is very informative. Therefore, when one is interested in outcomes such as death or the development of a disease, the time to event is much more informative and more powerful than only consider-ing the dichotomous outcome.

There are several ways to summarize time to event outcome variables, for example with the cumulative incidence at a certain time point t. The cumulative incidence of the event of interest, in the RA-cohort development of RA, at a certain time point t is estimated by one minus the Kaplan-Meier curve. Recall that the Kaplan-Meier curve is needed because some patients may not develop RA by the end of the follow-up period, this is called cen-soring (▶Sect. 2.2.3). The Kaplan-Meier curve estimates, at each time point t (until the last time an event was observed), the probability that the event does not occur before that time. This function of time is called the survival function, and is usually denoted by $S(t)$. The Kaplan-Meier curve and the one minus Kaplan-Meier curve for the RA-cohort can be found in ▶Chap. 2 (◐Fig. 2.3, ▶Sect. 2.2.3). In ▶Chap. 2, we only illustrated the Kaplan-Meier curve and the survival table. More in-depth information is needed to interpret the curve itself and the results. We provide this below, using the follow-up times and event out-comes of 10 fictive patients. ◐Figure 5.1 visualizes the observed data of these 10 patients.

An important fraction in the calculation of the Kaplan-Meier curve is the survival fraction at time t. This is the number of patients who 'survived', i.e., did not experience the event yet, up to time t, divided by the number of patients at risk of the event at that time. Let us denote the number of patients at risk at time t by n_t and the number of patients who experienced the event at time t by d_t. Then, the survival fraction is equal to

$$\text{survival fraction}(t) = \frac{n_t - d_t}{n_t} = 1 - \frac{d_t}{n_t}. \tag{E5.1}$$

The survival fraction is equal to one minus the probability that the event occurs exactly at time t. Probability theory then tell us that the probability that the event does not occur before time t is equal to the probability that the event does not occur before the previous event time times the survival fraction at time t. Formulated mathematically, this means that the Kaplan-Meier estimator for the survival function $S(t_i)$, denoted by $\hat{S}(t_i)$, at follow-up time t_i is equal to

$$\hat{S}(t_i) = \hat{S}(t_{i-1}) \times \text{survival fraction}(t_i). \tag{E5.2}$$

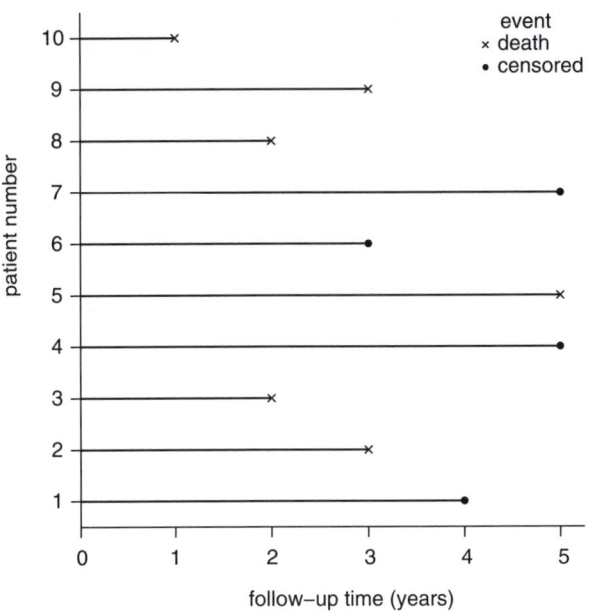

Fig. 5.1   Illustration of follow-up times and event outcomes of 10 fictive patients

To distinguish the current event time from the previous observed event time, we use the notation t_i and t_{i-1}, respectively. The Kaplan-Meier estimator always starts at the point $(0, 1)$, i.e., $\hat{S}(0) = 1$. After all, at baseline, or at time point zero, all patients are still at risk for the event. From ▶ Eqs. E5.1 and E5.2 it follows that the Kaplan-Meier curve only changes its value (i.e., 'jumps') at time points where at least one event was observed and not at time points where only patients were censored.

Now, let us look at the 10 patients in ◻Fig. 5.1, to see how we estimate the Kaplan-Meier curve with ▶ Eqs. E5.1 and E5.2. The first patient (number 10) died after 1 year, hence the survival fraction at time $t=1$ is equal to $1 - 1/10 = 0.9$ and the Kaplan-Meier estimator is equal to $\hat{S}(1) = \hat{S}(0) \times 0.9 = 1 \times 0.9 = 0.9$. After 2 years, two more patients (patients 3 and 8), of the remaining nine at risk, died. At time $t=2$, the survival fraction is equal to $1 - 2/9 = 7/9$ and the Kaplan-Meier estimator is equal to $\hat{S}(2) = \hat{S}(1) \times 7/9 = 0.9 \times 7/9 = 0.7$. After 3 years, seven patients are at risk, of which two patients died and one patient is censored (patient 6), e.g., lost to follow-up. The survival fraction at time $t=3$ is equal to $1 - 2/7 = 5/7$ and the Kaplan-Meier estimator is equal to $\hat{S}(3) = \hat{S}(2) \times 5/7 = 0.7 \times 5/7 = 0.5$. After 4 years, only four patients are at risk, and one patients is censored. Since no patient died at time $t=4$, the Kaplan-Meier curve does not change. After all, the survival fraction at time $t=4$ is equal to $1 - 0/4 = 1$ and consequently $\hat{S}(4) = \hat{S}(3) \times 1 = 0.5 \times 1 = 0.5$. Finally, after 5 years, one of the remaining three patients at risk dies and the other two are censored. Hence, at time $t=5$, the survival fraction is equal to $1 - 1/3 = 2/3$ and the Kaplan-Meier estimator is equal to $\hat{S}(5) = \hat{S}(3) \times 2/3 = 0.5 \times 2/3 = 0.33$. ◻Table 5.1 summarizes the survival probabilities and their calculations at each time point when at least one event (i.e., death) occurred.

◘ Table 5.1 The survival table for the 10 patients of ◘Fig. 5.1

Time point (t)	Number of patients at risk (n_t)	Number of patients with event (d_t)	Number of censored patients	Survival fraction	Kaplan-Meier estimator $\hat{S}(t)$
0	10	0	0	1	1.0
1	10	1	0	$1-9/10$	0.90
2	9	2	0	$1-2/9$	0.70
3	7	2	1	$1-2/7$	0.50
5	3	1	2	$1-1/3$	0.33

From ▶Eqs. E5.1 and E5.2 it also follows that small 'jumps' in the Kaplan-Meier curve indicate that only a few patients had the event at that time, while large 'jumps' could indicate two things. Either many patients had an event at that time or there are only very few patients still at risk for the event. Whichever of the two is the case, is checked by looking at the number of patients 'at risk' at that time in the survival table. The survival table is default SPSS output in the Kaplan-Meier query (Supplementary Information A.6.1). We already introduced the survival table in ▶Chap. 2 (◘Table 2.1, ▶Sect. 2.2.3). We used a part of that table to compute the Kaplan-Meier estimator for the time to development of RA in the RA-cohort in ▶Example 5.1

Example 5.1

Calculation of the Kaplan-Meier curve

In the RA-cohort, the first patient developed RA after 0.23 months. No other patient developed RA at exactly that time, and none of the patients were censored before. Hence $t_1 = 0.23$, $n_1 = 374$, $d_1 = 1$ and $\hat{S}(t_1) = (374-1)/374 \approx 0.997$. The second patient developed RA after 0.62 months, no other patient developed RA at exactly that time, and none of the remaining patients were censored. Hence, $t_2 = 0.26$, $n_2 = 373$, $d_2 = 1$ and $\hat{S}(t_2) = 0.997 \times (373-1)/373 \approx 0.994$.

5.2 In Case of a Dichotomous Determinant

We illustrate how to describe and compare time to event outcome variables between two groups with the following research question

❓ Is there a difference in time to development of RA between seropositive arthralgia patients with and without a first-degree relative (FDR) with RA?

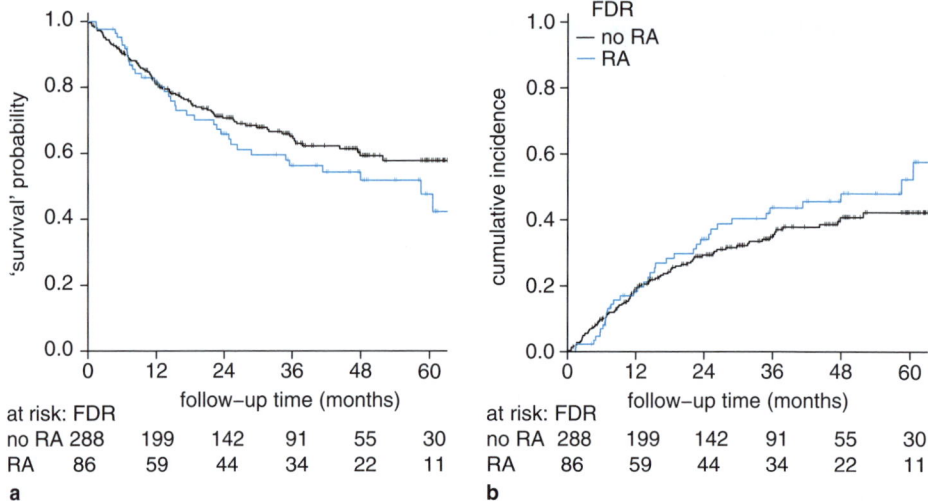

▫ Fig. 5.2   Kaplan-Meier curve (**a**) and one minus Kaplan-Meier curve (**b**) for the time to development of RA, for patients with and without an FDR with RA

The null and alternative hypothesis of the research question are

H0: there is no difference in time to development of RA between patients with an FDR
    with RA and without an FDR with RA;
H1: there is a difference in time to development of RA between patients with an FDR
    with RA and without an FDR with RA.

Before we illustrate how to answer this research question, we first provide different ways to summarize the time to event outcome variables for two different groups in a paper descriptively.

5.2.1 Descriptive Statistics

As already explained in ▶Chap. 2 and above, the Kaplan-Meier curve is used to visualize the survival probability at each time *t*. Moreover, one minus the Kaplan-Meier curve is used to calculate the cumulative incidence. The Kaplan-Meier curve can also be used to visually compare the time to event in the case of a dichotomous determinant (i.e., between two groups). ▫Figure 5.2 shows the Kaplan-Meier curve for the time to development of RA in the RA-cohort (▫Fig. 5.2a) and the one minus Kaplan-Meier curve for the same out-come variable (▫Fig. 5.2b) for patients with an FDR with RA and patients without an FDR with RA. The curves seem to cross twice in the first 12 months, then patients with an FDR with RA seem to develop RA slightly quicker than patients without an FDR with RA.

In addition to the graphical summary of the data by means of the Kaplan-Meier curve, several descriptive statistics could be derived: the cumulative incidence at a cer-tain time point, and the median time to development of RA. ▫Tables 5.2 and 5.3 are

◻ **Table 5.2** Part of the SPSS output of the survival table, separately for patients with and without an FDR with RA

Survival Table

FDR		Time	Status	Cumulative Proportion Surviving at the Time		N of Cumulative Events	N of Remaining Cases
				Estimate	Std. Error		
no RA	1	.230	arthritis	.997	.003	1	287
	84	11.729	arthritis	.811	.024	52	204
	93	12.025	arthritis	.807	.024	53	195
	147	23.688	arthritis	.706	.029	75	141
	162	25.561	arthritis	.701	.029	76	126
	249	51.844	arthritis	.578	.038	92	39
	275	64.854	arthritis	.536	.053	93	13
	288	79.310	no arthritis	.	.	93	0
RA	1	1.314	arthritis	.988	.012	1	85
	24	11.499	arthritis	.816	.043	15	62
	29	12.189	arthritis	.802	.045	16	57
	40	23.261	arthritis	.659	.055	26	46
	45	24.706	arthritis	.643	.056	27	41
	75	58.382	arthritis	.476	.071	35	11
	78	60.386	arthritis	.423	.080	36	8
	83	72.444	arthritis	.317	.110	37	3
	86	84.205	arthritis	.000	.000	38	0

◻ **Table 5.3** SPSS output of the estimated mean and median time to development of RA, separately for patients with and without an FDR with RA and for all patients together

Means and Medians for Survival Time

FDR	Mean[a]				Median			
	Estimate	Std. Error	95 % Confidence Interval		Estimate	Std. Error	95 % Confidence Interval	
			Lower Bound	Upper Bound			Lower Bound	Upper Bound
No RA	53.100	2.178	48.831	57.368	.	.	.	.
RA	48.718	4.101	40.681	56.756	58.382	12.574	33.738	83.026
Overall	53.516	2.141	49.319	57.713	72.444	9.210	54.392	90.496

[a]Estimation is limited to the largest survival time if it is censored

by default part of the SPSS output of the Kaplan-Meier curve query, and report the survival probability at each observed follow-up time (◘Table 5.2; the survival table) and the mean and median time in each group separately (◘Table 5.3). Both tables have been described in more detail in ▶Chap. 2 (▶Sect. 2.2.3).

The 95 % confidence interval (CI) for the cumulative incidence at a certain time t is computed using the standard form of the CI (▶Eq. (E2.2), ▶Sect. 2.3.3)

$$[\text{cumulative incidence} - 1.96 \times \text{SE; cumulative incidence} + 1.96 \times \text{SE}], \quad \text{(E5.3)}$$

where the standard error (SE) of the cumulative incidence is equal to the SE of the survival probability, which can be found in the survival table. In case the outcome of interest is not cumulative incidence but survival, the 95% CI for the survival probability is equal to ▶Eq. (E5.3), but with survival probability instead of cumulative incidence. In SPSS it is not possible to add the 95 % CI to the Kaplan-Meier curve, but with other statistical software, such as Stata and R, this is possible. In ▶Example 5.2, we illustrate how to compute the 95% CI for both groups.

Example 5.2

Calculation of 1- and 5-year cumulative incidence
Within the group of patients without an FDR with RA, the probability to not develop RA within 1 year is equal to 0.811 (SE 0.024), hence the cumulative incidence at 1 year is equal to 1 − 0.811 = 0.189, and the 95 % CI is equal to

$$[0.189 - 1.96 \times 0.024; 0.189 + 1.96 \times 0.024] \approx [0.14; 0.24].$$

Similarly, the 5-year cumulative incidence of RA within patients with an FDR with RA is equal to 1 − 0.476 = 0.524, and the 95 % CI is equal to

$$[0.524 - 1.96 \times 0.071; 0.524 + 1.96 \times 0.071] \approx [0.38; 0.66].$$

The SE at 5 years follow-up is larger than at 1 year follow-up, as the number of patients at risk to develop RA is much smaller further in time. Therefore, the 95 % CI at 5 years is wider compared to the 95 % CI at 1 year.

From ◘Table 5.3, we see that within the group of patients with an FDR with RA, the median time to development of RA is 58.4 months (in the row "RA"). For patients without an FDR with RA (in the row "no RA"), the Kaplan-Meier curve is never below 0.5, therefore the median time to development of RA cannot be estimated for that group and is left empty in the first row of the SPSS output. The median time to event is also reported for the whole study population (in the row "Overall"). The SE and the corresponding 95 % CI for the median time to development of RA are also reported, for patients with an FDR with RA and the whole study population. However, these are rarely reported in scientific papers. What is also not reported is the estimated mean time to development of RA, because a time to event outcome variable is never normally

◼ **Table 5.4** SPSS output of the log-rank test, comparing the time to development of RA between patients with and without an FDR with RA

Overall Comparisons			
	Chi-Square	df	Sig.
Log Rank (Mantel-Cox)	1.437	1	.231

Test of equality of survival distributions for the different levels of an FDR with RA

distributed. Recall that for non-normally distributed outcome variables, the median is reported instead of the mean. In addition, the median time to development of RA, estimated by SPSS, is not equal to the median time to development of RA within all patients that eventually developed RA. The median time to event in all patients with an event is sometimes reported as well, to describe features of the observed data. The median time to event within all patients who eventually developed RA can always be estimated.

The difference in time to development of RA between the two groups is tested statistically, either with the log-rank test or the Cox regression model

5.2.2 Log-Rank Test

The log-rank test compares the survival functions of the time to development of RA between the two groups. More specifically, it compares the expected number of events in both groups (under the null hypothesis of no difference) with the observed number of events in both groups over all time points in a similar way as the chi-square test for a dichotomous outcome variable. The definition of the test statistic is beyond the scope of this and not necessary to know to interpret the findings. We refer to the further readings (▶Sect. 5.6) for references with more information. The test statistic follows a chi-square distribution with 1 degree of freedom. Large differences between the number of expected and observed events, hence large values of the test statistic, are in favor of the alternative hypothesis and evidence against the null hypothesis, while small difference are not. Since the log-rank test does not have any assumptions with respect to the distribution of the time to event outcome (or equivalently the shape of the survival function or cumulative incidence function), it is also considered a non-parametric test.

◼Table 5.4 shows the SPSS output of the log-rank test, comparing the two Kaplan-Meier curves in ◼Fig. 5.2. SPSS reports the value of the test statistic (under "Chi-Square"), the degrees of freedom (under "df") and the p-value (under "Sig."). From this table, we conclude that there is not enough evidence to prove a difference in time to development of RA between patients with and without an FDR with RA ($p=0.23$). The 2-year cumulative incidence of RA was 29 % (95 % CI [65 %; 76 %]) among patients without an FDR with RA and 34 % (95 % CI [55 %; 77 %]) among patients with an FDR with RA (◼Table 5.2). Note that these percentages are slightly lower than the ones found when considering the dichotomous outcome variable development of RA within 2 years

(◻Table 4.2, ▶Sect. 4.2.2). This difference is explained by the fact that in the analyses with a time to event outcome variable, censoring is accounted for, leading to a larger sized study population, since all patients are included in the analyses, while patients who were censored before two years were excluded in the analyses of ▶Chap. 2. We could have also chosen to report the 1- or 5-year cumulative incidence instead. However, the cumulative incidence is only the effect at a single time point, and consequently taking the ratio of the incidences between the groups, is also still only an effect size at that specific time point.

5.2.3 Cox Regression Model

To quantify the effect of having an FDR with RA on the time to development of RA by one single effect size, we need to estimate a regression model, which includes the time component of the outcome variable. This model is called the Cox proportional hazards model (also shortened to Cox regression model). This model does not model the survival function $S(t)$, but the hazard function $h(t)$. The hazard function is mathematically related to the survival function: it is the derivative of the cumulative hazard function $H(t) = -\ln(S(t))$. The hazard at time t is the event rate at that time, given that the event did not occur yet. Loosely speaking, the hazard at time t is the instantaneous probability of the event at that time, under the condition that the event did not occur before time t. The Cox regression model models the ratio of the two hazard functions of the two groups, denoted by $h_0(t)$ and $h_1(t)$, in the following way

$$\ln(h_1(t)/h_0(t)) = b_1. \tag{M5.1}$$

The ratio of the two hazard functions, $h_1(t)/h_0(t)$, is called the hazard ratio (HR) and the model assumes that the HR is constant over time. Put differently, the two hazard functions $h_1(t)$ and $h_0(t)$ are assumed to be proportional to each other for all values of t, hence the proportionality in the name of the model. An HR larger than one indicates that the reference group has a shorter time to event (i.e., performs worst), while an HR smaller than one indicates that the reference group has a longer time to event (i.e., performs best). If the group without an FDR with RA is coded as zero and the group with an FDR with RA as one, the Cox regression model is equivalent to

$$\ln(h(t)) = \ln(h_0(t)) + b_1 \times \text{FDR}. \tag{M5.2}$$

This resembles the linear and logistic regression models, with the only difference that the regression coefficient b_0 is replaced by the natural logarithm (ln) transformation of the baseline hazard $h_0(t)$. In ▶Model M5.1, the regression coefficient b_1 is equal to $\ln(\text{HR})$ and consequently, the HR is obtained by taking its exponential (exp), i.e., $\exp(b_1)$. The Cox regression model tests the following null and alternative hypothesis

H0: $b_1 = 0$;
H1: $b_1 \neq 0$;

■ **Table 5.5** SPSS output of the Cox regression model, comparing time to development of RA between patients with and without an FDR with RA

Variables in the Equation								
	B	SE	Wald	df	Sig.	Exp(B)	95.0 % CI for Exp(B)	
							Lower	Upper
FDR	.233	.195	1.429	1	.232	1.262	.862	1.849

■Table 5.5 shows the SPSS output of the Cox regression model. This output is similar to the output of the logistic regression model, but since the baseline hazard function $h_0(t)$ is a function of time, there is no constant reported in the output. The estimated regression coefficient b_1 is given under "B" (with its SE under "SE"), the HR under "Exp(B)" and the 95 % CI for the HR under "95.0 % CI for Exp(B)". The 95 % CI is not default output of SPSS and has to be selected as an additional option in the Cox regression query (Supplementary Information A.6.2). The p-value is given in the column under "Sig.". The value of the Wald statistic (under "Wald") with one degree of freedom (under "df") is also reported. From this table, we again conclude that there is not enough evidence to prove that the time to development of RA differs between patients with and without an FDR with RA (HR 1.3, 95 % CI [0.86; 1.8], $p=0.23$).

The baseline hazard function $h_0(t)$, which is the hazard function of patients without an FDR with RA in our example, is estimated by SPSS, and is used to estimate the survival function or cumulative incidence function in each group separately (■Fig. 5.3). Note that the estimated cumulative incidence function of the Cox regression model differs from the one minus Kaplan-Meier curve in ■Fig. 5.2b. That is because the Cox regression model assumes the ratio of the two hazard function is constant over time (the proportionality assumption). In other words, the difference between the two cumulative incidence (or survival) curves increases at a constant rate. The Kaplan-Meier curve is a non-parametric estimator, which means that no assumptions at all are imposed to estimate the survival function in contrast to the Cox regression model. Consequently, the p-values of the log-rank test and the Cox regression model will always differ, although it could be only a small difference, as in our example. Before we draw a conclusion from ■Table 5.5 we formally have to test the proportionality assumption first.

5.2.4 Assumptions of the Cox Regression Model

The proportionality assumption can be investigated visually or tested statistically with different procedures. In the first place, the Kaplan-Meier curves (or the one minus Kaplan-Meier curves) for each group could be visually inspected. Proportionality of the

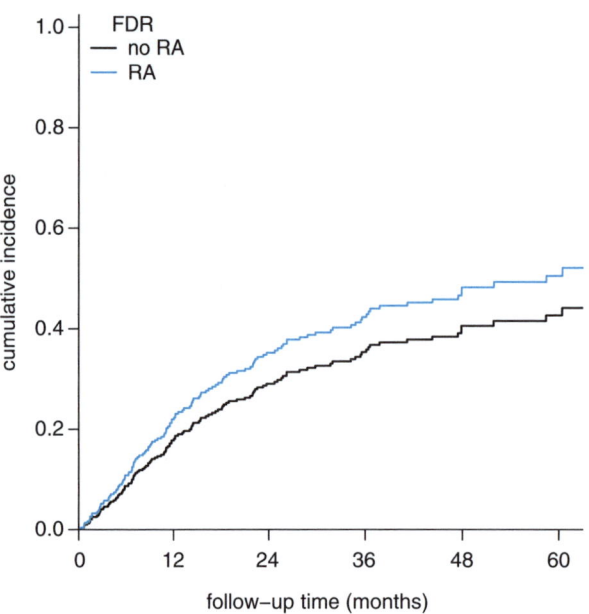

◻ Fig. 5.3   Estimated cumulative incidence of the development of RA, separately for patients with an FDR with RA and patients without an FDR with RA

curves of the two groups implies that they cannot cross. In ◻Fig. 5.2, we saw that the curves do cross after 8 or 9 months and are almost equal again around 12 months. From then on, patients with an FDR with RA tend to develop RA slightly quicker than patients without an FDR with RA. So, for the first year proportionality might not hold, but thereafter it may hold.

Another way to visually inspect the assumption is with a log-log plot. In this plot, the function $-\ln(-\ln(S(t)))=-\ln(H(t))$ is plotted on the y-axis for each group separately and time (or $\ln(t)$) is plotted on the x-axis. If the two curves of the groups are parallel, that is, if the difference between the curves is approximately equal at all times, proportionality seems valid. For references for more information on the mathematics behind this plot, we refer to the further readings (▶Sect. 5.6). ◻Figure 5.4a shows the log-log plot of the Kaplan-Meier curve. This log-log plot could be compared to the estimated log-log plot resulting from the Cox regression model (◻Fig. 5.4b). The latter one is only plotted for illustrative purposes, as the Cox regression model assumes proportionality, hence the log-log curves are parallel by definition. The log-log plot of the Kaplan-Meier curves are not parallel, since they cross as well.

Besides visual inspection of the Kaplan-Meier curve and the log-log plot, we could also test the proportionality assumption statistically. First of all, we could let the regression coefficient b_1 vary over time. In that case, the Cox regression model is referred to as a Cox regression model with a time-dependent covariate, and the model would be as follows

$$\ln(h(t)) = \ln(h_0(t)) + b_1(t) \times \text{FDR, with} \tag{M5.3}$$

$$b_1(t) = c_0 + c_1 \times f(t).$$

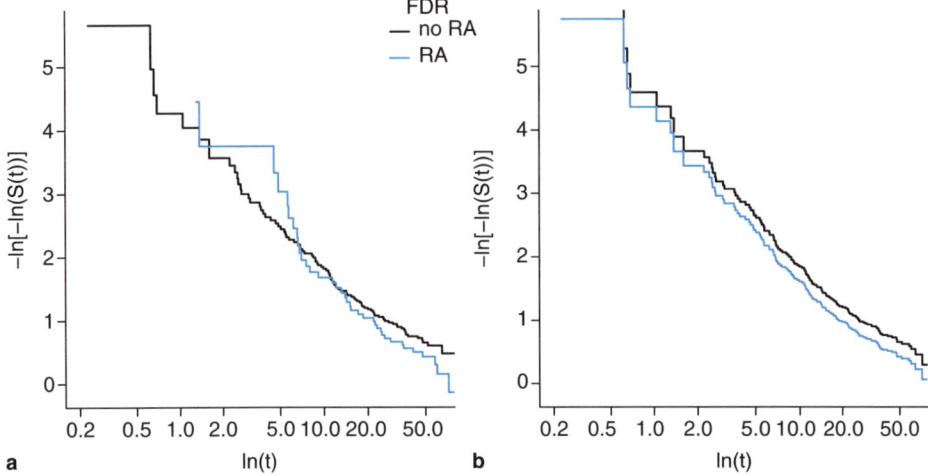

◻ **Fig. 5.4** Log-log plot of the Kaplan-Meier curve (**a**) and the estimated survival function of the Cox regression model (**b**), to assess the proportionality assumption

The function $f(t)$ could be any function of time t. Commonly used functions are $f(t)=t$, $f(t)=\ln(t)$ or $f(t)=d_T(t)$ where for a certain cut-off time T the function $d_T(t)$ is zero for all $t \leq T$, and one for all $t > T$. Different functions $f(t)$ have different interpretations: $f(t)=t$ assumes that the HR increases (or decreases, depending on the sign of c_1) constantly, while $f(t)=d_T(t)$ assumes that there are two different HRs (one for the time up to time T, and one for the time after time T). If the Kaplan-Meier curves cross, this function might be the best choice. Since the curves of patients with and without an FDR with RA cross around 8 to 9 months, and then come together again just after 12 months, we choose the cut-off T equal to 12 months in our example. The Cox regression model is then split in two parts:

$$\ln(h(t)) = \ln(h_0(t)) + c_0 \times \text{FDR, for } t \leq 12, \tag{M5.4}$$

$$\ln(h(t)) = \ln(h_0(t)) + (c_0 + c_1) \times \text{FDR, for } t > 12. \tag{M5.5}$$

Hence, the HR for $t \leq 12$ is equal to $\exp(c_0)$, and the HR for $t > 12$ is equal to $\exp(c_0+c_1)$. In the Cox regression model with a time-dependent covariate, two null and alternative hypotheses are tested. The first hypothesis is whether the new regression coefficient c_0 is equal to zero or not (i.e., whether there is a difference in time to development of RA between patients with and without an FDR with RA during the first 12 months of follow-up)

H0: $c_0 = 0$;
H1: $c_0 \neq 0$;

□ Table 5.6   SPSS output of the Cox regression model with time-dependent covariate to test the proportionality assumption

Variables in the Equation

	B	SE	Wald	df	Sig.	Exp(B)	95.0 % CI for Exp(B)	
							Lower	Upper
FDR	−.036	.293	.015	1	.903	.965	.543	1.714
FDR*T_COV_	.514	.395	1.693	1	.193	1.673	.771	3.629

The second hypothesis is whether or not the 'time-dependent' coefficient c_1 is zero or not (i.e., whether the proportionality assumptions holds or not)

H0: $c_1 = 0$;
H1: $c_1 \neq 0$;

To test the proportionality assumption we are only interested in the second test. □Table 5.6 shows the SPSS output of the Cox regression model with the time-dependent covariate. The output is similar as a Cox regression model with proportional hazards. The result for the regression coefficient c_1 is printed in the second row ("FDR*T_COV_"). The estimate for c_1 is given in the column labeled "B", the corresponding p-value against the null hypothesis under "Sig.". From this table, we conclude that there is no evidence to reject the null hypothesis, and we can assume proportionality holds. Note that this conclusion could depend on our choice of the cut-off point $T = 12$. We tested this, but other cut-off points did not provide any evidence against the null hypothesis either (data not shown).

If the p-value for c_1 would have been significant, the results in the first row of □Table 5.6 would provide the HR for the time to development of RA (and corresponding 95 % CI) of patients with FDR with RA compared to patients without FDR with RA for the first 12 months. The HR for the time to development of RA after 12 months is obtained directly from the SPSS output, which is the product of the two HRs under column "Exp(B)", since $\exp(c_0) \times \exp(c_1) = \exp(c_0 + c_1)$. This multiplication, however, does not hold for the 95 % CI. Hence, to obtain the 95 % CI for the HR after 12 months follow-up, the time-dependent covariate has to be recoded in SPSS, such that d_T is zero for all $t > 12$ and one for all $t \leq 12$.

A second statistical test to assess the proportionality, is based on the Schoenfeld residuals. These residuals, which are only computed for patients who developed RA, can be saved in SPSS (Supplementary Information A.6.2); the sum of these residuals add up to one. If the Schoenfeld residuals do not depend on time, proportionality holds. This is visualized with a scatterplot with time to development of RA on the x-axis and the Schoenfeld residuals on the y-axis (□Fig. 5.5). Separation of the dots is caused by the two groups that are compared: the Schoenfeld residuals of patients with an FDR with RA are all positive (and slightly lower than 0.75) while the Schoenfeld residuals of patients without an FDR

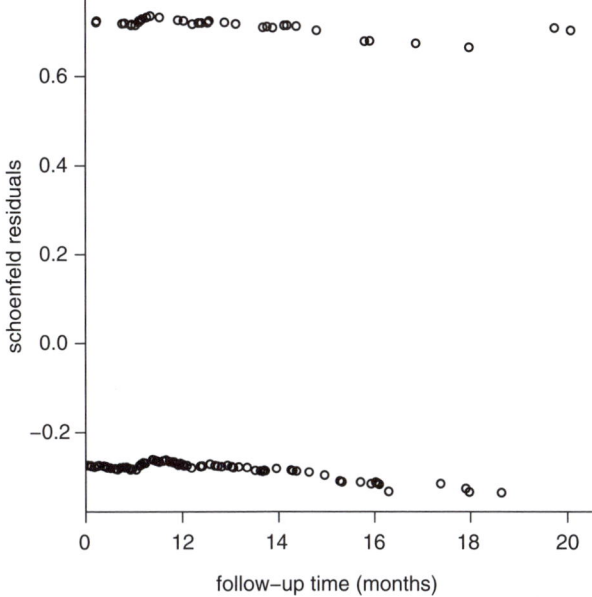

□ **Fig. 5.5** Scatterplot of Schoenfeld residuals against time, to investigate the proportionality assumption

□ **Table 5.7** SPSS output of the linear regression model, testing the proportionality assumption

Coefficients[a]

Model		Unstandardized Coefficients		Standardized Coefficients	t	Sig.
		B	Std. Error	Beta		
1	(Constant)	−.051	.057		−.885	.378
	follow-up time (months)	.003	.002	.106	1.211	.228

[a]Dependent Variable: Partial residual for FDR

with RA are all negative (and slightly lower than −0.25). Proportionality is then equivalent to the slope of a regression line through all dots, being equal to zero. Whether the slope of the regression line is equal to zero, could be tested with a linear regression, with time to development of RA as continuous determinant and the Schoenfeld residuals as the outcome variable. □Table 5.7 shows the SPSS output of this linear regression model, from which we conclude that the proportionality assumption is valid: the estimated slope of the linear regression model is 0.003 (under "B" in the second row), which does not differ significantly from zero ($p = 0.23$).

□ **Table 5.8** SPSS output of the Cox regression model, comparing time to development of RA between patients that received treatment A or B

Variables in the Equation

	B	SE	Wald	df	Sig.	Exp(B)	95.0 % CI for Exp(B)	
							Lower	Upper
treatment	.202	.178	1.290	1	.256	1.224	.864	1.733

5.2.5 Non-inferiority and Equivalence

Non-inferiority (or equivalence) of treatment B compared to treatment A is proven similarly for a time to event outcome variable as for a continuous outcome variable. A priori, a non-inferiority margin is set, i.e., a non-inferiority HR (HR_{inf}). Whether this non-inferiority HR is smaller or larger than one, depends on the type of the event: for some events, an HR below one indicates better results compared to the reference group, while for another event an HR above one indicates better results. For illustrative purposes, assume the RA-cohort was set up as an randomized controlled trial (RCT), designed to prove non-inferiority of treatment B compared to treatment A. For illustrative purposes, we simulated the data on treatment. The exemplary research question would then be

❓ Is treatment B non-inferior compared to treatment A in time to development of RA in seropositive arthralgia patients?

In this case (with treatment A as the reference group), an HR below one indicates that time to development of RA in patients treated with treatment B is longer that in patients treated with treatment A. Non-inferiority of treatment B is then means that the true HR is not much larger than one, so the HR_{inf} needs to be larger than one. For a non-inferiority margin of $HR_{inf}=1.25$ in this exemplary study (where, for illustrative purposes all 374 patients in the RA-cohort were randomly divided in two treatment groups), the corresponding null and alternative hypothesis are

H0: HR ≥ 1.25;
H1: HR < 1.25.

Hence, non-inferiority is proven (at the significance level α of 0.025), if the upper bound of the 95 % CI for the HR is below 1.25. □Table 5.8 shows the SPSS output of the Cox regression model, comparing treatment B to treatment A. From this output, we conclude that there is not enough evidence to prove treatment B is non-inferior compared to treatment A in prolonging the time to development of RA (HR 1.22, 95 % CI [0.86; 1.7]), as the upper bound of the CI (i.e., 1.7) is above the predefined margin of 1.25. Note that the *p*-value is not reported, because the null hypothesis of the Cox regression model (in terms of the HR) is equal to

H0: $HR = 1$.

To study equivalence between treatment A and B with respect to time of development of RA, two a priori fixed HRs need to be set: the lower and upper bound for equivalence (HR_L and HR_U). Since the HR is a ratio, which is anti-symmetric, these two bounds need to be anti-symmetric as well, i.e., $HR_L = 1/HR_U$. If we keep the upper bound HR_U equal to 1.25, the lower bound HR_L should be equal to $1/1.25 = 0.8$, to be anti-symmetric. The corresponding null and alternative hypothesis for the research question

? Is treatment B equivalent compared to treatment A in time to development of RA in seropositive arthralgia patients?

are that the true HR lies between HR_L and HR_U, i.e.,

H0: $HR \leq 0.8$ or $HR \geq 1.25$;
H1: $0.8 < HR < 1.25$.

The 95 % CI for the HR would need to fall completely within the interval $[HR_L; HR_U]$ to prove equivalence. The 95 % CI for the HR in our example (◻Table 5.8) is equal to [0.86; 1.7]. The lower bound of the 95 % CI is larger than HR_L, but the null hypothesis cannot be rejected, since the upper bound is not smaller than HR_U.

5.3   In Case of a Categorical Determinant

The association between a time to event outcome variable and a categorical determinant is also tested with a log-rank test and with the Cox regression model. We illustrate both with the following research question

? Is there a difference in time to development of RA between seropositive arthralgia patients with different antibody status at baseline?

The null and alternative hypothesis for this research question are

H0: there is no difference in the time to development of RA between patients with different antibody status at baseline;
H1: there is a difference in the time to development of RA between at least two groups of patients with different antibody status at baseline.

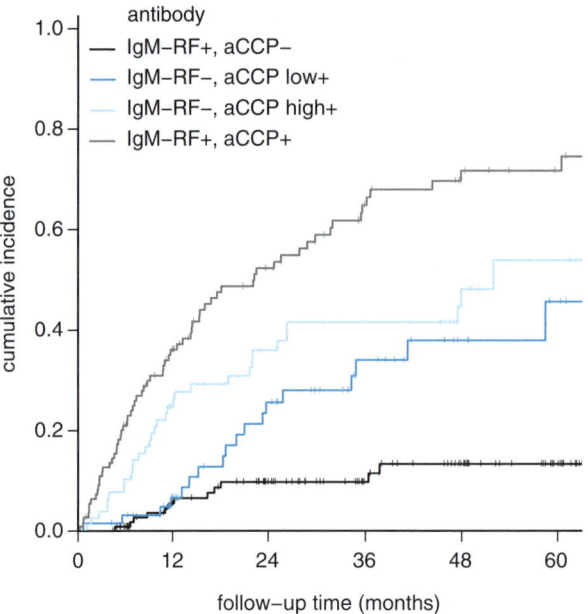

◻ Fig. 5.6   One minus Kaplan-Meier curve for the time to development of RA, for patients with different antibody status at baseline

Similar to the association between a continuous outcome variable and a categorical determinant (with more than two groups), the alternative hypothesis only states a difference in time to development of RA between at least two groups, not between all groups.

5.3.1 Descriptive Statistics

The Kaplan-Meier curves for each group provides a good visualization of the (potential) differences in time to development of RA between patients with different antibody status at baseline. ◻Figure 5.6 shows the one minus Kaplan-Meier curves for each of the four groups. Patients who are rheumatoid factor type immunoglobulin M (IgM-RF) positive but anticyclic citrullinated peptide (aCPP) negative have the lowest risk to develop RA: their median time to develop RA could not be estimated (◻Table 5.9), and the 5-year cumulative incidence of development of RA is equal to 13 % (95 % CI [5.8 %; 21 %]; ◻Table 5.10). Patients who are positive for both IgM-RF and aCPP have the highest risk to develop RA: their estimated median time to develop RA is 22.3 months and 5-year cumulative incidence of 72 % (95 % CI [62 %; 82 %]). The 95 % CIs are computed with ▶Eq. E5.3 (▶Sect. 5.2.1).

▪ **Table 5.9** SPSS output of the estimated mean and median time to development of RA, separately for patients with different antibody status at baseline, and for all patients together

Means and Medians for Survival Time

Antibody	Mean[a]					Median			
	Estimate	Std. Error	95 % Confidence Interval			Estimate	Std. Error	95 % Confidence Interval	
			Lower Bound	Upper Bound				Lower Bound	Upper Bound
IgM-RF +, aCCP −	66.462	1.999	62.543	70.381		.	.	.	.
IgM-RF −, aCCP low +	52.227	3.893	44.597	59.858		72.444	.000	.	.
IgM-RF −, aCCP high +	50.030	4.583	41.046	59.014		51.844	5.472	41.119	62.568
IgM-RF +, aCCP +	32.758	3.169	26.547	38.969		22.275	5.229	12.027	32.524
Overall	53.516	2.141	49.319	57.713		72.444	9.210	54.392	90.496

[a]Estimation is limited to the largest survival time if it is censored

◻ **Table 5.10**   Part of the SPSS output of the survival table, separately for patients with different antibody status at baseline

Survival Table

Antibody	Time		Status	Cumulative Proportion Surviving at the Time		N of Cumulative Events	N of Remaining Cases
				Estimate	Std. Error		
IgM-RF +, aCCP −	1	4.370	No arthritis	.	.	0	119
	21	11.499	Arthritis	.945	.022	6	99
	28	12.189	Arthritis	.935	.024	7	92
	36	18.070	Arthritis	.903	.029	10	84
	70	36.370	Arthritis	.885	.034	11	50
	74	37.749	Arthritis	.867	.038	12	46
	120	73.823	No arthritis	.	.	12	0
IgM-RF −, aCCP low +	1	.624	Arthritis	.985	.015	1	64
	13	11.729	Arthritis	.934	.032	4	52
	21	13.109	Arthritis	.914	.037	5	44
	30	23.688	Arthritis	.744	.062	13	35
	35	25.758	Arthritis	.720	.064	14	30
	58	58.382	Arthritis	.544	.099	18	7
	65	72.444	Arthritis	.000	.000	19	0
IgM-RF −, aCCP high +	1	1.051	Arthritis	.987	.013	1	77
	22	11.236	Arthritis	.752	.049	19	56
	27	12.025	Arthritis	.738	.050	20	51
	40	22.012	Arthritis	.641	.057	26	38
	45	25.068	Arthritis	.622	.059	27	33
	78	84.205	Arthritis	.000	.000	33	0
IgM-RF +, aCCP +	1	.230	Arthritis	.991	.009	1	110
	50	11.729	Arthritis	.640	.047	38	61
	54	12.550	Arthritis	.629	.048	39	57
	71	22.538	Arthritis	.477	.051	52	40
	74	24.706	Arthritis	.465	.052	53	37
	97	47.836	Arthritis	.283	.052	65	14
	102	60.386	Arthritis	.255	.054	66	9
	111	79.310	No arthritis	.	.	67	0

◻ **Table 5.11** SPSS output of the log-rank test, comparing the time to development of RA between patients with different antibody status at baseline

Overall Comparisons			
	Chi-Square	df	Sig.
Log Rank (Mantel-Cox)	72.189	3	.000

Test of equality of survival distributions for the different levels of antibody

5.3.2 Log-Rank Test

The log-rank test is also used to compare the survival functions of more than two groups. The only difference with the log-rank test for comparing two groups, is the number of degrees of freedom, which is equal to 3 in this case. Similar to the chi-square test for a dichotomous outcome variable, the degrees of freedom is equal to $k - 1$ when k groups are compared. ◻Table 5.11 shows the SPSS output of the log-rank test, from which we conclude that there is an overall difference in time to the development of RA between patients with different antibody status at baseline ($p < 0.001$).

The post hoc analysis, to investigate which groups differ from each other, could be done in SPSS manually, or as an additional option in the log-rank test (Supplementary Information A.6.1.). ◻Table 5.12 shows the post hoc analyses for the log-rank test with a categorical determinant. For each pairwise comparison, the value of the test-statistic is reported under "Chi-Square" and the corresponding p-value under "Sig.". For instance, the test statistic of the pairwise comparison between patients who are IgM-RF positive but aCCP negative and patients who are IgM-RF negative but aCCP low positive is equal to 11.058, and the corresponding p-value to 0.001. However, the p-values in this table are not corrected for multiple testing with, for example, the Bonferroni correction. To apply the Bonferroni correction manually, each p-value needs to be multiplied by 6 (the total number of comparisons) in our example. When doing so, we find that the time to development of RA differs between all groups, except between the patients who are IgM-RF negative but aCCP low positive at baseline and patients who are IgM-RF negative but aCCP low positive at baseline ($p = 1.0$ after Bonferroni correction). A p-value can never be exactly equal to zero, but also not larger than one, so if the multiplication results in a p-value above one, this needs to be reported as $p = 1.0$.

5.3.3 Cox Regression Model

Effect sizes, to quantify the differences in the time to development of RA between the different groups are again obtained with a Cox regression model. As in the linear and logistic regression model, dummy variables need to be created for the different groups. This is done automatically in SPSS with the 'Categorical' button in the Cox regression

☐ **Table 5.12** SPSS output of the pairwise comparisons in the post hoc analysis, comparing time to development of RA between patients with different antibody status at baseline

Pairwise Comparisons

	Antibody	IgM-RF +, aCCP −		IgM-RF −, aCCP low +		IgM-RF −, aCCP high +		IgM-RF +, aCCP +	
		Chi-Square	Sig.	Chi-Square	Sig.	Chi-Square	Sig.	Chi-Square	Sig.
Log Rank (Mantel-Cox)	IgM-RF +, aCCP −			11.058	.001	26.179	.000	68.547	.000
	IgM-RF −, aCCP low +	11.058	.001			1.780	.182	16.239	.000
	IgM-RF −, aCCP high +	26.179	.000	1.780	.182			8.112	.004
	IgM-RF +, aCCP +	68.547	.000	16.239	.000	8.112	.004		

> **Table 5.13** SPSS dummy variable coding table for the Cox regression model, comparing the time to development of RA between patients with different antibody status at baseline

Categorical Variable Codings[a]

		Frequency	(1)	(2)	(3)
Antibody[b]	1 = IgM-RF +, aCCP −	120	0	0	0
	2 = IgM-RF −, aCCP low +	65	1	0	0
	3 = IgM-RF −, aCCP high +	78	0	1	0
	4 = IgM-RF +, aCCP +	111	0	0	1

[a]Category variable: antibody
[b]Indicator Parameter Coding

query (Supplementary Information A.6.2). One group is set as the reference group, for which all dummy variables are equal to zero. For all other groups, exactly one dummy variable is equal to one for that group and zero for the other groups. For this example, we set antibody status 'IgM-RF positive but aCCP negative' as the reference group. ▢Table 5.13 shows the dummy coding for the different dummy variables.

With these dummy variables, the Cox regression model is equal to

$$\ln(h(t)) = \ln(h_0(t)) + b_1 \times d_1 + b_2 \times d_2 + b_3 \times d_3. \qquad \text{(M5.6)}$$

Here $h_0(t)$ is the hazard function for the reference group. Then it follows that
- the natural logarithm of the hazard function of group 2 (IgM-RF negative but aCCP low positive) is equal to

$$\ln(h_0(t)) + b_1 \times 1 + b_2 \times 0 + b_3 \times 0 = \ln(h_0(t)) + b_1;$$

- the natural logarithm of the hazard function of group 3 (IgM-RF negative but aCCP high positive) is equal to

$$\ln(h_0(t)) + b_1 \times 0 + b_2 \times 1 + b_3 \times 0 = \ln(h_0(t)) + b_2; \text{ and}$$

- the natural logarithm of the hazard function of group 3 (IgM-RF positive and aCCP positive) is equal to

$$\ln(h_0(t)) + b_1 \times 0 + b_2 \times 0 + b_3 \times 1 = \ln(h_0(t)) + b_3.$$

In other words, the HR of group 2 compared to group 1 is equal to $\exp(b_1)$, the HR of group 3 compared to group 1 is equal to $\exp(b_2)$, and the HR of group 4 compared to group 1 is equal to $\exp(b_3)$. ▢Table 5.14 shows the SPSS output of the Cox regression model. The HR for the time to development of RA for patients who are IgM-RF positive but aCCP negative compared to patients who are IgM-RF negative but aCCP low positive' (the reference group) is 3.2 (95 % CI [1.6; 6.6]). The HR for patients who are

Table 5.14 SPSS output of the Cox regression model, comparing time to development of RA between patients with different antibody status at baseline

Variables in the Equation									
	B	SE	Wald	df	Sig.	Exp(B)	95.0 % CI for Exp(B)		
								Lower	Upper
antibody			55.907	3	.000				
antibody(1)	1.169	.369	10.042	1	.002	3.220		1.562	6.636
antibody(2)	1.555	.339	21.047	1	.000	4.735		2.437	9.201
antibody(3)	2.182	.314	48.250	1	.000	8.865		4.789	16.409

IgM-RF negative but aCCP high positive compared to the reference group is 4.7 (95 % CI [2.4; 9.2]). And the HR for patients who are IgM-RF positive and aCCP positive compared to the reference group is 8.9 (95 % CI [4.8; 16.4]).

5.3.4　Assumptions of the Cox Regression Model

Before we finalize our conclusion with respect to the time to development of RA of groups 2 to 4 compared to group 1, we need the check the proportionality assumption of the Cox regression model. From the log-log plot (■Fig. 5.7a), it seems that the curves are not really proportional: for larger values of $\ln(t)$, the curves are closer to each other than for smaller values of $\ln(t)$. Also from the Schoenfeld residuals (■Fig. 5.7b) it seems that proportionality is not valid: for antibody dummy 3 (i.e., patients who are positive for both IgM-RF and aCCP) the Schoenfeld residuals tend to increase over time, while for antibody dummies 1 and 2, the Schoenfeld residuals tend to decrease over time. Note that for each dummy variable the Schoenfeld residuals are computed separately, comparing the time to development of RA of patients in that dummy-group to all other groups together. ■Table 5.15 shows the SPSS output of the three linear regression models testing whether the Schoenfeld residuals depend on time or not. From this table, we conclude that the proportionality assumption does not hold: the slope of the regression model for the partial residual of antibody(1) is significant ($p=0.012$). Therefore, we need to include a time-dependent covariate in the Cox regression model.

From the Kaplan-Meier curves in ■Fig. 5.6 it is difficult to select a cut-off time point T, but after 10 months the curves seem to become further apart from each other than before. Therefore, a cut-off time point T at 10 months is chosen. The Cox regression model with a time-dependent covariate is

$$\ln(h(t)) = \ln(h_0(t)) + b_1(t) \times d_1 + b_2(t) \times d_2 + b_3(t) \times d_3, \text{with} \qquad \text{(M5.7)}$$
$$b_1(t) = c_{1,0} + c_{1,1} \times d_T(t), b_2(t) = c_{2,0} + c_{2,1} \times d_T(t), \text{and}$$
$$b_3(t) = c_{3,0} + c_{3,1} \times d_T(t),$$

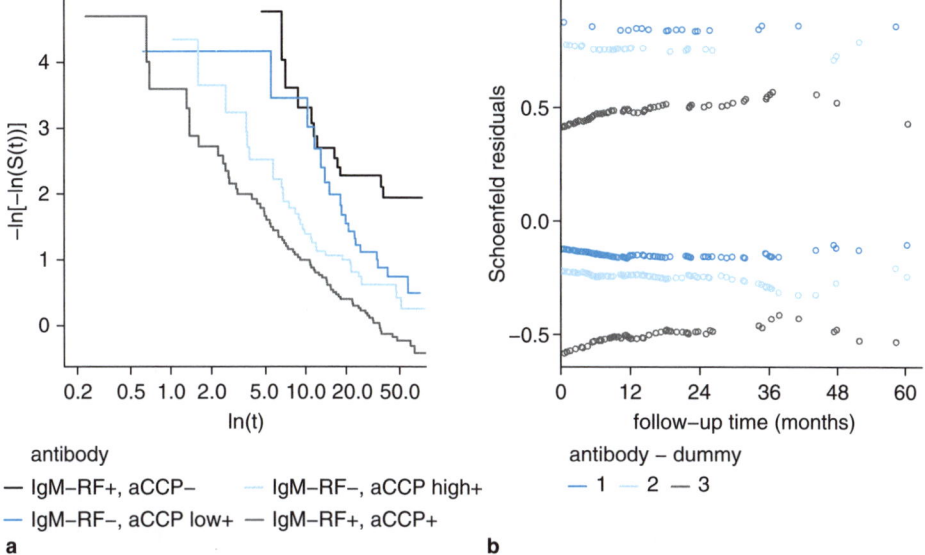

○ **Fig. 5.7** Log-plot of the Kaplan-Meier curve (**a**) and scatterplot of the Schoenfeld residuals against time (**b**), to assess the proportionality assumption

○ **Table 5.15** Combined SPSS output of three linear regression models, testing the proportionality assumption in a categorical determinant

Coefficients

Model		Unstandardized Coefficients		Standardized Coefficients	t	Sig.
		B	Std. Error	Beta		
1[a]	(Constant)	−.082	.044		−1.860	.065
	follow-up time (months)	.005	.002	.219	2.545	.012
1[b]	(Constant)	.043	.055		.774	.441
	follow-up time (months)	−.003	.002	−.093	−1.058	.292
1[c]	(Constant)	.028	.063		.440	.661
	follow-up time (months)	−.002	.003	−.053	−.602	.548

[a]Dependent Variable: Partial residual for antibody(1)
[b]Dependent Variable: Partial residual for antibody(2)
[c]Dependent Variable: Partial residual for antibody(3)

where d_T is zero for all $t \leq 10$, and one for all $t > 10$. ○Table 5.16 shows the SPSS output of
▶ Model M5.7. Since we have three dummy variables, three null and alternative hypotheses are tested

Table 5.16   SPSS output of the Cox regression model with time-dependent covariate to test the proportionality assumption, d_T is zero for $t \leq 10$

Variables in the Equation

	B	SE	Wald	df	Sig.	Exp(B)	95.0 % CI for Exp(B) Lower	Upper
antibody			29.409	3	.000			
antibody(1)	−.084	.866	.009	1	.923	.920	.168	5.022
antibody(2)	1.927	.556	12.019	1	.001	6.867	2.310	20.407
antibody(3)	2.377	.530	20.141	1	.000	10.771	3.814	30.412
antibody*T_COV_			7.830	3	.050			
antibody(1)*T_COV_	1.612	.967	2.783	1	.095	5.014	.754	33.337
antibody(2)*T_COV_	−.665	.708	.883	1	.347	.514	.128	2.059
antibody(3)*T_COV_	−.330	.660	.249	1	.617	.719	.197	2.621

H0: $c_{1,1} = 0$ versus H1: $c_{1,1} \neq 0$,
H0: $c_{2,1} = 0$ versus H1: $c_{2,1} \neq 0$, and
H0: $c_{3,1} = 0$ versus H1: $c_{3,1} \neq 0$.

However, there is also an overall p-value reported in the row "antibody*T_COV", corresponding to the null hypothesis

H0: the proportionality assumption is valid;
H1: the proportionality assumption is not valid.

This overall p-value is equal to 0.050. To check if this p-value is smaller than the significance level α of 0.05, we need to check the decimals, by double clicking on the output table and then double clicking on the cell with the p-value. It turns out that $p = 0.0497$, which is indeed smaller than α, hence the null hypothesis is rejected. In other words, the proportionality assumption does not hold, and we need to report HRs for the time to development of RA within the first 10 months, and after 10 months separately. Note that the significance level α of 0.05 is arbitrarily chosen. So although a significant result is found, it does not mean this result is also clinically relevant.

By the choice of d_T, the HRs (with corresponding 95 % CIs) for the first 10 months are obtained from ◻Table 5.16. For example, the HR for the time to develop RA between patients who are IgM-RF positive but aCCP negative and patients who are IgM-RF negative but aCCP low positive after 10 months is equal to 4.6 (i.e., $\exp(−0.084 + 1.612) = \exp(1.528)$). To obtain the 95 % CIs of the HRs after 10 months follow-up, we recoded d_T to be equal to zero for all $t \geq 10$ and one for all $t < 10$. ◻Table 5.17 shows the SPSS output of that Cox regression model.

Table 5.17 SPSS output of the Cox regression model with time-dependent covariate to test the proportionality assumption, d_T is zero for $t > 10$

Variables in the Equation

	B	SE	Wald	df	Sig.	Exp(B)	95.0 % CI for Exp(B)	
							Lower	Upper
antibody			28.777	3	.000			
antibody(1)	1.529	.429	12.689	1	.000	4.613	1.989	10.697
antibody(2)	1.261	.439	8.269	1	.004	3.531	1.494	8.341
antibody(3)	2.047	.394	27.048	1	.000	7.746	3.581	16.755
antibody*T_COV_			7.830	3	.050			
antibody(1)*T_COV_	−1.612	.967	2.783	1	.095	.199	.030	1.326
antibody(2)*T_COV_	.665	.708	.883	1	.347	1.945	.486	7.790
antibody(3)*T_COV_	.330	.660	.249	1	.617	1.390	.381	5.068

Table 5.18 Summary of the analyses comparing time to development of RA between patients with different antibody status at baseline

	5-yr cum. inc. [95 % CI]	HR [95 % CI]		p-value
		Up to 10 months	After 10 months	
Antibody status				< 0.001
IgM-RF +, aCCP −	13 % [5.8 %; 21 %]	1	1	
IgM-RF −, aCCP low +	46 % [26 %; 65 %]	0.92 [0.17; 5.0]	4.6 [2.0; 10.7]	
IgM-RF −, aCCP high +	54 % [38 %; 70 %]	6.9 [2.3; 20.4]	3.5 [1.5; 8.3]	
IgM-RF +, aCCP +	72 % [62 %; 82 %]	10.8 [3.8; 30.4]	7.7 [3.6; 16.8]	

Cum. inc. cumulative incidence, *HR* hazard ratio, *yr* years

Our final conclusion with respect to the research question is that there is a significant difference in time to development of RA between patients with different antibody status at baseline ($p < 0.001$). Table 5.18 shows an example of how the results of these analyses could be reported in a scientific paper. The results of the post hoc analysis are generally only reported in the text of the manuscript, not in a table.

5.4   In Case of a Continuous Determinant

The only way to investigate the association between a time to event outcome variable and a continuous determinant is with a Cox regression model. We illustrate this with the following research question

❓ Is the time to development of RA associated with the visual analogue scale (VAS) pain score at baseline?

The null and alternative hypothesis corresponding to this research question are

H0: there is no association between time to development of RA and the VAS pain score at baseline;

H1: there is an association between time to development of RA and the VAS pain score at baseline.

In the RA-cohort, VAS pain was only recorded as a dichotomous variable: below or above 50. For illustrative purposes, we simulated for each patient the original VAS pain score ('VAS_pain') in such a way that the simulated score matched with the official recorded dichotomous VAS pain score.

5.4.1 Cox Regression Model

The Cox regression model to investigate this research question is as follows

$$\ln(h_{\text{VAS\_pain}}(t)) = \ln(h_0(t)) + b_1 \times \text{VAS\_pain}. \tag{M5.8}$$

The baseline hazard function $h_0(t)$ is now the hazard function for a patient with a VAS pain score of zero at baseline. The effect size, the HR per increase of one point in VAS pain score at baseline, is equal to $\exp(b_1)$. After all, for two patients who differ in a VAS pain score at baseline by one point, for example with VAS pain scores of 30 and 31 at baseline,

$$b_1 = \ln(h_{31}(t)) - \ln(h_{30}(t)) = \ln(h_{31}(t)/h_3(t)) = \ln(\text{HR}).$$

In our research question, a VAS pain score of zero is clinically meaningful, but this is not always the case. If, for example, age would have been the continuous determinant, the baseline hazard function $h_0(t)$ would be the hazard function of patients with an age of zero. This is only clinically meaningful for newborns, but not for the research question we are investigating. In case of a non-meaningful baseline hazard function, centralizing the determinant can yield a clinical meaningful baseline hazard function (▶ Sect. 3.1).

The null and alternative hypothesis, in terms of the regression coefficient b_1, of our research question are

H0: $b_1 = 0$;
H1: $b_0 \neq 0$;

⬛ **Table 5.19** SPSS output of the Cox regression model, relating time to development of RA to the VAS pain score at baseline

Variables in the Equation

	B	SE	Wald	df	Sig.	Exp(B)	95.0 % CI for Exp(B)	
							Lower	Upper
VAS	.025	.004	31.127	1	.000	1.025	1.016	1.034

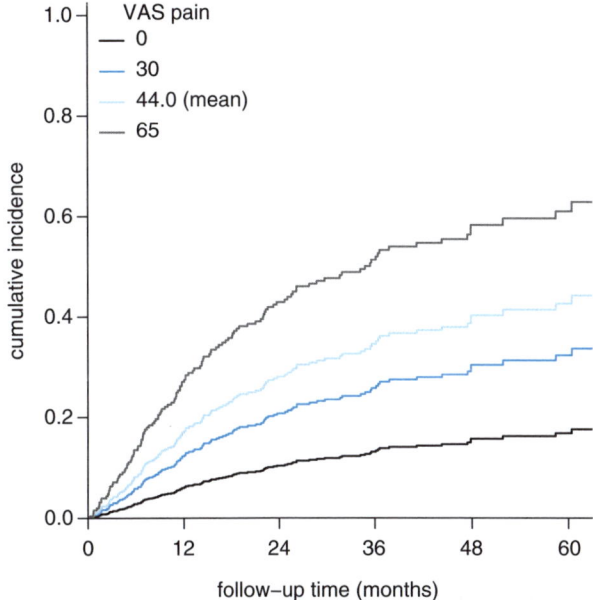

⬛ **Fig. 5.8** Estimated cumulative incidence of the development of RA, for patients with different VAS pain scores at baseline

⬛Table 5.19 shows the SPSS output of the Cox regression model for ▶model (M5.8). The output is equal to the output of a Cox regression model with a dichotomous determinant, however, the value under "Exp(B)" is the HR per 1 point increase in the VAS pain score at baseline. To obtain the HR per increase of 5 or 10 points in the VAS pain score at baseline, the HR per 1 point is taken to the power 5 or 10, as we did for a dichotomous outcome variable (▶Example 4.2, ▶Sect. 4.4.1). From ⬛Table 5.19 we conclude that the time to development of RA is associated with the VAS pain score at baseline: patients with a higher VAS pain score tend to develop RA faster than patients with a lower VAS pain score (HR 1.025 per 1 point in VAS pain, 95 % CI [1.016; 1.034], $p < 0.001$). From the estimated baseline hazard function $h_0(t)$ we could also estimate the cumulative incidence for patients with different a VAS pain scores at baseline, for example for patients with a VAS pain score of zero (i.e., the 'baseline' cumulative incidence), 30, 44 (mean VAS pain score) or 65 at baseline (⬛Fig. 5.8). Indeed, patients with a higher VAS pain

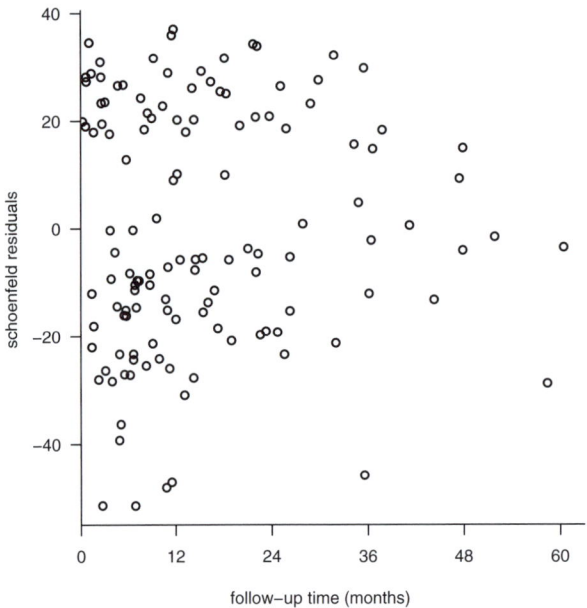

Fig. 5.9   Scatterplot the Schoenfeld residuals against time, to assess proportionality

score at baseline have a higher chance to develop RA more quickly than patients with a low VAS pain score at baseline. Patients with a VAS pain score of zero at baseline have approximately 18 % chance to develop RA within 5 years, while patients with a VAS pain score of 65 at baseline have approximately 65 % chance to develop RA within 5 years.

5.4.2 Assumptions of the Cox Regression Model

The Cox regression model with a continuous determinant also assumes that the hazard functions, corresponding to two different VAS pain scores at baseline, are proportional. This assumption is again checked with the Schoenfeld residuals (▶ Sect. 5.2.4), which can be tested with a linear regression model (▣ Fig. 5.9 and ▣ Table 5.20). The slope of the regression line does not differ significantly from zero ($p = 0.58$), so the proportionality assumption seems valid.

However, as within a linear and a logistic regression model with a continuous determinant, the Cox regression model also assumes a linear relation between the outcome of the model, i.e., $\ln(h(t))$, and the continuous determinant. That is, the $\ln(HR)$ increases or decreases linearly as the VAS pain score at baseline increases constantly. In other words, the HR between two patients, one with a VAS pain score of 30 and one of 31 at baseline, is equal to the HR between two patients, one with a VAS score of 50 and one with a VAS score of 51 at baseline. This assumption is investigated with the Martingale residuals. The Martingale residuals are derived from the estimated cumulative hazard at the follow-up

◻ **Table 5.20**   SPSS output of the linear regression model, testing the proportionality assumption

Coefficients[a]

Model		Unstandardized Coefficients		Standardized Coefficients	t	Sig.
		B	Std. Error	Beta		
1	(Constant)	−1.173	2.869		−.409	.683
	follow-up time (months)	.070	.125	.049	.559	.577

[a]Dependent Variable: Partial residual for VAS

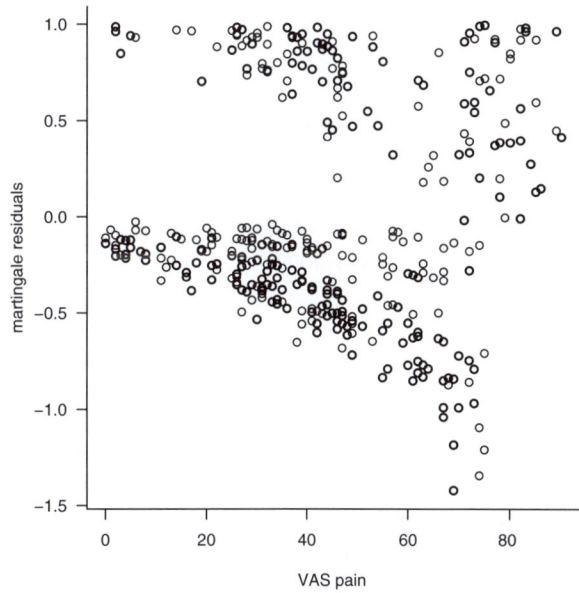

◻ **Fig. 5.10**   Scatterplot of the Martingale residuals against the VAS pain score at baseline, to investigate linearity of the association

time of each patient. The estimated cumulative hazard can be saved as a new variable in the Cox regression query (Supplementary Information A.6.2). Then, the Martingale residual of a patient is equal to his/her status (0 for no event, 1 for an event) minus his/her estimated cumulative hazard (▶ Example 5.3). Linearity is then checked with a scatterplot where these residuals are plotted on the *y*-axis and the continuous determinant on the *x*-axis (◻ Fig. 5.10). If there is no association between the Martingale residuals and the determinant, linearity is valid. In our case, the Martingale residuals tend to decrease as the VAS pain score at baseline increases, indicating the linearity assumption might not be valid.

◻ **Table 5.21**   SPSS output of the Cox regression model relating time to development of RA to VAS pain score at baseline in quartiles (NVAS)

Variables in the Equation

	B	SE	Wald	df	Sig.	Exp(B)	95.0 % CI for Exp(B)	
							Lower	Upper
NVAS			26.103	3	.000			
NVAS(1)	.317	.293	1.166	1	.280	1.373	.772	2.440
NVAS(2)	.373	.285	1.716	1	.190	1.452	.831	2.538
NVAS(3)	1.132	.258	19.241	1	.000	3.103	1.871	5.146

Example 5.3

Calculation of the Martingale residual
Patient A developed RA after 10.4 months follow-up, with an estimated cumulative hazard at 10.4 months of 0.344. Because this patient developed RA, the status is equal to 1 and the Martingale residual to $1 - 0.344 = 0.656$.
Patient B did not develop RA within 61.3 months, with an estimated cumulative hazard at 61.3 months of 0.330. Because this patient did not develop RA, the status is equal to 0 and the Martingale residual to $0 - 0.330 = -0.330$.

Besides checking the Martingale residuals, linearity could also be investigated similarly as in the linear and logistic regression model. The first option is to add a quadratic/cubic/etc. term to the Cox regression model and test whether the regression coefficients are unequal to zero or not. The other option is to divide the VAS pain score at baseline in quartiles and check the differences in regression coefficients between two consecutive groups. The latter option is advised, for the same reasons as in a linear regression model (▸Sect. 3.4.4). ◻Table 5.21 shows the SPSS output of the Cox regression model, where VAS pain score at baseline in quartiles is included as categorical determinant. ◻Table 5.22 shows the categorical dummy coding created by SPSS. The consecutive differences between all groups are all positive ($0.317 - 0 = 0.317$; $0.373 - 0.317 = 0.056$, and $1.132 - 0.373 = 0.759$), indicating that the association could be linear, although the difference between the second and third group differs from the difference between the first and second, and the third and fourth group. This could be due to the fact that the VAS pain score at baseline was divided into four groups of approximately the same size, not of approximately the same width. Therefore, we plot the regression coefficients again at the mid-point of the groups (◻Fig. 5.11).

Based on ◻Fig. 5.11, it seems that the difference between the second and third group is lower than expected under the linearity assumption. Hence, we conclude that the linearity assumption is not valid and therefore divide VAS pain score at baseline in clinical meaningful categories: below 30 (set as reference group), between 30 and 49 (dummy 1),

Table 5.22 SPSS categorical variable coding table, indicating the dummies of a categorical variable in the Cox regression model

Categorical Variable Codings[a]

		Frequency	(1)	(2)	(3)
NVAS[b]	1	95	0	0	0
	2	90	1	0	0
	3	95	0	1	0
	4	94	0	0	1

[a]Category variable: NVAS (Percentile Group of VAS)
[b]Indicator Parameter Coding

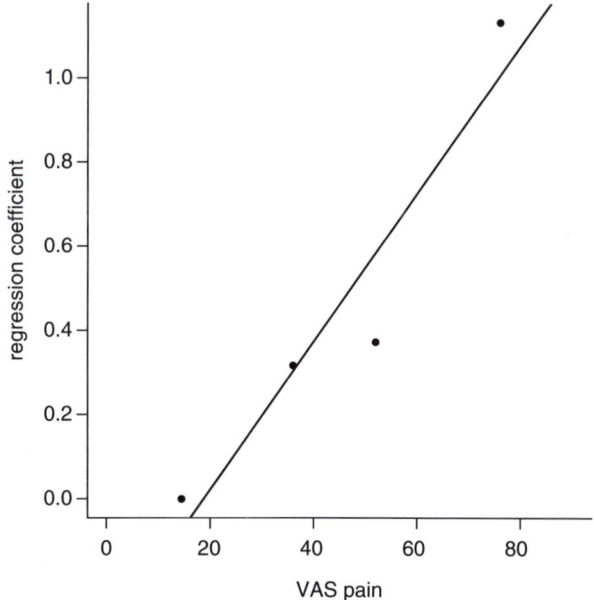

Fig. 5.11 Scatterplot of the midpoints of the four VAS groups and the corresponding regression coefficients in that group

or 50 and above (dummy 2). **Table 5.23** shows the SPSS output of the Cox regression model with this new categorical determinant included. The conclusion with regard to the research question is that the time to development of RA is associated with the VAS pain score at baseline ($p=0.001$): patients with a VAS pain score of 50 or above have a higher risk to develop RA faster than those with a VAS pain score below 30 (HR 2.5, 95 % CI [1.5; 4.0]).

□ Table 5.23   SPSS output of a Cox regression model, relating time to development of RA to the VAS pain score at baseline in three meaningful groups (VAS3)

Variables in the Equation

	B	SE	Wald	df	Sig.	Exp(B)	95.0 % CI for Exp(B)	
							Lower	Upper
VAS3			14.391	2	.001			
VAS3(1)	.423	.260	2.644	1	.104	1.526	.917	2.541
VAS3(2)	.903	.254	12.595	1	.000	2.467	1.498	4.062

□ Table 5.24   Summary of the statistical test with the corresponding effect sizes and assumptions, to investigate associations with a time to event outcome variable

		Non-parametric	Regression model
Dichotomous determinant	Statistical test	Log-rank test	Cox regression model
	Effect size	Kaplan-Meier curve/cumulative incidence	HR
	Assumptions	None	Proportionality
Categorical determinant	Statistical test	Log-rank test	Cox regression model
	Effect size	Kaplan-Meier curve/cumulative incidence	HR (one group set as reference)
	Assumptions	None	Proportionality
Continuous determinant	Statistical model		Cox regression model
	Effect size		Exponential of regression coefficient (HR; per increase of 1 unit)
	Assumptions		Proportionality
			Linearity

5.5   Summary of Analyses

In □Table 5.24 the effect sizes and assumptions for all statistical tests described in this chapter are summarized.

5.6   Further Readings

The standard textbooks on medical statistics and epidemiology all provide more information on the analyses of time to event outcome variables [2–5]. Clark and Bradburn co-authored a (short) tutorial on survival analysis in the British Journal of Cancer: parts I and III can be read for more information on the analyses described in this chapter [6, 7].

Kleinbaum & Klein wrote an illustrative book on survival analyses [8]. Another applied introduction on survival analyses in medical research is written by Collet [9].

The analyses described in this chapter, assume that the time to event is either observed, or right censored. This means that the event of interest is only known to be larger than the follow-up time. There are other types of censoring, for example left truncation or interval censoring. More information on these types of censoring, and how to deal with them, can be found in the textbooks written by Kleinbaum & Klein and by Collet [8, 9]. Furthermore, the analyses described in this chapter also assume that the censoring is non-informative. That is, for example, lost to follow-up of a patient is unrelated to the study [10]. Sometimes the event of interest is censored by the occurrence of another important event. In bone marrow transplanted patients, relapse of leukemia is, for example, censored because the patient died before relapse. When a multiple of such events are of interest, but occurrence of one event prevents occurrence of the other events, we find ourselves in the area of competing risks. It is important to account for these competing risks, otherwise the cumulative incidence or survival function is under- or overestimated. Putter et al. wrote a clear, not too technical tutorial on how to analyze the time to event with competing risks [11]. Competing risks cannot be analyzed in SPSS, instead R or Stata needs to be used.

Note that the Kaplan-Meier curve or the cumulative incidence at one or more times are the most common descriptive statistics for a time to event outcome variable, sometimes the incidence rate is reported. We introduced the incidence rate in ▶Chap. 2 (▶Sect. 2.2.3) and did not discuss it further in this chapter. For more information on comparing incidence rates, we refer to the book written by Kirkwood & Sterne [5].

References

1. van de Stadt LA, Witte BI, Bos WH, van Schaardenburg D. A prediction rule for the development of arthritis in seropositive arthralgia patients. Ann Rheum Dis. 2013;72(12):1920–6. ▶https://doi.org/10.1136/annrheumdis-2012-202127.
2. Altman DG. Practical statistics for medical research. London: Chapman & Hall; 1991.
3. Rothman KJ, Lash TL, Greenland S. Modern epidemiology. 3rd ed. Philadelphia: Lippincott-Raven; 2012.
4. Armitage P, Berry G, Matthews JNS. Statistical methods in medical research. Oxford: Blackwell Science Ltd; 2002.
5. Kirkwood BR, Sterne JAC. Essential medical statistics. 2nd ed. Oxford: Blackwell Science Ltd; 2003.
6. Clark TG, Bradburn MJ, Love SB, Altman DG. Survival analysis part I: basic concepts and first analyses. Br J Cancer. 2003;89(2):232–8. ▶https://doi.org/10.1038/sj.bjc.6601118.
7. Bradburn MJ, Clark TG, Love SB, Altman DG. Survival analysis part III: multivariate data analysis – choosing a model and assessing its adequacy and fit. Br J Cancer. 2003;89(4):506–11. ▶https://doi.org/10.1038/sj.bjc.6601120.
8. Kleinbaum DG, Klein M. Survival analysis. New York: Springer; 2012.
9. Collet D. Modelling survival data in medical research. London: Chapman & Hall/CRC; 2004.
10. Clark TG, Bradburn MJ, Love SB, Altman DG. Survival analysis part IV: further concepts and methods in survival analysis. Br J Cancer. 2003;89(5):781–6. ▶https://doi.org/10.1038/sj.bjc.6601117.
11. Putter H, Fiocco M, Geskus RB. Tutorial in biostatistics: competing risks and multi-state models. Stat in Med. 2007;26:2389–430. ▶https://doi.org/10.1002/sim.

Variables Influencing the Association

Abstract

The overall aim of investigating an association, is to assess the true effect of one central determinant on the outcome variable. However, the association is always influenced by other influencing variables, such that the true effect of the determinant might be different. These potential influencing variables must be corrected for. In this chapter, we quantify the influence of other variables, measured in the study, on the association between the outcome variable and the determinant. We explain and discuss three types of influencing effects: confounding, effect modification, and mediation. We also explain how the joint influence of multiple determinants on the outcome variable is assessed in multiple regression models.

6.1 Confounding

A variable is considered a confounder when part of the association between the outcome variable and the central determinant is explained by this third variable. We specifically state the central determinant, as that is the variable of interest. A confounder is also called an independent variable or a determinant. So to prevent misunderstanding, we use the terms central determinant, outcome variable and confounder(s).

If the association is not corrected for, the effect could be biased and the true effect under- or overestimated. Assume, for example, we investigate the difference in cholesterol levels between males and females, but unfortunately the males in the study population are younger than the females. It is known that cholesterol levels change with increasing age, so the question is whether the difference in cholesterol levels we would find is indeed the 'true' difference between males and females, or if it is partly explained by differences in age. This would not be an issue, if males and females were of the same age, or if cholesterol is not associated with age. Therefore, from a theoretical point of view, a confounder can only be considered a potential confounder if it is associated with the determinant, and if it influences the outcome variable. ■Figure 6.1 visualizes the concept of confounding, in which the confounder influences the central determinant (and vice versa) as well as the outcome variable.

The association of the potential confounder with the central determinant, as well as with the outcome variable, is tested as explained in ▶Chaps. 3–5. To assess the influence of the potential confounder on the association between the central determinant and the outcome variable, the original (or crude) effect is compared with the effect after correcting for the potential confounder. The potential confounder is considered to be a true confounder, if the effect changes by 10 % or more. The 10 % in this rule of thumb is arbitrarily chosen, just as the significance level α of 0.05. Therefore, it is important to keep in mind that a change of 9 % in the effect might be clinically very relevant, but a change of 15 % might not be.

In clinical practice, the associations between the potential confounder on the one side and the outcome variable and central determinant on the other side, are rarely tested. The disadvantage of this theoretical approach is that many variables are ignored as potential confounders, although they could influence the estimated effect. There is no consensus approach on how to check and correct for confounding. It is of most importance to always report the method used to correct for confounding. We discuss checking for confounding by stratification, as well as with regression models, only by considering a change of 10 % in the effect to define confounding.

6.1.1 Confounding Through Stratification

To gain more insight in the concept of confounding, we investigate the difference between males and females in the chance to reach a low disease activity score of 44 joints (DAS44; yes/no) after 52 weeks of treatment in the COmbinatie Behandeling Reumatoïde Artritis (COBRA)-light trial [1]. A low DAS44 is defined as a DAS44 score below 1.6. The research question is as follows

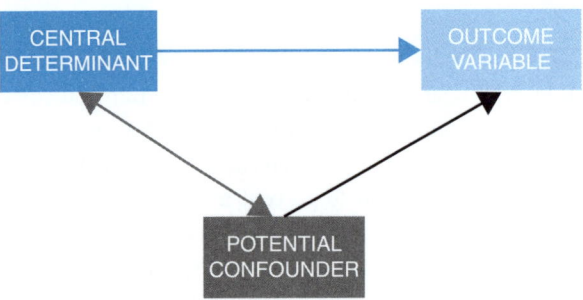

◻ **Fig. 6.1**   Visualization of the concept of confounding

◻ **Table 6.1**   Crosstab for the association between low DAS44 after 52 weeks of treatment and gender

	DAS44 after 52 weeks		Total
	≥1.6	<1.6	
Female	67	37	104
Male	18	32	50
Total	85	69	154

❓ Is there a difference in the risk to reach a low DAS44 after 52 weeks of treatment between males and females?

The corresponding null and alternative hypothesis for this research question are

H0: there is no difference in risk to reach a low DAS44 between males and females;
H1: there is a difference in risk to reach a low DAS44 between males and females.

The research question is always translated into a null and alternative hypothesis as has been done in ▸Chaps. 3–5. For this chapter, we decided not to provide the null and alternative hypothesis as these remain the same, even when checking for potential influencing variables.

Having a low DAS44 after 52 weeks of treatment is a dichotomous outcome variable, hence the effect of gender on reaching a low DAS44 is quantified by the odds ratio (OR). ◻Table 6.1 summarizes the number of males and females that reached a high (i.e., ≥1.6) or a low DAS44 (i.e., <1.6) after 52 weeks of treatment. From this table (or with SPSS), we calculate the OR and the 95 % confidence interval (CI). The OR for having a low DAS44 after 52 weeks of treatment in males compared to females is 0.31 (95 % CI [0.15; 0.63]). In other words, the odds to reach a low DAS44 after 52 weeks of treatment is 0.31 times higher in males than the odds to reach a low DAS44 after 52 weeks of treatment in females, or $1/0.31 = 3.2$ (95 % CI [1.6; 6.7]) times higher in females than in males. This effect is referred to as the crude effect (or uncorrected or unadjusted effect).

Now assume we want to assess whether smoking is a confounder, we first need to stratify the 2 × 2 crosstab for smoking status. To stratify an analysis in SPSS, we use the

■ **Table 6.2** Crosstab for the association between low DAS44 after 52 weeks of treatment and gender, stratified for smokers and non-smokers

		DAS44 after 52 weeks		Total
		≥1.6	<1.6	
Smokers	Female	15	8	23
	Male	7	13	20
	Total	22	21	43
Non-smokers	Female	52	29	81
	Male	11	19	30
	Total	63	48	111

split file query (Supplementary Information A.2). Two separate 2 × 2 crosstabs are then created: one for smokers and one for non-smokers (■Table 6.2).

Forty-nine percent of the smokers (i.e., 21/43) and 43 % of the non-smokers (i.e., 48/111) reach a low DAS44 after 52 weeks of treatment. The OR to reach a low DAS44 after 52 weeks of treatment (of females compared to males) in smokers is 3.1 and 3.3 in non-smokers. These two ORs are pooled together for an overall OR, to study the influence of smoking on the association between gender and reaching a low DAS44. The pooled OR, corrected for smoking status, is calculated with the Mantel-Haenszel pooled OR. The pooled OR is a weighted average of the ORs for each stratum of a dichotomous determinant. The weighted average of the ORs is calculated by multiplying the OR in each stratum with the number of patients in that stratum divided by the size of the total study population, which is then summed over all strata.

The Mantel-Haenszel test for trend (▶Sect. 4.3.1) is used for testing an association between a dichotomous outcome variable and an ordinal categorical determinant. The Mantel-Haenszel pooled OR is an additional option in the crosstabs query of SPSS (Supplementary Information A.5.1). ■Table 6.3 shows the SPSS output for the Mantel-Haenszel pooled OR. The pooled OR is reported in the row "Estimate", its corresponding 95 % CI in the rows "Commons Odds Ratio" in "Asymp. 95 % Confidence Interval", and is equal to 3.2 (95 % CI [1.6; 6.6]). The pooled OR is similar to the crude effect, (i.e., OR 3.2, 95 % CI [1.6; 6.7]) hence we conclude that smoking is not a confounder (in the association between reaching a low DAS44 after 52 weeks of treatment and gender). SPSS also reports the natural logarithm (ln) of the pooled OR (in the row "ln(Estimate)", its standard error (SE) (in the row "Std. Error of the ln(Estimate)") and corresponding 95 % CI (in the rows "ln(Common Odds Ratio)"). SPSS also tests the null hypothesis that the pooled OR is equal to one against the alternative hypothesis that the pooled OR is unequal to one; the p-value of this test is reported in the row "Asymp. sig. (2-sided)".

For the analyses of a continuous outcome variable and a time to event outcome variable, the pooled estimates of the effect need to be calculated manually. However, confounding can also be investigated easily with regression models. This is a more common approach then stratification of the analyses, and is explained in the following sections.

□ **Table 6.3**   SPSS output of the Mantel-Haenszel pooled OR for smoking status

The Mantel-Haenszel common odds ratio estimate			
Estimate			3.217
ln(Estimate)			1.169
Std. Error of the ln(Estimate)			.365
Asymp. sig. (2-sided)			.001
Asymp. 95 % Confidence Interval	Common Odds Ratio	Lower Bound	1.573
		Upper Bound	6.580
	ln(Common Odds Ratio)	Lower Bound	.453
		Upper Bound	1.884

The Mantel-Haenszel common odds ratio estimate is asymptotically normally distributed under the common odds ratio of 1.000 assumption. So is the natural log of the estimate

6.1.2 Confounding in a Linear Regression Model

Let us reassess the association between the change in DAS44 after 52 weeks of treatment ('dDAS44') and erythrocyte sedimentation rate (ESR) at baseline (categorized as low, moderate and high), as studied in ▶Model M3.5 (▶Sect. 3.4.3). This association was analyzed with a linear regression model, in which two dummy variables d_1 (for moderate ESR at baseline) and d_2 (for high ESR at baseline) were created for the categorical determinant (□Table 3.18, ▶Sect. 3.4.3). The linear regression model for this association is equal to

$$\text{mean dDAS44} = b_0 + b_1 \times d_1 \times d_1 + b_2 \times d_2. \tag{M6.1}$$

□Table 6.4 shows the SPSS output of this crude model, with low ESR set as reference group, which is equal to □Table 3.19 (▶Sect. 3.4.3). The mean difference in change in DAS44 after 52 weeks of treatment between patients with moderate and low ESR at baseline is −0.47. In other words, the change in DAS44 score is 0.47 points lower in patients with moderate ESR at baseline compared to patients with low ESR at baseline. The mean difference in change in DAS44 after 52 weeks of treatment between patients with high and low ESR at baseline is −0.98. These differences are defined as the crude differences.

To report the result of this association as accurately as possible, we need to investigate whether the association is influenced by a potential confounder. To illustrate this, we investigate the total swollen joint count (TSJC) at baseline as a potential confounder. We should first actually investigate whether TSJC at baseline is associated with ESR at baseline, with an analysis of variance (ANOVA) or non-parametric Kruskal-Wallis test (▶Sect. 3.3.2). We skip this step for illustrative purposes, and assume (for illustrative purposes) that there is a significant association. TSJC is added to the crude linear regression model. The model corrected for TSJC is then equal to

$$\text{mean dDAS44} = b_0 + b_1 \times d_1 + b_2 \times d_2 + b_3 \times \text{TSJC}. \tag{M6.2}$$

■ **Table 6.4** SPSS output of a linear regression model comparing change in DAS44 between patients with low, moderate and high ESR at baseline

Coefficients[a]

Model		Unstandardized Coefficients		Standardized Coefficients	t	Sig.	95 % Confidence Interval for B	
		B	Std. Error	Beta			Lower Bound	Upper Bound
1	(Constant)	−1.808	.132		−13.665	.000	−2.069	−1.547
	d1	−.465	.200	−.194	−2.321	.022	−.861	−.069
	d2	−.983	.205	−.401	−4.786	.000	−1.389	−.577

[a]Dependent Variable: change in DAS44

■ **Table 6.5** SPSS output of a linear regression model for the association between the change in DAS44 and ESR at baseline, corrected for TSJC

Coefficients[a]

Model		Unstandardized Coefficients		Standardized Coefficients	t	Sig.	95 % Confidence Interval for B	
		B	Std. Error	Beta			Lower Bound	Upper Bound
1	(Constant)	−1.808	.132		−13.665	.000	−2.069	−1.547
	d1	−.465	.200	−.194	−2.321	.022	−.861	−.069
	d2	−.983	.205	−.401	−4.786	.000	−1.389	−.577
2	(Constant)	−.596	.197		−3.020	.003	−.986	−.206
	d1	−.395	.172	−.165	−2.303	.023	−.734	−.056
	d2	−.770	.178	−.314	−4.326	.000	−1.122	−.418
	TSJC	−.097	.013	−.493	−7.496	.000	−.123	−.072

[a]Dependent Variable: change in DAS44

If the regression coefficients b_1 or b_2 change by more than 10 %, TSJC is considered a confounder.

■Table 6.5 shows the SPSS output of the crude and corrected model. Model 2 was obtained in SPSS with the 'Next' button in the linear regression query in SPSS (Supplementary Information A.4.3). It is important to use this option, because SPSS will then run both models on the same group of patients. When patients with missing values on the potential confounder are excluded from the analysis in the crude model, the regression coefficients of the central determinant could already change with more than 10 %. To keep the comparison of the crude and corrected model as fair as possible, the same group of patients need to be used to estimate the models. The regression coefficients of the crude model are reported in model "1" and of the corrected model in model "2". The first regression coefficient b_1 changed from -0.465 to -0.395 (a decrease of 15 %), the second coefficient b_2 from -0.983 to -0.770 (a decrease of 22 %). Both coefficients changed by more than 10 %, therefore we conclude that TSJC is a confounder.

The regression coefficients b_0, b_1 and b_2 in this new model are interpreted as follows:

- b_0 (the intercept) is equal to the mean change in DAS44 for patients with a low ESR at baseline and a TSJC at baseline of zero. After all, for these patients ▶ Model M6.2 yields

$$\text{mean dDAS44} = b_0 + b_1 \times 0 + b_2 \times 0 + b_3 \times 0 = b_0;$$

- b_1 is equal to the mean difference in change in DAS44 between a patient with moderate ESR at baseline and a patient with low ESR as baseline, but with the same TSJC at baseline. After all, for two patients, for example, both with 15 swollen joints at baseline, but one patient with low ESR and one with moderate ESR at baseline, ▶ Model M6.2 yields

$$\text{mean dDAS44} = b_0 + b_1 \times 0 + b_2 \times 0 + b_3 \times 15 = b_0 + b_3 \times 15,$$

$$\text{mean dDAS44} = b_0 + b_1 \times 1 + b_2 \times 0 + b_3 \times 15 = b_0 + b_1 + b_3 \times 15.$$

Hence, their difference is equal to b_1;

- b_2 is equal to the mean difference in change in DAS44 between a patient with high ESR at baseline and a patient with low ESR as baseline, irrespective of TSJC.

The regression coefficient b_3 has an interpretation as well, which we provide in ▶ Sect. 6.5.1. When checking for confounding, the regression coefficient of the confounder itself is not of interest because we are only interested in the change of the regression coefficient(s) of the central determinant.

Because TSJC is a confounder, we need to report that patients with a moderate ESR at baseline have a stronger decrease in DAS44 after 52 weeks of treatment compared to patients with a low ESR at baseline after correcting for TSJC (mean difference -0.40, 95 % CI $[-0.73; -0.56]$, $p = 0.023$), and patients with a high ESR at baseline have an even stronger decrease (mean difference -0.77, 95 % CI $[-1.1; -0.42]$, $p < 0.001$). In other words, the effect of ESR at baseline on the change in DAS44 after 52 weeks of treatment is overestimated if we do not correct for TSJC. Irrespective of the type of outcome variable, the crude and the corrected effect (or adjusted effect) are always reported in the scientific paper, for example in a table such as ◻Table 6.6.

In our example, both regression coefficients changed by more than 10 %. If only one of the regression coefficients changed by more than 10 %, the added variable is still considered a confounder. This always holds for a categorical determinant: at least one of the regression coefficients of the central determinant has to change by more than 10 %. Note that all the above mentioned p-values are not corrected for multiple testing.

6.1.3 Confounding in a Logistic or Cox Regression Model

Confounding for a dichotomous or a time to event outcome variable with a logistic or Cox regression model is investigated in the same way as for a continuous outcome

▣ **Table 6.6** Final results for the association between change in DAS44 after 52 weeks of treatment and ESR at baseline

	Mean difference[a]	95 % CI	p-value
Crude model			
Moderate ESR	−0.47	−0.86; −0.069	0.022
High ESR	−0.98	−1.4; −0.58	<0.001
Corrected model[b]			
Moderate ESR	−0.40	−0.73; −0.056	0.023
High ESR	−0.77	−1.1; −0.42	<0.001

[a]Compared to low ESR at baseline
[b]Corrected for TSJC

variable with a linear regression model. The type of potential confounder, i.e., whether the variable is dichotomous, categorical or continuous, does not matter either for the procedure. We illustrate this by re-examining the example of ▶ Sect. 4.4.1 in which the association between the development of rheumatoid arthritis (RA) within 2 years and the pain score at baseline, measured with a visual analogue scale (VAS; 'VAS_pain'), was assessed in the RA-cohort [2]. All determinants considered in ▶ Chap. 4 did not have missing values, however, some other variables, that we use in this chapter, do. Therefore, for illustrative purposes, we used one of the imputed datasets (▶ Chap. 8) and ignore the missing data for the moment. The logistic regression model for this association is equal to

$$\ln(\text{odds for RA within 2 years}) = b_0 + b_1 \times \text{VAS\_pain}. \tag{M6.3}$$

Although we know the linearity assumption of the logistic regression model does not hold, which we assessed in ▶ Sect. 4.4.2, we ignore this for now, also for illustrative purposes. ▣ Table 6.7 shows the SPSS output of this model, which is the same as ▣ Table 4.12 (▶ Sect. 4.4.1).

We now investigate whether antibody status is a potential confounder, which we need to correct for. Antibody status is a categorical variable, with four groups: (i) rheumatoid factor type immunoglobulin M (IgM-RF) positive but anticyclic citrullinated peptide (aCCP) negative, (ii) IgM-RF negative but aCCP low positive, (iii) IgM-RF negative but aCCP high positive, and (iv) both IgM-RF positive and aCCP positive. For illustrative purposes, we assume that VAS pain score at baseline and antibody stated are significantly associated without further testing this assumption. We set the antibody status IgM-RF positive but aCCP negative group as the reference group, so that the logistic regression model corrected for antibody status is equal to

$$\ln(\text{odds for RA within 2 years}) = b_0 + b_1 \times \text{VAS\_pain} + b_2$$
$$\times \text{antibody}(1) + b_3 \times \text{antibody}(2) \tag{M6.4}$$
$$+ b_4 \times \text{antibody}(3).$$

> ◻ **Table 6.7** SPSS output of a logistic regression model relating development of RA within 2 years to VAS pain score at baseline

Variables in the Equation

		B	SE	Wald	df	Sig.	Exp(B)	95 % C.I. for EXP(B)	
								Lower	Upper
Step 1ª	VAS	.024	.006	15.684	1	.000	1.024	1.012	1.037
	Constant	−1.719	.321	28.670	1	.000	.179		

ªVariable(s) entered on step 1: VAS

The interpretation of the regression coefficients b_0 and b_1 are as follows:
- b_0 is the ln(odds) to develop RA within 2 years for a patient with a VAS pain score of zero at baseline who is IgM-RF positive but aCCP negative;
- b_1 is the difference in ln(odds) to develop RA within 2 years between two patients who differ by 1 point in the VAS pain score at baseline, with the same antibody status. Again, b_1 is independent of the value of the confounder.

This means that the OR to develop RA within 2 years between two patients who differ in the VAS pain score at baseline by one point, irrespective of antibody status, is equal to the exponential (exp) of b_1, i.e., $\exp(b_1)$. The interpretation of b_2, b_3 and b_4 is skipped again because we are only interested in the effect of the VAS pain score at baseline on the development of RA (the central determinant and outcome variable).

◻Table 6.8 shows the SPSS output of the corrected model. We used the 'Next' button in the logistic regression query in SPSS (Supplementary Information A.5.2), to estimate the model. This is required, because SPSS then estimates both models on the same group of patients, i.e., patients with missing values on the potential confounder are excluded in the crude model as well as the in the corrected model. SPSS does not report the models in the same output. Instead, two different blocks are generated. This does not matter, as we are only interested in the change in the regression coefficient b_1. The regression coefficient was 0.024 in the crude model (◻Table 6.7) and increased to 0.030 in the corrected model, i.e., an increase in b_1 of 25 %. Therefore, we conclude that antibody status is a confounder. After correcting for antibody status, the development of RA within 2 years is associated with the VAS pain score at baseline, with an OR of 1.03 per increase of 1 point in the VAS pain score at baseline (95 % CI [1.02; 1.04], $p < 0.001$). The OR per increase of 5 or 10 points in the VAS pain score at baseline could be calculated the same way as illustrated in ▶Example 4.2 (▶Sect. 4.4.1), by taking b_1 to the power 5 or 10. The results in a scientific paper are reported in a table similar to ◻Table 6.6.

Investigating confounding in a study with a time to event outcome variable is done in exactly the same way as with a dichotomous outcome variable. The interpretation of the exponential of the regression coefficient(s) is the corrected hazard ratio (HR). Important to note is that in the logistic and Cox regression model, the rule of thumb has to be applied to the regression coefficient and not to the OR and the HR.

◻ **Table 6.8** SPSS output of a logistic regression model relating development of RA within 2 years to the VAS pain score at baseline, corrected for antibody status at baseline

Variables in the Equation

		B	SE	Wald	df	Sig.	Exp(B)	95 % C.I. for EXP(B)	
								Lower	Upper
Step 1ᵃ	VAS	.030	.007	18.330	1	.000	1.030	1.016	1.044
	antibody			37.658	3	.000			
	antibody(1)	.957	.481	3.962	1	.047	2.604	1.015	6.683
	antibody(2)	1.714	.439	15.245	1	.000	5.553	2.348	13.130
	antibody(3)	2.445	.419	34.089	1	.000	11.528	2.074	26.192
	Constant	−3.438	.509	45.632	1	.000	.032		

ᵃVariable(s) entered on step 1: antibody

6.1.4 Regression to the Mean

A different form of confounding is regression to the mean. This phenomenon describes the fact that patients with more extreme values at the first measurement are more likely to have a value closer to the mean at the second measurement. The other way around is also true: if the second measurement is more extreme, it is more likely that the first measurement was closer to the mean.

◻Figure 6.2 shows the phenomenon of regression to the mean for measuring blood pressure. In this figure, blood pressure is a normally distributed variable, with a mean of 120/80 millimeters of mercury (mmHg) and a standard deviation (SD) of 20 mmHg. The probability that a patient with a blood pressure of 160/120 mmHg at the first measurement will have a lower blood pressure at the second measurement is 98 %, while the probability that his/her blood pressure is even higher at the second measurement is just 2 %. If a patient has a blood pressure of 100/60 mmHg at the first measurement, the chance of having a lower blood pressure at the second measurement is 16 %, opposed to 84 % of having a higher blood pressure at the second measurement. The values of the second measurement will regress to the mean. For this reason, blood pressure is measured three times nowadays and the mean of these measurements is recorded.

Regression to the mean is especially important in experimental studies or trials, such as in a randomized controlled trial (RCT). In the COBRA-light study, patients in the COBRA arm had a somewhat higher DAS44 at baseline (mean 4.1, SD 0.74) compared to the patients in the COBRA-light arm (mean 4.0, SD 0.90), although not statistically significant. Due to regression to the mean, the DAS44 at a second measurement is likely to be lower in the COBRA arm than in the COBRA-light arm. To account for the difference at baseline, the DAS44 at baseline ('DAS44_wk0') was added to a linear regression model to assess the differences in change in DAS44 between both treatment arms. ◻Table 6.9 shows the SPSS output of the crude and corrected model. The uncorrected mean difference in the change in

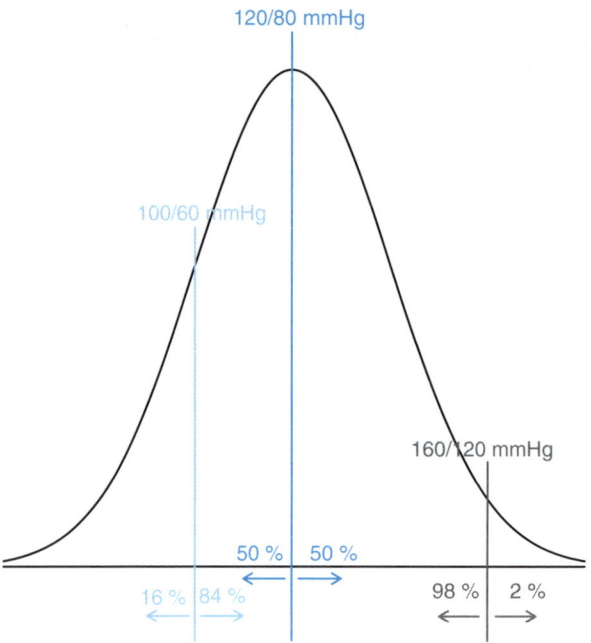

Fig. 6.2 Visualization of the phenomenon regression to the mean

Table 6.9 SPSS output of a linear regression model to correct for regression to the mean in the COBRA-light study

Coefficients[a]

Model		Unstandardized Coefficients		Standardized Coefficients	t	Sig.	95 % Confidence Interval for B	
		B	Std. Error	Beta			Lower Bound	Upper Bound
1	(Constant)	−2.405	.125		−19.165	.000	−2.653	−2.157
	treatment	.343	.177	.155	1.932	.055	−.008	.694
2	(Constant)	.411	.390		1.055	.293	−.359	1.181
	treatment	.232	.153	.105	1.517	.131	−.070	.533
	DAS44_wk0	−.686	.091	−.518	−7.519	.000	−.866	−.505

[a]Dependent Variable: change in DAS44 after 52 weeks

the DAS44 after 52 weeks of treatment between the COBRA and COBRA-light arm is 0.34 (95 % CI [−0.008; 0.69], $p = 0.055$). The corrected mean difference decreased to 0.23 (95 % CI [−0.070; 0.53], $p = 0.13$). From this, we see that the effect of treatment on the change in the DAS44 is influenced by regression to the mean. Therefore, one should always correct for the baseline value of the outcome variable of interest in medical research, especially in trials.

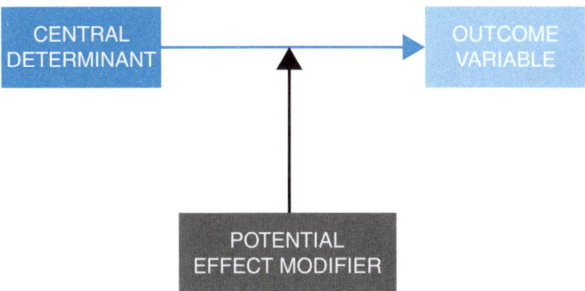

◻ **Fig. 6.3** Visualization of the concept of effect modification

6.2   Effect Modification

The association between the outcome variable and central determinant could also be influenced by effect modification. A variable is considered to be an effect modifier if the effect of the association is different for different groups (called strata) within the study population. ◻Figure 6.3 visualizes the concept of effect modification. A known example of effect modification is the difference in gender for the association between cardiovascular risk and cholesterol level. Confounding is bias that needs to be eliminated, whereas effect modification is a stand-alone result. This implies that a variable cannot be an effect modifier and a confounder in the same association.

6.2.1 Effect Modification Through Stratification

Although the concept of effect modification is different from confounding, it could be assessed through stratification as well by taking the following steps:
1. Calculate the crude effect size.
2. Stratify the analyses for the strata of the potential effect modifier, and calculate the stratum specific effect size with the corresponding 95 % CI.
3. Compare the stratum specific effect sizes:
   a) if the 95 % CIs of the stratum specific effect sizes do not overlap, effect modification is present and the stratum specific effect sizes should be reported.
   b) If the effect size of one stratum lies in the 95 % CI of the other stratum (and/or vice versa), effect modification is not present.
   c) If the 95 CIs overlap but the effect size of one stratum does not lie within the 95 % of the other stratum, effect modification cannot be ruled out or confirmed.

To explain these steps, we investigate whether the association between ESR after 52 weeks of treatment and treatment arm is different for males and females. Since ESR is not normally distributed (▶Sect. 3.2.1), the natural logarithm (ln) of ESR is used in the analyses. The crude effect size in step 1 is calculated with the independent samples *t*-test. ◻Table 6.10 shows the SPSS output of this test for the whole study population (see also ◻Table 3.2, ▶Sect. 3.2.1). The mean difference in ln(ESR) after 52 weeks of treatment is −0.29, in favor of the COBRA-light treatment arm.

◘ Table 6.10 SPSS output of the independent samples t-test, comparing the ln-transformed ESR after 52 weeks of COBRA treatment with COBRA-light treatment

Independent Sample Test

		Levene's Test for Equality of Variances		t-test for Equality of Means					95 % Confidence Interval of the Difference	
		F	Sig.	t	df	Sig. (2-tailed)	Mean Difference	Std. Error Difference	Lower	Upper
ln(ESR) after 52 weeks	Equal variances assumed	.816	.638	−1.949	152	.053	−.28905	.14833	−.58210	.00399
	Equal variances not assumed			−1.949	150.791	.053	−.28905	.14833	−.58212	.00401

For step 2, the analyses need to be stratified. ◨Table 6.11 shows the SPSS output of the independent samples t-test stratified by gender. The mean difference in ln(ESR) between COBRA-light and COBRA in female patients is -0.47 (95 % CI $[-0.83; -0.10]$), and in male patients 0.079 (95 % CI $[-0.38; 0.54]$). The effect size within female patients does not lie within the 95 % CI for the effect size within male patients, and vice versa. Therefore, we conclude that gender is an effect modifier in the association between ESR after 52 weeks and treatment arm. The conclusion to the research question is that within female patients, the ESR after 52 weeks of COBRA-light treatment is lower than COBRA treatment (relative difference 0.63, 95 % CI $[0.44; 0.90]$, $p = 0.012$), but within males there is no difference between the two treatment arms (relative difference 1.1, 95 % CI $[0.68; 1.7]$, $p = 0.73$). The mean difference in ln(ESR) is transformed to a relative difference between the two arms with the exponential of the mean differences in ln(ESR), as explained in ▶ Sect. 3.2.1.

This procedure can only be performed for a dichotomous or categorical potential effect modifier. Moreover, no definite conclusion can be drawn if the 95 % CIs of the stratum specific effect sizes overlap while the effect sizes of the other stratum(s) are not contained in its 95 % CI. Therefore, we advise to assess effect modification with regression models, just like investigating confounding. Moreover, this also allows for investigating effect modification of a continuous variable.

6.2.2 Effect Modification in a Linear Regression Model

In general, the potential effect modifier and its interaction with the central determinant are added to the regression model. The interaction (or interaction term) is the product of the potential effect modifier and the central determinant. This interaction has to be computed manually for a linear regression model in SPSS (Supplementary Information A.2), but is created automatically in a logistic or Cox regression model (Supplementary Information A.5.2 and A.6.2).

We illustrate how to check for effect modification with a continuous outcome variable and a continuous determinant with the following research question

> ❓ Is the decrease in DAS44 after 52 weeks of COBRA-light or COBRA treatment associated with the general well-being (measured with a VAS) at baseline in patients with early RA?

The linear regression model for this association is

$$\text{mean dDAS44} = b_0 + b_1 \times \text{VAS\_general.} \tag{M6.5}$$

To investigate if gender is an effect modifier, we add the variable gender (where females are coded as zero and males as one) and the interaction of gender with VAS general well-being ('VAS_general') to the linear model:

$$\text{mean dDAS44} = b_0 + b_1 \times \text{VAS\_general} + b_2 \times \text{gender}$$
$$+ b_3 \times \text{VAS\_general} \times \text{gender.} \tag{M6.6}$$

Table 6.11 SPSS output of the independent samples *t*-test, comparing the ln-transformed ESR after 52 weeks of COBRA treatment with COBRA-light treatment stratified by gender

Independent Sample Test

		Levene's Test for Equality of Variances		t-test for Equality of Means					95 % Confidence Interval of the Difference	
		F	Sig.	t	df	Sig. (2-tailed)	Mean Difference	Std. Error Difference	Lower	Upper
females										
ln(ESR) after 52 weeks	Equal variances assumed	.625	.431	−2.550	102	.012	−.46585	.18266	−.82816	−.10355
	Equal variances not assumed			−2.550	101.411	.012	−.46585	.18266	−.82819	−.10352
males										
ln(ESR) after 52 weeks	Equal variances assumed	3.328	.074	.342	48	.734	.07870	.23029	−.38433	.54173
	Equal variances not assumed			.342	42.236	.734	.07870	.23029	−.38565	.54305

To explain how effect modification is tested with ▶Model M6.6, we first provide the interpretation of the regression coefficients in this model:

- b_0 is the mean change in DAS44 for a female patient with a VAS general well-being score of zero at baseline. After all, for a female patient with a VAS general well-being score of zero at baseline, ▶Model M6.6 yields

$$\text{mean dDAS44} = b_0 + b_1 \times 0 + b_2 \times 0 + b_3 \times 0 \times 0 = b_0;$$

- b_1 is the mean change in DAS44 after 52 weeks of treatment between two female patients who differ by one point in the VAS general well-being score at baseline. For example, for two female patients, one with score of 48 and one with a score of 49, ▶Model M6.6 yields

$$\text{mean dDAS44} = b_0 + b_1 \times 48 + b_2 \times 0 + b_3 \times 48 \times 0 = b_0 + b_1 \times 48,$$

$$\text{mean dDAS44} = b_0 + b_1 \times 49 + b_2 \times 0 + b_3 \times 49 \times 0 = b_0 + b_1 \times 49.$$

Hence, their difference is equal to b_1;

- b_2 is the mean change in DAS44 after 52 weeks of treatment between a male and a female both with a VAS general well-being score of zero at baseline. After all, for a male patient with a VAS general well-being score of zero at baseline ▶Model M6.6 yields

$$\text{mean dDAS44} = b_0 + b_1 \times 0 + b_2 \times 1 + b_3 \times 0 \times 1 = b_0 + b_2.$$

Hence, the difference between a female and male patient (both with a VAS general well-being score of zero at baseline) is equal to b_2;

- b_3 is the additional mean change in DAS44 after 52 weeks of treatment between two males who differ by one point in the VAS general well-being score at baseline, compared to the mean change in DAS44 after 52 weeks of treatment between two females who differ by one point in the VAS general well-being score at baseline. For example, for two male patients, one with score of 48 and one with a score of 49, ▶Model M6.6 yields

$$\text{mean dDAS44} = b_0 + b_1 \times 48 + b_2 \times 1 + b_3 \times 48 \times 1$$
$$= b_0 + b_1 \times 48 + b_2 + b_3 \times 48,$$

$$\text{mean dDAS44} = b_0 + b_1 \times 49 + b_2 \times 1 + b_3 \times 49 \times 1$$
$$= b_0 + b_1 \times 49 + b_2 + b_3 \times 49.$$

Hence, their difference is equal to $b_1 + b_3$ and b_3 is the additional difference compared to females.

It is important to add both the potential effect modifier itself to the model as well as the interaction with the central determinant, otherwise the interpretation of the regression coefficients is incorrect.

■ **Table 6.12**   SPSS output of a linear regression model relating the change in DAS44 after 52 weeks of treatment to the VAS general well-being at baseline with gender as potential effect modifier

Coefficients[a]

Model		Unstandardized Coefficients		Standardized Coefficients	t	Sig.	95 % Confidence Interval for B	
		B	Std. Error	Beta			Lower Bound	Upper Bound
1	(Constant)	−1.904	.242		−7.851	.000	−2.383	−1.425
	VASgeneral	−.006	.004	−.118	−1.464	.145	−.013	.002
2	(Constant)	−1.320	.304		−4.350	.000	−1.920	−.721
	VASgeneral	−.012	.005	−.258	−2.623	.010	−.021	−.003
	gender	−1.384	.480	−.585	−2.886	.004	−2.331	−.436
	VASgeneral_gender	.014	.008	.383	1.873	.063	−.001	.030

[a]Dependent Variable: change in DAS44

If the effect of the VAS general well-being score at baseline on the change in DAS44 after 52 weeks of treatment is not modified by gender, b_3 should be equal to zero. Hence, testing effect modification is the same as testing the following null and alternative hypothesis

H0: $b_3 = 0$;
H1: $b_3 \neq 0$.

The significance level α for testing effect modification is usually set at 0.10, instead of at 0.05, especially in smaller sized study populations. This is because a small study population does not have enough power to detect effect modification at the 0.05 significance level.

■Table 6.12 shows the SPSS output of the ▶models M6.5 and M6.6, in models "1" and "2" respectively. The variable gender and its interaction with VAS general well-being at baseline were both added to the model with only the VAS general well-being at baseline with the 'Next' button in the linear regression query in SPSS (Supplementary Information A.4.3). From this output, we conclude that without taking gender into account, there is not enough evidence for an association between the change in DAS44 after 52 weeks of treatment and the VAS general well-being at baseline (mean difference −0.006 points per increase of 1 point, 95 % CI [−0.013; 0.002], $p = 0.15$). However, since the interaction term in the last row ('VASgeneral_gender') is statistically significant at the level α of 0.1, we conclude that the association between the change in DAS44 after 52 weeks of treatment and the VAS general well-being at baseline is modified by gender ($p = 0.063$). In the results of the scientific paper, the crude effect is reported in the text and the stratified results are referred to in a table

▪ **Table 6.13** Final result of the association between the change in DAS44 after 52 weeks and the VAS general well-being at baseline, for males and females separately

	B	95 % CI	p-value
Crude effect	−0.006	−0.013; 0.002	0.15
Females			
VAS general well-being	−0.012	−0.021; −0.003	0.010
Males			
VAS general well-being	0.002	−0.010; 0.015	0.72

(▪Table 6.13), irrespective of the type of outcome variable. The effect size for this association in females is obtained directly from 'VASgeneral' in model "2" of ▪Table 6.12. Within females, the mean decrease in change of DAS44 is a 0.012 per point increase in the VAS general well-being at baseline (95 % CI [0.003; 0.021], $p = 0.010$). The effect size for males could be derived from ▪Table 6.12 as well, it is equal to 0.002 (i.e., $b_1 + b_3 = -0.012 + 0.014$). However, the 95 % CI could only be obtained from a linear regression model stratified by gender (SPSS output not shown). For males there is no evidence for an association between the change in DAS44 and the VAS general well-being at baseline (mean increase 0.002 per 1 point, 95 % CI [−0.010, 0.015], $p = 0.72$).

6.2.3 Effect Modification in a Logistic or Cox Regression Model

The procedure to check for effect modification is similar for a continuous, a dichotomous or a time to event outcome variable, through a linear, logistic or a Cox regression model, respectively. However, the interaction between the central determinant and the potential effect modifier does not have to be computed manually in a logistic or Cox regression model. We illustrate the procedure to check for effect modification in a logistic regression model in the RA-cohort with the following research question

? Is there a difference in odds to develop RA within 2 years between patients with arthralgia who use alcohol and those who do not?

The logistic regression model is

$$\ln(\text{odds for RA within 2 years}) = b_0 + b_1 \times \text{alcohol},$$ (M6.7)

where alcohol use is coded as zero and no alcohol use as one. ▪Table 6.14 shows the SPSS output of this logistic regression model. From this output, we conclude that patients who use alcohol have higher odds to develop RA within 2 years than patients who do not use alcohol (OR 1.9, 95 % CI [1.1; 3.1], $p = 0.015$).

□ **Table 6.14**   SPSS output of the logistic regression model for the association between development of RA within 2 years and alcohol use

Variables in the Equation

		B	SE	Wald	df	Sig.	Exp(B)	95 % C.I. for EXP(B)	
								Lower	Upper
Step 1ª	alcohol	.621	.255	5.924	1	.015	1.861	1.129	3.068
	Constant	−.831	.163	25.996	1	.000	.435		

ªVariable(s) entered on step 1: alcohol

□ **Table 6.15**   SPSS output of the logistic regression model to test effect modification of VAS pain score (dichotomized, 'VAS50') in the association between development of RA within 2 years and alcohol use

Variables in the Equation

		B	SE	Wald	df	Sig.	Exp(B)	95 % C.I. for EXP(B)	
								Lower	Upper
Step 1ª	alcohol	1.191	.338	12.417	1	.000	3.292	1.697	6.385
	VAS50	1.187	.345	11.823	1	.001	3.276	1.666	6.443
	VAS50 by alcohol	−1.525	.528	8.357	1	.004	.218	.077	.612
	Constant	−1.258	.218	33.275	1	.000	.284		

ªVariable(s) entered on step 1: alcohol, VAS50, VAS50 * alcohol

Whether having a VAS pain score of 50 points or higher ('VAS50'), modifies the effect in this association, is assessed in the second step. The variable VAS50 (with a VAS score below 50 coded as zero and a VAS score of 50 or higher as one) as well as the interaction between VAS50 and alcohol use, are added to the logistic regression model

$$\ln(\text{odds for RA within 2 years}) = b_0 + b_1 \times \text{alcohol} + b_2 \times \text{VAS50} \qquad \text{(M6.8)}$$
$$+ b_3 \times \text{alcohol} \times \text{VAS50}.$$

The interaction between alcohol use and VAS50 does not have to be created manually as with linear regression (see Supplementary Information A.5.2), but do not forget to include the VAS pain score to the model as well and not only the interaction. The interpretation of the regression coefficients is similar as in a linear regression model. The only difference is the outcome of the model, which is now ln(odds). □Table 6.15 shows the SPSS output of ▶Model (M6.8). We conclude that VAS pain score is indeed an effect modifier ($p = 0.004$). Therefore, we need to stratify the analyses and report the ORs for

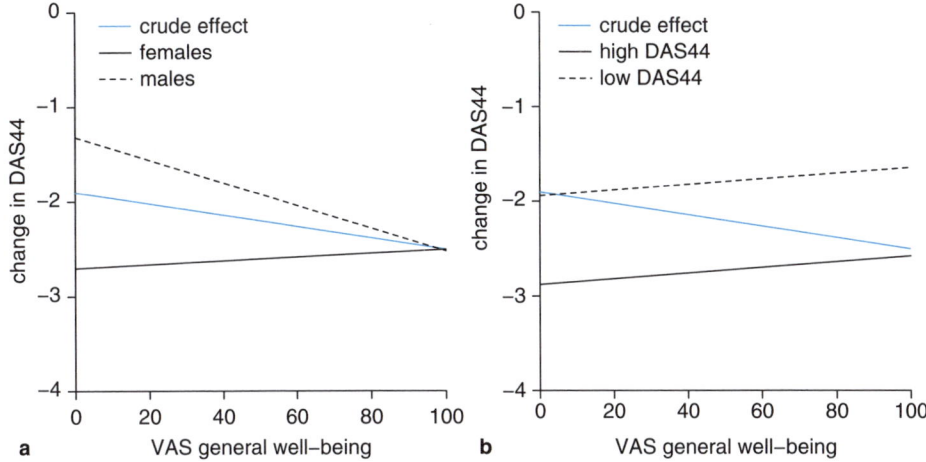

◻ **Fig. 6.4** Visualization of the difference between effect modification (**a**) and confounding (**b**).
Blue line is crude effect

development of RA within 2 years for patients who use alcohol compared to those that do not use alcohol, separately for patients with a VAS pain score below 50 and with a VAS pain score of 50 or higher (just as in ◻Table 6.13). For patients with a VAS pain score below 50, the odds to develop RA within 2 years differ significantly between patients who use alcohol and those who do not (OR 3.3, 95 % CI [1.7; 3.4], $p < 0.001$, ◻Table 6.15). However, there is no evidence for such a difference in patients with a VAS pain score of 50 or higher (OR 0.72, 95 % CI [0.32; 1.6], $p = 0.79$, data not shown).

Note that the crude effect was not statistically significant; normally no further analyses would be necessary. However, as is seen in this example, effect modification could still occur. So if we had not checked for effect modification, we would have concluded that there was no evidence for an association between the development of RA within 2 years and alcohol consumption. This is however incorrect: there is a significant association in patients with a VAS pain score below 50. So, always check for the presence of effect modification, even if there is no statistical significant result in the crude analysis.

6.2.4 Difference Between Confounding and Effect Modification

The effect of confounding is often quite difficult to understand, in contrast to the effect of effect modification. ◻Figure 6.4 visualizes the difference between confounding and effect modification for the association between change in DAS44 after 52 weeks of treatment and the VAS general well-being at baseline (▶ Sect. 6.2.2). The crude effect size (i.e., b_1 in ▶Model M6.5) of this association was −0.006 (95 % CI [−0.013; 0.002], $p = 0.15$; blue line). Gender modified this effect (◻Fig. 6.4a): the effect size in females was −0.012 (95 % CI [−0.021; −0.003], $p = 0.009$; black solid line) and in males 0.002 (95 %CI [−0.010; 0.015], $p = 0.72$; black dashed line). Both the intercept and the slope differ between females and males.

The DAS44 score at baseline, dichotomized as low (i.e., a score below 4.0, and coded as zero) versus high (i.e., a score of 4.0 or higher, and coded as one), confounded the effect (◘Fig. 6.4b). The crude effect size is still -0.006 (95 % CI $[-0.013; 0.002]$, $p = 0.15$; blue line). After correcting for DAS44 at baseline, the effect size changed to 0.003 (95 % CI $[-0.004; 0.011]$, $p = 0.40$). Only the intercept differs between patients with a low (black dashed line) and a high DAS44 (black solid line) at baseline, but their slopes are the same. However, the new slope differs from the slope of the crude model. That is the difference in confounding and effect modification: with confounding, the intercept differs between two groups, but the slopes are the same. With effect modification, both the intercept and slope differ between two groups.

6.3   Multiple Confounders and/or Effect Modifiers

In all medical research, multiple variables are measured besides the central determinant and the outcome variable. All these variables could potentially be a confounder or an effect modifier. Many different strategies exist to correct for multiple confounders and effect modifiers, and no one of them is necessarily the best. The choice of a specific strategy is often based on what experts in the field tend to do, to make sure the results are comparable to existing literature. No matter what strategy is chosen, the crude effect of the determinant on the outcome variable is always investigated first.

6.3.1 Multiple Effect Modifiers

One possible approach to check for multiple effect modifiers, is with a stepwise approach. In this approach, all potential effect modifiers are analyzed individually, and in the first step the strongest effect modifier, i.e., the effect modifier with the lowest p-value of the interaction with the central determinant, is selected. The analyses are then stratified for this effect modifier. In the next step, all remaining potential effect modifiers are analyzed in the stratified regression models one by one. Again, the strongest effect modifier is selected and stratified for in further analysis. Within the different strata, different effect modifiers could be identified in the further analyses. This is repeated until no more effect modifiers are found. Then, potential confounders are added to each of the stratified regression models. This strategy is unfavorable in case of many significant effect modifiers because the study population will be stratified in various subgroups, containing only a limited number of patients. A minimum of 10 patients per stratum is advised in the case of a continuous outcome variable and a minimum of 20 patients, with at least 10 events and 10 non-events, is advised in the case of a dichotomous or time to event outcome variable.

Another strategy that could be used is only to stratify for known or biological plausible effect modifiers. However, this strategy does not work if there is no or little evidence known on biological plausible effect modifiers in the literature.

Note that in case of an continuous effect modifier, the study population cannot be stratified. In the scientific paper, one then writes that the effect of the determinant on the outcome variable was even stronger for higher values of the effect modifier (or weaker, depending on the influence of the effect modifier).

Although effect modification is a result on its one and confounding is bias which needs to be eliminated, in general confounding is checked first and potential effect modifiers are then investigated in the final corrected model.

6.3.2 Multiple Confounders

Hierarchical Approach

Correcting for potential confounders could also be done through several strategies. The stepwise approach for effect modification can also be used for confounding. In the first step, each potential confounder is added to the crude model individually, one by one. The strongest confounder, i.e., the confounder with the largest change in the regression coefficient of the central determinant, is added to the model. The new 'base' model is then the model corrected for this confounder. In the second step, each remaining potential confounder is added to this new base model one by one. And again, the strongest confounder (with the highest relative change compared to the new base model, not the crude model) is selected and added. This is repeated until none of the remaining variables are considered a confounder. In the final corrected model, effect modification is then checked. The analyses will not be stratified, but the influence of the effect modifier on the adjusted model is described in the results section of the scientific paper, for each effect modifier separately.

In ▶ Sect. 6.1.3, we concluded that antibody status was a confounder in the association between the development of RA within 2 years and the VAS pain score at baseline, with a 25 % change in the regression coefficient of the central determinant VAS pain. Other potential confounders were also present: adding duration of symptoms (dichotomized as shorter than 12 months or at least 12 months) resulted in a change of 13 % of the regression coefficient of the central determinant VAS pain. Antibody status was the strongest confounder, and was therefore added to the model first. Each remaining potential confounder was then added to the model including the central determinant VAS pain and antibody status, but none changed the regression coefficient of the central determinant VAS pain by more than 10 %.

In the following step, potential effect modifiers were checked in the model corrected for antibody status. Both alcohol use and arthralgia in the small joints appeared to be an effect modifier ($p = 0.071$ and $p = 0.052$, respectively). In a scientific paper, the crude and corrected effects are presented in a table such as ◻Table 6.16, while the influence of the effect modifiers is only reported in the results section, for example as follows: in patients who use alcohol the (corrected) effect is somewhat stronger than in patients who do not use alcohol (OR 1.039, 95 % CI [1.020; 1.058], $p < 0.001$ and OR 1.015, 95 % CI [0.99; 1.036], $p = 0.18$, respectively). Also in patients with arthralgia in the small

□ Table 6.16   Final results for the association between the development of RA within 2 years and the VAS pain score at baseline (dichotomized)

	OR	95 % CI	p-value
Crude model	1.024	1.012; 1.037	<0.001
Adjusted model[a]	1.030	1.016; 1.044	<0.001

[a]Adjusted for antibody status

joints the (corrected) effect is somewhat stronger than in patients without arthralgia in the small joints (OR 1.037, 95 % CI [1.021; 1.054], $p < 0.001$ and OR 1.009, 95 % CI [0.98; 1.039], $p = 0.54$).

Clinical Approach

The hierarchical approach is time-consuming in case of many potential confounders. Another strategy is to only correct for the known or biological plausible confounders, either with the stepwise approach or by just adding them all at once to the model and ignoring the rule of thumb for a change in the regression coefficient by more than 10 %. However, this strategy does not work if there is no or only little evidence available on known or biological plausible confounders in the literature. Instead, grouping potential confounders is a better option, again ignoring the rule of thumb. The (final) corrected model is then checked for effect modification, such as in the previous strategy. In ▶ Sect. 6.1.2, we investigated the association between change in DAS44 after 52 weeks of treatment and the ESR status at baseline, categorized as low, moderate or high. We first correct for demographic variables (e.g., gender and age). Then, we add lifestyle factors (e.g., smoking habit) and finally add antibody status (e.g., being IgM-RF positive and being aCCP positive). The results of these models are presented in □Table 6.17. We conclude that the change in DAS44 after 52 weeks of treatment is associated with ESR at baseline: patients with a moderate or high ESR at baseline have a stronger decrease in DAS44 after 52 weeks of treatment than patients with a low ESR at baseline, even after correcting for age, gender and smoking status (mean difference 0.47, 95 % CI [0.075; 0.86], $p = 0.020$ and mean difference 1.0, 95 % CI [0.59; 1.4], $p < 0.001$, respectively). After correcting also for IgM-RF and aCPP status, there was no evidence of a difference between patients with a low or moderate ESR (mean difference 0.34, 95 % CI [−0.013; 0.81], $p = 0.057$, i.e., minus the difference between moderate to low), but patients with high ESR at baseline had a stronger decrease than patients with a low ESR at baseline (mean difference 0.96, 95 % CI [0.54; 1.4], $p < 0.001$). Effect modification would then be investigated in the final model, and reported similarly as in the stepwise approach illustrated above.

A disadvantage of this strategy is that the effect of the central determinant on the outcome variable is estimated less precisely due to the inclusion of many variables in the model. Secondly, the crude effect is adjusted for variables that might not in fact be a true confounder, as the change in the regression coefficient is not so large. And lastly, this strategy cannot be applied if there are many potential confounders or only a few patients, because of overfitting.

▣ **Table 6.17** Estimated effects of the association between the change in DAS44 after 52 weeks of treatment and ESR at baseline in categories for different models

	Mean difference[a]	95 % CI	p-value
Crude model			
Moderate ESR	−0.47	−0.86; −0.069	0.022
High ESR	−0.98	−1.4; −0.58	<0.001
Corrected model 1[b]			
Moderate ESR	−0.47	−0.86; −0.076	0.020
High ESR	−1.0	−1.4; −0.59	<0.001
Corrected model 2[c]			
Moderate ESR	−0.47	−0.86; −0.075	0.020
High ESR	−1.0	−1.4; −0.59	<0.001
Corrected model 3[d]			
Moderate ESR	−0.34	−0.81; 0.013	0.057
High ESR	−0.96	−1.4; −0.54	<0.001

[a]Compared to low ESR at baseline
[b]Corrected for age and gender
[c]Corrected for age, gender, and smoking status
[d]Corrected for age, gender, smoking status, being RF positive, and being aCPP positive

In conclusion, different strategies result in different models and could potentially lead to different conclusions. It is important to bear this in mind when correcting for potential influencing factors. The most important thing is that the applied method should always be described in the scientific paper.

6.4 Mediation

The aim of some medical research is to find a causal association between the outcome variable and the central determinant. This is also known as causal inference. A causal association, i.e., an association with a causal pathway, could also be influenced by influencing variables. These variables are then called mediators and moderators. Moderation is basically effect modification in a causal association. It is investigated the same way as effect modification, and therefore not illustrated further.

The difference between a confounder and a mediator is that the mediator lies in the causal pathway while a confounder does not. ▣Figure 6.5 visualizes the concept of mediation. The (crude) association between the outcome variable and the central determinant is called the total effect (denoted by c). In case of mediation, the central determinant influences the mediator (its effect is denoted by a) which in turn influences the outcome variable (its effect is denoted by b). There is also a direct effect of the central determinant on

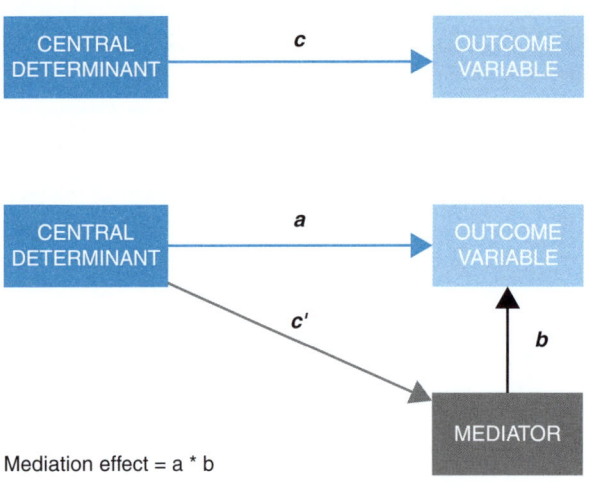

Mediation effect = a * b

■ Fig. 6.5   Visualization of the concept of mediation

the outcome variable in the mediated model (denoted by c'). The indirect effect of the central determinant on the outcome variable through the mediator can be calculated in two ways: by $c - c'$, or by $a \times b$. These two methods yield the same estimated indirect effect when the mediator and outcome variable are both continuous but not when the mediator and/or outcome variable is dichotomous. In the latter case, $a \times b$ is preferred to estimate the indirect effect. The indirect effect is interpreted as the difference in outcome variable for one unit difference in the central determinant that is explained by the mediator.

The values of the different effects (i.e., a, b, c and c') are obtained from three different regression models: one for the total effect of the central determinant on the outcome variable, one for the effect of the central determinant on the mediator and one for the effects of the central determinant and the mediator on the outcome variable. We illustrate the mechanism of mediation by investigating the association between change in the Health Assessment Questionnaire (HAQ) score after 52 weeks of treatment ('dHAQ'), and ESR at baseline, as a continuous determinant. However, we think that the change in the HAQ score after 52 weeks of treatment in not influenced by ESR at baseline, but by the HAQ score at baseline ('HAQ_wk0') since higher ESR might lead to a higher HAQ score, which could lead to a higher or smaller change in the HAQ score. In other words, the HAQ score at baseline might be a possible mediator in the association between ESR at baseline and the change in the HAQ score after 52 weeks of treatment. In this example, the three regression models to estimate the different effects are

$$\text{mean dHAQ} = b_{0,1} + c \times \text{ESR}, \tag{M6.9}$$

$$\text{mean HAQ\_wk0} = b_{0,2} + a \times \text{ESR}, \tag{M6.10}$$

□ **Table 6.18** Combined SPSS output to investigate mediation of the causal association between the change in the HAQ score after 52 weeks of treatment and ESR at baseline by the HAQ score at baseline

Coefficients

Model		Unstandardized Coefficients		Standardized Coefficients	t	Sig.	95 % Confidence Interval for B	
		B	Std. Error	Beta			Lower Bound	Upper Bound
1[a]	(Constant)	−.374	.080		4.647	.000	−.533	−.215
	ESR	−.012	.000	−.447	−6.120	.000	−.016	−.008
2[b]	(Constant)	.899	.081		11.138	.000	.741	1.050
	ESR	.014	.002	.509	7.109	.000	.011	.018
3[a]	(Constant)	.122	.091		1.337	.183	−.058	.301
	ESR	−.004	.002	−.160	−2.266	.025	−.008	−.001
	HAQ_wk0	−.551	.068	−.572	−8.099	.000	−.686	−.417

[a]Dependent Variable: change in HAQ score
[b]Dependent Variable: HAQ score at baseline

$$\text{mean dHAQ} = b_{0,3} + c' \times ESR + b \times \text{HAQ\_wk0}, \quad\quad (M6.11)$$

where $b_{0,1}$, $b_{0,2}$ and $b_{0,3}$ are the intercepts of the different regression models. A variable is considered to be a mediator if all regression coefficients (a, b, c and c') in these models differ statistically significantly from zero. If one of the regression coefficients does not differ significantly from zero, mediation is not present.

□Table 6.18 shows the SPSS outputs of these three models. The estimate of the total effect (the c-path) is found in model "1": the total effect of ESR at baseline on the change in HAQ after 52 weeks is −0.012 (95 % CI [−0.016; −0.008]), $p < 0.001$). The estimate of the a-path is found in model "2": 0.014 (95 % CI [0.011; 0.018], $p < 0.001$). The estimates of the b- and c'-path are found in model "3": −0.55 (95 % CI [−0.69; 0.42], $p < 0.001$) and −0.004 (95 % CI [−0.008; −0.001], $p = 0.025$), respectively. Because all associations are statistically significant at the significance level α of 0.05, we conclude that the association between the change in the HAQ score after 52 weeks and ESR at baseline is mediated by the HAQ score at baseline. To quantify the effect of mediation, the indirect effect is calculated by

1. $c - c' = -0.012 - -0.004 = -0.008$, or by
2. $a \times b = 0.014 \times -0.551 \approx -0.008$

In other words, the effect of ESR at baseline on the change in the HAQ score was −0.012 (per increase of 1 mm/h increase in ESR), but two-thirds of this effect (i.e., 0.008 / 0.012) is mediated by the HAQ score at baseline.

◻ Table 6.19 Estimated direct and indirect effect of HAQ at baseline on the causal association between change in HAQ after 52 weeks and ESR at baseline, with a boostrapped 95 % CI for the indirect effect

Direct effect of ESR at baseline on change in HAQ score		
Variable	Effect	95 % CI
ESR at baseline	−0.012	−0.016; −0.008
Indirect effect of ESR at baseline on change in HAQ score		
Variable	Effect	Bootstrapped 95 % CI
ESR at baseline	−0.008	−0.011; −0.005

A 95 % CI for the indirect effect cannot be computed using the standard form of a CI (▶ Eq. E2.2, ▶ Sect. 2.3.3) because the indirect effect depends on two estimates. Instead, the bootstrap procedure needs to be used. With the bootstrap procedure, a predefined number of new samples is created by random sampling the same number of patients from the original study population with replacements. For each bootstrap sample, the three regression models are re-estimated to calculate the indirect effect in that sample. This is repeated many times (1,000 times is commonly used), and the 95 % bootstrap CI is then obtained by taking the 2.5th and 97.5th percentile of the bootstrapped indirect effects. This could be done in SPSS with several macros, but other statistical software such as R or Stata could also be used. We used R (version 3.4.2) to compute the 95 % bootstrap CI for the indirect effect of HAQ score at baseline on the association between the change in the HAQ score after 52 weeks of treatment and ESR at baseline (◻Table 6.19, with 1,000 bootstrapped samples). From the 95 % CI we conclude that with 95 % confidence the true indirect effect in the research population lies between −0.011 and −0.005.

There are other methods to investigate mediation, such as the method of MacKinnon et al. [3–5, 12], and structural equation modelling (path analyses) [6].

6.5   Multiple Regression Models

In all examples up to now, a research question with one outcome variable and one central determinant was studied, and corrected for potential confounder(s) and/or effect modifier(s). Sometimes a researcher is more interested in the joint influence of several variables on the outcome variable, in which all these variables of interest are added to a regression model at once. Regression models with multiple variables are called multiple regression models (or multivariable regression models), as opposed to simple regression models (or univariable regression models) with one single variable. An incorrect term for multiple regression models, yet frequently used in scientific papers, is multivariate regression models (and univariate regression models for simple regression models).

However, from a statistical point of view, multivariate regression models refer to regression models with multiple outcome variables modeled at the same time, and consequently, univariate models refer to regression models with one single outcome variable but with one or multiple determinants.

6.5.1 Interpretation of a Multiple Linear Regression Model

In multiple regression models, multiple regression coefficients are estimated. We first explain how to analyze a multiple linear regression model, with DAS44 after 52 weeks of treatment ('DAS44_wk52') in the COBRA-light trial as outcome variable, with the research question

> ❓ Is the DAS44 after 52 weeks of treatment associated with treatment arm (i.e., COBRA-light versus COBRA strategy), the DAS44 at baseline, ESR at baseline and being aCCP positive at baseline in patients with early RA?

The regression model consists of four determinants: the received treatment (with COBRA coded as zero and COBRA-light as one), the DAS44 at baseline ('DAS44_wk0'), ESR at baseline ('ESR_wk0') and aCCP status (with negative coded as zero and positive coded as one). The multiple linear regression model equals

$$\text{mean DAS44\_wk52} = b_0 + b_1 \times \text{treatment} + b_2 \times \text{DAS44\_wk0} \\ + b_3 \times \text{ESR\_wk0} + b_4 \times \text{aCCP}. \tag{M6.12}$$

The linear regression model now has five regression coefficients:

- b_0 is the mean DAS44 after 52 weeks of treatment when all determinants are equal to zero, i.e., for patients treated with the COBRA strategy; a DAS44 score at baseline of zero; an ESR value at baseline of zero; and who are aCCP negative. After all, for such a patient ▶ Model M6.12 yields

$$\text{mean DAS44\_wk52} = b_0 + b_1 \times 0 + b_2 \times 0 + b_3 \times 0 + b_4 \times 0 = b_0.$$

- b_1 is the difference in mean DAS44 after 52 weeks of treatment between patients treated with COBRA-light and COBRA strategy, but with the same DAS44, ESR and aCCP status at baseline. For example, for two patients, one treated with COBRA and one with COBRA-light, both with a DAS44 score at baseline of 3.5; an ESR at baseline of 30 mm/h, and both aCCP positive, ▶ Model M6.12 yields

$$\text{mean DAS44\_wk52} = b_0 + b_1 \times 0 + b_2 \times 3.5 + b_3 \times 30 + b_4 \times 1,$$

$$\text{mean DAS44\_wk52} = b_0 + b_1 \times 1 + b_2 \times 3.5 + b_3 \times 30 + b_4 \times 1.$$

Hence the difference between these patients is equal to b_1.
- b_2 is the difference in mean DAS44 after 52 weeks of treatment between two patients who differ by one point in the DAS44 at baseline, but with the same treatment (could be either one), ESR level and aCCP status at baseline.

▫ **Table 6.20**   SPSS output of a multiple linear regression model, relating the DAS44 after 52 weeks of treatment to treatment arm, the DAS44 score at baseline, ESR at baseline and aCCP status at baseline

Coefficients[a]

Model		Unstandardized Coefficients		Standardized Coefficients	t	Sig.	95.0 % Confidence Interval for B	
		B	Std. Error	Beta			Lower Bound	Upper Bound
1	(Constant)	.657	.452		1.452	.149	−.237	1.551
	treatment	.232	.152	.119	1.526	.129	−.069	.533
	DAS44_wk0	.322	.113	.274	2.834	.005	.097	.546
	ESR_wk0	−.002	.004	−.049	−.511	.610	−.010	.006
	aCCP	−.324	.164	−.158	−1.970	.051	−.649	.001

[a]Dependent Variable: DAS44 (after 52 weeks)

- b_3 is the difference in mean DAS44 after 52 weeks of treatment between two patients who differ by 1 mm/h in ESR at baseline, but with the same treatment (could be either one), the same DAS44 score and the same aCCP status at baseline.
- b_4 is the difference in mean DAS44 after 52 weeks of treatment between two patients of which one is aCCP positive and one is aCCP negative, but treated according to the same strategy and with the same DAS44 score and ESR level at baseline.

The interpretation of b_0 has no clinical meaning in this example: patients with a DAS44 score of zero at baseline and an ESR level of 0 mm/h are not included in this trial. As for the simple linear regression model, the continuous determinant(s) could be centralized so that b_0 has a meaningful interpretation.

▫Table 6.20 shows the SPSS output of this model, each regression coefficients b_0 to b_4 in a different row. SPSS also calculates the standardized regression coefficients. These are the regression coefficients of a model in which all variables, i.e., the outcome variable and all determinants, are standardized (▶ Sect. 3.1). This allows for an easy comparison of all regression coefficients: all are interpreted as the mean increase in outcome variable (measured in SD) for an increase of 1 SD in each of the determinants. The standardized regression coefficients range between −1 and 1: the closer to zero, the weaker the effect of the determinant on the outcome variable. An increase of the outcome variable measured on the SD level, however is clinically difficult to interpret, so usually these regression coefficients are not reported in the scientific paper.

For each regression coefficient the null hypothesis, i.e., the estimate is equal to zero, is tested against the alternative hypothesis, i.e., the estimate is unequal to zero. A p-value smaller than the significance level α of 0.05 indicates that the determinant is associated with the outcome variable, i.e., influences the outcome variable, while a p-value larger than α indicates that there is no evidence of an influence on the outcome. So in our example model, only the DAS44 at baseline significantly influences the DAS44. The higher the DAS44 at baseline, the higher the DAS44 after 52 weeks, with an increase of 0.32 points after 52 weeks of treatment per increase of 1 point at baseline (95 % CI [0.97; 0.55], $p=0.005$). For this study, patients treated with the COBRA-light strategy had on average a 0.23 point higher DAS44 after 52 weeks of treatment than patients treated with the COBRA strategy, but this was not statistically significant (95 % CI [−0.069; 0.53], $p=0.13$). There was also no influence of ESR at baseline (mean difference −0.002 per 1 mm/h increase, 95 % CI [−0.010; 0.006], $p=0.61$) and of aCCP status (mean difference −0.32, 95 % CI [−0.65; 0.001], $p=0.051$).

6.5.2 Interpretation of a Multiple Logistic Regression Model

A multiple logistic regression model is interpreted similarly as a multiple linear regression model. We illustrate this by assessing the association of development of RA within 2 years in the RA-cohort with three determinants: age at baseline, having a first-degree relative (FDR) with RA (with having no FDR with RA coded as zero and having an FDR with RA as one), and duration of morning stiffness ('stiffness', with less than one hour coded as zero and at least one hour as one). The multiple logistic regression equals

$$\ln(\text{odds for RA within 2 years}) = b_0 + b_1 \times \text{age} + b_2 \times \text{FDR}$$
$$+ b_3 \times \text{stiffness}. \tag{M6.13}$$

This logistic regression model has four regression coefficients:
- b_0 is the baseline $\ln(\text{odds})$ to develop RA within 2 years for a patient of age zero, who does not have an FDR with RA and reports having morning stiffness for less than one hour. After all, for that patient ▶Model M6.13 yields

$$\ln(\text{odds for RA within 2 years}) = b_0 + b_1 \times 0 + b_2 \times 0 + b_3 \times 0 = b_0.$$

- b_1 is the difference in $\ln(\text{odds})$ between two patients who differ by 1 year in age, but either both have an FDR with RA or they both do not have an FDR with RA, and with the same duration of morning stiffness. For example, for two patients, one aged 50 and one aged 51, but both without an FDR with RA and both reported having morning stiffness for at least one hour, ▶Model M6.13 is equal to

$$\ln(\text{odds for RA within 2 years}) = b_0 + b_1 \times 50 + b_2 \times 0 + b_3 \times 1,$$

$$\ln(\text{odds for RA within 2 years}) = b_0 + b_1 \times 51 + b_2 \times 0 + b_3 \times 1.$$

Hence the difference in $\ln(\text{odds})$ between these patients is equal to b_1, and the OR per increase of 1 year in age (with equal FDR with RA and morning stiffness duration) is equal to $\exp(b_1)$.
- b_2 is the difference in $\ln(\text{odds})$, i.e., $\exp(b_2)$ is the OR for development of RA within 2 years, between two patients, one with and one without an FDR with RA but of the same age and with the same duration of morning stiffness.

◘ **Table 6.21** SPSS output of a multiple logistic regression model, relating development of RA within 2 years to age, having an FDR with RA and duration of morning stiffness

Variables in the Equation

		B	SE	Wald	df	Sig.	Exp(B)	95 % C.I.for EXP(B)	
								Lower	Upper
Step 1ª	age	−.010	.012	.747	1	.388	.990	.968	1.013
	FDR	.218	.294	.549	1	.459	1.244	.699	2.214
	stiffness	.982	.320	9.441	1	.002	2.670	1.427	4.997
	Constant	−.356	.584	.371	1	.542	.701		

ªVariable(s) entered on step 1: age, FDR, stiffness

- b_3 is the difference in ln(odds), i.e., $\exp(b_3)$ is the OR for development of RA within 2 years, between two patients, one reports having duration of morning stiffness for at least one hour and one for less than one hour, but of the same age and either both with an FDR with RA or both without an FDR with RA.

The interpretation of $\exp(b_0)$ has no clinical meaning in this example: patients with an age of zero at baseline are not included in this cohort. As for the simple logistic regression model, centralized continuous determinant(s) provide $\exp(b_0)$ with a meaningful interpretation.

◘Table 6.21 shows the SPSS output of this model. Only the 283 patients with at least 2 years of follow-up were included in the analysis. The regression coefficient for each determinant is reported in different rows. For each regression coefficient separately the null hypothesis, i.e., that the coefficient is equal to zero, is tested against the alternative hypothesis, i.e., that the coefficient is unequal to zero. In our exemplary model, only the duration of morning stiffness influences the odds to develop RA within 2 years. Patients who report having morning stiffness for at least one hour have higher odds to develop RA within 2 years compared to patients who report morning stiffness lasts for less than one hour (OR 2.7, 95 % CI [1.4; 5.0], $p=0.002$). The odds to develop RA within 2 years does not depend on age at baseline (OR 0.99 per increase of 1 year, 95 % CI [0.97; 1.01], $p=0.39$) and also not on having an FDR with RA (OR 1.2, 95 % CI [0.70; 2.2], $p=0.46$). The OR for age per increase of 5 or 10 years instead of per year, can be computed for the OR per increase of 1 year in the same way as in a simple logistic regression model (▶Example 4.2, ▶Sect. 4.4.1).

6.5.3 Interpretation of a Multiple Cox Regression Model

A multiple Cox regression model is interpreted similarly as a multiple linear and logistic regression model. We illustrate this by studying the association between the time to development of RA and the same three determinants as in the multiple logistic regression model: age at baseline, having an FDR with RA, and duration of morning stiffness (▶ Sect. 6.5.2). The multiple Cox regression model equals

$$\ln(h(t)) = \ln(h_0(t)) + b_1 \times \text{age} + b_2 \times \text{FDR} + b_3 \times \text{stiffness}. \qquad \text{(M6.14)}$$

The function $h_0(t)$ is the baseline hazard function, i.e., the hazard function for the time to development of RA for a patient of age zero, without an FDR with RA and in whom morning stiffness lasts for less than one hour. After all, for that patient ▶ Model M6.14 yields

$$\ln(h(t)) = \ln(h_0(t)) + b_1 \times 0 + b_2 \times 0 + b_3 \times 0 = \ln(h_0(t)).$$

The interpretation of the three regression coefficients are as follows:

- b_1 is the difference in $\ln(h(t))$ between two patients who differ by 1 year in age, but either both with an FDR with RA or both without an FDR with RA and the same duration of morning stiffness. For example, for two patients, one aged 50 and one aged 51, but both without an FDR with RA and both reported having morning stiffness for at least one hour, ▶ Model M6.14 yields

$$\ln(h(t)) = \ln(h_0(t)) + b_1 \times 50 + b_2 \times 0 + b_3 \times 1,$$

$$\ln(h(t)) = \ln(h_0(t)) + b_1 \times 51 + b_2 \times 0 + b_3 \times 1.$$

  Hence the difference in $\ln(h(t))$ between these patients is equal to b_1, and the HR per increase of 1 year in age (either both with or both without an FDR with RA and equal morning stiffness duration) is equal to $\exp(b_1)$.
- b_2 is the difference in $\ln(h(t))$, i.e., $\exp(b_2)$ is the HR for the time to development of RA, between two patients, one with and one without an FDR with RA, but of the same age and with the same duration of morning stiffness.
- b_3 is the difference in $\ln(h(t))$, i.e., $\exp(b_3)$ is the HR for the time to development of RA, between two patients, one who reports having morning stiffness for at least one hour and one who reports having mornings stiffness for less than one hour, but of the same age and either both with an FDR with RA or both without an FDR with RA.

The interpretation of the baseline hazard function $h_0(t)$ has no clinical meaning in this example: patients aged zero at baseline are not included in this cohort. As for the simple Cox regression model, centralizing the continuous determinant(s) provides the $h_0(t)$ with a meaningful interpretation.

▢Table 6.22 shows the SPSS output for this model. In this analysis all 374 patients of the RA-cohort were included. Only the duration of morning stiffness influences the time to development of RA. Patients in whom morning stiffness is present for more than one hour developed RA faster compared to patients in whom morning stiffness is present for less than one hour (HR 2.0, 95 % CI [1.3; 3.0], $p=0.001$). The time to development of RA does not depend on the age at baseline (HR 0.99 per increase of 1 year, 95 % CI [0.98; 1.0], $p=0.25$) and also not on having an FDR with RA (HR 1.3, 95 % CI [0.92; 2.0], $p=0.13$). The HR for age per increase of 5 or 10 years instead of per 1 year, is computed from the HR per increase of 1 year in the same way as in a simple logistic or Cox regression model (▶ Example 4.4, ▶ Sect. 4.4.1).

□ **Table 6.22**   SPSS output of a multiple Cox regression model, relating time to development of RA to age, having an FDR with RA and duration of morning stiffness

Variables in the Equation

	B	SE	Wald	df	Sig.	Exp(B)	95.0 % CI for Exp(B)	
							Lower	Upper
age	−.009	.008	1.312	1	.252	.991	.976	1.006
FDR	.299	.197	2.297	1	.130	1.348	.916	1.984
stiffness	.702	.210	11.176	1	.001	2.018	1.337	3.045

6.5.4 Checking Assumptions in a Multiple Regression Model

Most of the assumptions that need to be checked for the simple regression models also need to be checked for multiple regression models. First of all, linearity between the outcome of the model (i.e., ln(odds) for the logistic regression model and $\ln(h(t))$ for the Cox regression model) and any continuous determinant needs to be checked. For all three models, this assumption is tested in exactly the same way as in the simple regression models: either by adding a square term, or by dividing the determinant into quartiles and compare the differences between the consecutive regression coefficients. They should be more or less equal (or more specifically, lie more or less on a straight line, ▶Sects. 3.4.4, 4.4.2, and 5.4.2). Below, we describe how to assess the other assumptions in a multiple linear and multiple Cox regression model.

Multiple Linear Regression Model

In addition to the linearity assumption, the normality and homoscedasticity assumptions of the linear regression model have to be checked. The extension of the general simple linear regression model (▶Model M3.3, ▶Sect. 3.4.2) for k determinants $x_1, x_2, ..., x_k$ is

$$Y = b_0 + b_1 \times x_1 + b_2 \times x_2 + ... + b_k \times x_k + \varepsilon. \tag{M6.15}$$

The assumptions of this model are

1. ε is normally distributed with mean equal to zero (normality);
2. the variance of ε does not depend on any of the determinants $x_1, x_2, ..., x_k$ (homoscedasticity);
3. the association between Y and any continuous determinant is linear (linearity).

Normality of the error variable ε is investigated with a histogram (or QQ-plot) of the saved residuals. If this assumption is violated, transforming the outcome variable could be a solution. Unfortunately, there is no alternative for multiple linear regression models if the transformation does not result in normally distributed residuals. Note that the normality assumption is formulated for the error variable and not for the outcome variable

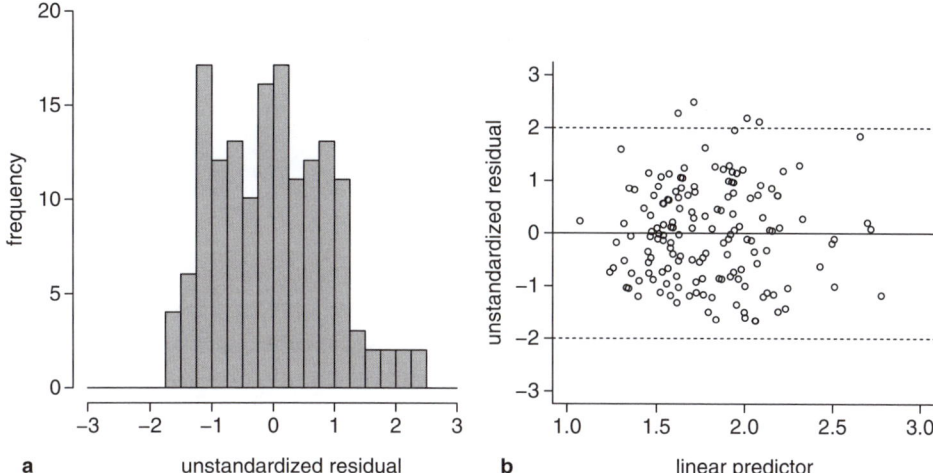

      unstandardized residual   **b**   linear predictor

■ **Fig. 6.6** Histogram of the residuals (**a**) and residual-versus-predictor plot (**b**) of a multiple linear regression model for the DAS44 after 52 weeks of treatment

nor for a continuous determinant. Finally, homoscedasticity is investigated with the residual-versus-predictor plot. Instead of plotting such a plot for each determinant separately, the predictor plotted on the x-axis is the linear predictor (LP):

$$\mathrm{LP} = b_0 + b_1 \times x_1 + b_2 \times x_2 + \ldots + b_k \times x_k. \hspace{2cm} \text{(E6.1)}$$

■ Figure 6.6 shows the histogram of the residuals (**a**) and the residual-versus-predictor (**b**) of the multiple linear regression model for DAS44 after 52 weeks. The linear predictor using the results of ■ Table 6.20 was computed as follows

$$0.657 + 0.232 \times \text{treatment} + 0.322 \times \text{DAS44\_wk0} - 0.002$$
$$\times \text{ESR\_wk0} - 0.324 \times \text{aCCP}.$$

Based on the histogram and residual-versus-predictor plot, the assumptions of normality and homoscedasticity seem valid. We did not investigate the linearity assumption between DAS44 after 52 weeks of treatment and DAS44 or ESR at baseline for illustrative purposes. We assumed it is valid, though this should have been checked first.

Multiple Cox Regression Model

In a multiple Cox regression model, the proportionality assumption for each determinant needs to be checked individually. For each parameter in the model (i.e., including the dummy variables of a categorical determinant), the Schoenfeld residuals are plotted against time (■ Fig. 6.7). For each parameter, proportionality holds if the slope of the regression line through the residuals is equal to zero. This is tested with a linear regression model, for each parameter separately (■ Table 6.23). The residuals for age (■ Fig. 6.7a) seem to bounce randomly around the value zero. The residuals for having an FDR with RA (■ Fig. 6.7b) seem to increase over time, and for duration of morning

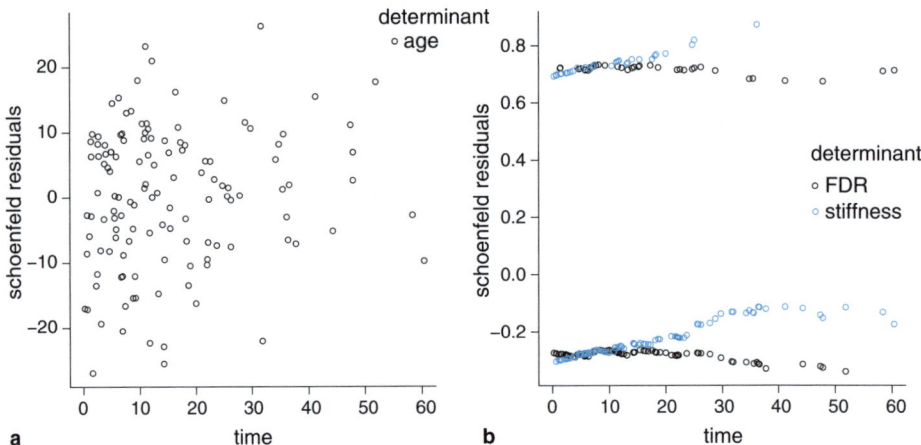

○ **Fig. 6.7** Scatterplot of the Schoenfeld residuals against time, to investigate the proportionality assumption for each determinant (**a**: age; **b**: FDR and stiffness) in a multiple Cox regression model

○ **Table 6.23**   Combined SPSS output of three linear regression models, testing the proportionality assumption in each of the determinants in a multiple Cox regression model

Coefficients[a]

Model		Unstandardized Coefficients		Standardized Coefficients	t	Sig.
		B	Std. Error	Beta		
1[a]	(Constant)	−.675	1.366		−.494	.622
	follow-up time (months)	.040	.059	.059	.676	.500
1[b]	(Constant)	−.052	.057		−.918	.360
	follow-up time (months)	.003	.002	.110	1.256	.211
1[c]	(Constant)	.045	.053		.847	.398
	follow-up time (months)	−.003	.002	−.102	−1.159	.248

[a]Dependent Variable: Partial residual for age
[b]Dependent Variable: Partial residual for FDR
[c]Dependent Variable: Partial residual for stiffness

stiffness (○Fig. 6.7b) seem to decrease over time. However, none of the *p*-values of the follow-up time are significant ($p=0.50$ for age, $p=0.21$ for having an FDR with RA, and $p=0.25$ for duration of morning stiffness). Hence, the slope of the three linear regression models can be assumed to be zero. We therefore conclude that the proportionality assumption holds for each of the determinants in the multiple Cox regression model.

6.6 Further Readings

Extensive information on confounding and effect modification, which is sometimes also referred to as interaction, can be found in the classical textbooks written by Kirkwood & Sterne and by Rothman et al. [7, 8]. They cover regression models as well as stratified analyses, including the Mantel-Haenszel pooled OR. The Mantel-Haenszel pooled OR is also described in more detail by Armitage et al. [9]. More information on the interpretation of multiple regression models can be found in these classical textbooks as well [7–9]. Multiple Cox regression models are also described in the tutorials on survival analysis in the British Journal of Cancer, parts II and III [10, 11].

References

1. ter Wee MM, den Uyl D, Boers M, Kerstens P, Nurmohamed M, van Schaardenburg D, et al. Intensive combination treatment regimens, including prednisolone, are effective in treating patients with early rheumatoid arthritis regardless of additional etanercept: 1-year results of the COBRA-light open-label, randomised, non-inferiority trial. Ann Rheum Dis. 2015;74(6):1233–40. ▶https://doi.org/10.1136/annrheumdis-2013-205143.
2. van de Stadt LA, Witte BI, Bos WH, van Schaardenburg D. A prediction rule for the development of arthritis in seropositive arthralgia patients. Ann Rheum Dis. 2013;72(12):1920–6. ▶https://doi.org/10.1136/annrheumdis-2012-202127.
3. MacKinnon DP, Fairchild AJ, Fritz MS. Mediation analysis. Annu Rev Psychol. 2007;58:593–614. ▶https://doi.org/10.1146/annurev.psych.58.110405.085542.
4. MacKinnon DP, Krull JL, Lockwood CM. Equivalence of the mediation, confounding and suppression effect. Prev Sci. 2000;1(4):173–81. ▶https://doi.org/10.1023/a:1026595011371.
5. MacKinnon DP, Lockwood CM, Hoffman JM, West SG, Sheets V. A comparison of methods to test mediation and other intervening variable effects. Psychol Methods. 2002;7(1):83–104. PMC: 2819363.
6. Gunzler D, Chen T, Wu P, Zhang H. Introduction to mediation analysis with structural equation modeling. Shanghai Arch Psychiatry. 2013;25(6):390–4. ▶https://doi.org/10.3969/j.issn.1002-0829.2013.06.009.
7. Kirkwood BR, Sterne JAC. Essential Medical Statistics. 2nd ed. Oxford: Blackwell Science Ltd; 2003.
8. Rothman KJ, Lash TL, Greenland S. Modern epidemiology. 3rd ed. Philadelphia: Lippincott-Raven; 2012.
9. Armitage P, Berry G, Matthews JNS. Statistical methods in medical research. Oxford: Blackwell Science Ltd; 2002.
10. Bradburn MJ, Clark TG, Love SB, Altman DG. Survival analysis part II: multivariate data analysis – an introduction to concepts and methods. Br J Cancer. 2003;89(3):431–6. ▶https://doi.org/10.1038/sj.bjc.6601119.
11. Bradburn MJ, Clark TG, Love SB, Altman DG. Survival analysis part III: multivariate data analysis – choosing a model and assessing its adequacy and fit. Br J Cancer. 2003;89(4):506–11. ▶https://doi.org/10.1038/sj.bjc.6601120.
12. MacKinnon DP. Introduction to statistical mediation analyses. New York: Routledge; 2008.

To Predict or not to Predict?

Abstract

In published research, many expressions such as 'predictor', 'association', 'relation with' or 'prognostic factor', are used to describe the interpretation of results. Often, these terms are randomly applied, ignoring the correct context in which they have to be used. In the interpretation of results, it is important to always keep in mind whether the analyses are based on an association model or a prediction model. In this chapter we explain the difference between association and prediction, as well as how to build a prediction model, assess its quality and how to compare different prediction models.

© Bohn Stafleu van Loghum is een imprint van Springer Media B.V., onderdeel van Springer Nature 2019
M. M. ter Wee and B. I. Lissenberg-Witte, *A Quick Guide on How to Conduct Medical Research*,
https://doi.org/10.1007/978-90-368-2248-0_7

7.1 Association Versus Prediction

In ▶Chap. 6 (except for ▶Sect. 6.5), all examples focused on the association between one outcome variable and one central determinant. The main aim was to estimate the association as precisely as possible. This is considered an association model. All research questions considered in ▶Chap. 3–6 are examples of an association model. The results of such models should always be reported focusing on the association between the outcome variable and the central determinant of interest, and include both the crude analyses (▶Chap. 3–5) as well as the corrected analyses (▶Chap. 6).

The aim of a prediction model is to build the best but simplest regression model, consisting of a combination of determinants, to predict the future outcome of a new patient. Famous examples of a prediction model are the Framingham model [1, 2], and the test to predict the possibility of a fetus having Down syndrome [3, 4]. Important differences between an association and a prediction model are

1. the formulation of the research question;
2. no hypotheses are defined in a prediction model;
3. the interpretation of the results.

All these differences are explained in the following sections.

7.2 Building Prediction Models

The research question of a study designed to build a prediction model, does not follow the PICO(t) model as there is usually no comparison (C) and no intervention (I) group. This means that in the research question involving a prediction model, no central determinant is specified as the focus is on finding the best combination of variables (from now on referred to as predictors) that predict the outcome the most accurately. Moreover, since the study does not focus on the effect of one central determinant on the outcome variable, no hypotheses are formulated in such studies either. ▶Example 7.1 illustrates two different research question for the two different types of models.

Example 7.1

Different research questions for an association and a prediction model

Association model: Is there a difference between the COBRA-light strategy (the intervention, I) compared to the COBRA strategy (the comparison, C) in decrease of the disease activity score (the outcome, O) in patients with early rheumatoid arthritis (the patient, P) after 52 weeks of treatment (the time, T)?

Prediction model: Which combination of variables measured at baseline can predict having a low disease activity score (the outcome, O) in patients with early rheumatoid arthritis (the patient, P), after 52 weeks of treatment in the COBRA-light trial (the time, T)?

To build a prediction model, several selection procedures are available to choose from. The two simplest procedures are the backward and the forward selection procedure. We describe and illustrate these procedures below. Prediction models can be developed for a continuous, a dichotomous, and a time to event outcome variable; the steps to take in the selection procedure are equal for the three types of outcome variables.

7.2.1 Selection of Predictors

Before the selection procedure is run to build a prediction model, a predefined inclusion criterion is set. The inclusion criterion is a criterion for the p-value of the predictor. Predictors are included in the model (in the forward procedure) or excluded from the model (in the backward procedure) as long as their p-values fullfil this criterion. The criterion often depends on the size of the study population: the larger the study population, the smaller the p-value for inclusion in the model. P-values smaller than 0.05, 0.1 or 0.2 are commonly used. The inclusion criterion in a backward selection procedure is referred to as p-removal; the criterion in a forward selection procedure as p-entry.

In most research, the database contains many variables which are considered potential predictors. It is impossible to include all variables in the selection procedure and therefore, possible predictors are pre-selected with univariable analyses in case of many potential predictors. In that case, only those predictors with a p-value smaller than 0.05 (i.e., significantly associated with the outcome variable), are entered in the selection procedure (either the forward or the backward selection). Sometimes, depending on the size of the study population, variables with a p-value smaller than 0.1 or 0.2 in the pre-selection procedure are entered in the selection procedure.

7.2.2 Number of Predictors in the Model

The number of predictors that can be included in a prediction model is limited. There is a rule of thumb for the number of predictors in a prediction model, depending on the type of outcome variable, to prevent overfitting. For a continuous outcome variable, this rule of thumb states that at least 10 patients per included predictor in the model are required in the study population. For a dichotomous or time to event outcome variable, this rule of thumb states that at least 10 events and 10 non-events per predictor are required. Keep in mind that for a categorical predictor with k categories k-1 dummy variables are (or need to be) created, so that this predictor actually counts for k-1 predictors instead of 1. Sometimes a stricter rule of thumb is used: at least 15 patients per included predictor for a continuous outcome variable and at least 15 events and 15 non-events for a dichotomous or time to event outcome variable. Note that these rules of thumb also apply to an association model when correcting for confounding and effect modification.

For example, based on a study population of 160 patients, a prediction model for a continuous outcome can contain at most 16 predictors and if one predictor is a categorical determinant with four groups, at most 13 other predictors (i.e., $16 - 3$) could be included. The maximum number of predictors in a prediction model for a dichotomous or time to event outcome variable, is determined by the smallest group of patients with or without the event. For example, in a study population of 160 patients of which 60 patients have (or develop) an event and 100 do not, the prediction model can contain at most 6 predictors.

7.2.3 Backward Selection Procedure

The backward selection procedure starts with a full regression model including all potential predictors. In the first step of the procedure, the predictor with the highest p-value is removed. In the next step of the procedure, a new regression model is estimated, excluding the removed variable. Again, the predictor with the highest p-value is removed from the regression model. These steps are repeated until all of the remaining predictors fulfill the predefined inclusion criterion (i.e., their p-values are all below p-removal).

We illustrate this procedure with the following research question, using data from the COmbinatie Behandeling Reumatoïde Artritis (COBRA)-light trial [5]

> ❓ Which variables measured at baseline predict the disease activity score of 44 joints (DAS44) in early rheumatoid arthritis (RA) patients after 52 weeks of treatment in the COBRA-light trial?

The outcome variable in this case is the DAS44 after 52 weeks of treatment, which is a continuous outcome variable, hence we use a linear regression model to answer this research question. The DAS44 after 52 weeks of treatment was available for 154 patients included in the trial, therefore we set p-removal at 0.05.

The following variables measured at baseline are included in the backward selection procedure: age at baseline, gender (with female coded as zero and male as one), body mass index (BMI), smoking status ('smoking', with current non-smoker coded as zero and current smoker as one), treatment arm (with COBRA treatment coded as zero and COBRA-light treatment coded as one), disease duration ('duration', in weeks), rheumatoid factor type immunoglobulin M (IgM-RF) status (with IgM-RF negative coded as zero and IgM-RF positive as one), anticyclic citrullinated peptide (aCCP) status (with aCCP negative coded as zero and aCCP positive as one), C-reactive protein (CRP; in mg/L), total tender and swollen joint count ('TJC' and 'SJC', respectively), DAS44 at baseline ('DAS44_wk0'), fatigue (with not fatigue coded as zero and being fatigue as one), morning stiffness ('stiffness', with no morning stiffness coded as zero and morning stiffness coded as one), Health Assessment Questionnaire (HAQ) score, general wellbeing, pain and disease activity measured by visual analogue scale (VAS; 'VAS_general', 'VAS_pain', and 'VAS_RA', respectively), and the disease activity of the patient as judged by the physician, also measured with a VAS score ('VAS_physician').

In the first step of the backward selection procedure, all variables are entered to the linear regression model with DAS44 after 52 weeks of treatment as outcome variable. ◨Table 7.1 shows the SPSS output of the full model. The predictor with the highest p-value is the first removed, in this case age ($p = 0.92$).

□ **Table 7.1**   SPSS output of the first step in the backward selection procedure to predict DAS44 after 52 weeks of treatment

Coefficients[a]

Model		Unstandardized Coefficients		Standardized Coefficients	t	Sig.	95.0 % Confidence Interval for B	
		B	Std. Error	Beta			Lower Bound	Upper Bound
1	(Constant)	.490	.868		.565	.574	−1.236	2.217
	age	−.001	.009	−.012	−.107	.915	−.019	.017
	gender	−.428	.214	−.199	−1.998	.049	−.853	−.002
	BMI	.016	.017	.094	.972	.334	−.017	.050
	smoking	.390	.221	.171	1.763	.082	−.050	.830
	treatment	.235	.198	.116	1.189	.238	−.158	.629
	duration	.003	.005	.056	.590	.556	−.007	.012
	IgM_RF	−.065	.264	−.032	−.246	.806	−.589	.459
	aCCP	−.380	.293	−.182	−1.297	.198	−.962	.203
	CRP	.003	.004	.086	.744	.459	−.005	.012
	TJC	.015	.018	.116	.866	.389	−.020	.051
	SJC	−.071	.026	−.371	−2.694	.009	−.124	−.019
	DAS44_wk0	.345	.261	.263	1.322	.190	−.174	.864
	fatigue	.335	.235	.150	1.426	.157	−.132	.803
	stiffness	−.146	.308	−.044	−.473	.637	−.757	.466
	HAQ	.202	.181	.133	1.115	.268	−.158	.563
	VAS_general	.002	.007	.035	.236	.814	−.012	.015
	VAS_pain	.010	.007	.215	1.356	.179	−.005	.024
	VAS_RA	−.010	.007	−.218	−1.442	.153	−.025	.004
	VAS_physician	−.002	.008	−.028	−.257	.798	−.019	.014

[a]Dependent Variable: DAS44 (after 52 weeks)

This step is repeated until all predictors included in the model have a p-value smaller than 0.05. After removal of the predictor age, the following predictors were removed (in chronological order): VAS general well-being ($p = 0.82$), VAS physician ($p = 0.81$), IgM-RF ($p = 0.71$), morning stiffness ($p = 0.64$), disease duration ($p = 0.54$), CRP ($p = 0.42$), total tender joint count ($p = 0.38$), BMI ($p = 0.36$), smoking ($p = 0.12$), VAS disease activity ($p = 0.14$), VAS pain ($p = 0.42$), treatment arm ($p = 0.15$), gender ($p = 0.12$), and HAQ score ($p = 0.056$). Important to note is that in the model from which gender was removed, both fatigue and gender had the same p-value. In the case of equal p-values for two or more potential predictors, the value of the test statistic

	Mean difference	95 % CI	p-value
Intercept	0.54		
Being aCCP positive	−0.48	−0.84; −0.12	0.010
Swollen joint count	−0.074	−0.11; −0.033	<0.001
DAS44 (at baseline)	0.40	0.030; 0.78	0.035
Being fatigue	0.57	0.30; 0.85	<0.001

◘ **Table 7.2** Final prediction model for the DAS44 after week 52 of treatment

(the t-statistic under "t") is predominate: the higher the absolute value of the t-statistic, the smaller the p-value. For this reason gender was removed (with a t-statistic of -1.551 versus 1.553 for fatigue). Another possibility is to look at the exact p-values in SPSS, by double clicking on the output table and double clicking on the specific cells containing the p-value.

It took 16 steps to build the final prediction model. ◘Table 7.2 presents the results of the final prediction model as it would be reported in a scientific paper. In general, the intercept (i.e., b_0) is only reported for prediction models and not for association models. In a prediction model, the intercept is needed to predict the outcome of a new patient (▶ Sect. 7.3). The conclusion to our research question is that the DAS44 after 52 weeks of treatment is predicted by being aCCP positive, amount of swollen joints, DAS44 at baseline and being fatigued at baseline. Having a higher DAS44 at baseline as well as being fatigued at baseline increases the DAS44 score after 52 weeks of treatment while being aCCP positive and having a higher swollen joint count at baseline decreased the DAS44 score.

Two remarks need to be made about this example. First of all, for any continuous predictor, the linearity assumption (of the relation between the predictor and the outcome variable) always needs to be checked before including it as a continuous predictor in the selection procedure. For illustrative purposes, we skipped this check as, in clinical practice, a continuous predictor is often included without checking the linearity assumption. Secondly, based on the rule of thumb, we were only allowed to include 15 predictors in the first step of the selection procedure because our study population consisted of 154 patients. However, in this example we included 19 predictors. We could have first tested which of these 19 variables were associated with DAS44 after 52 weeks of treatment in a simple linear regression model (or univariable linear regression model) for each potential predictor separately. We would only then include those variables with a p-value smaller than 0.05, for example, in the first step of the backward selection procedure. This would have shortened the procedure, and is the preferred procedure to follow in the case of many potential predictors.

7.2.4 Forward Selection Procedure

The forward selection procedure starts with an empty prediction model (the null model, or 'base case' model). In the first step of this procedure, each possible predictor is added individually to the null model as a simple regression model. After the first step, the predictor with the lowest p-value is then included in the model. This model is then considered the new 'base case' model, to which each of the remaining predictors are added, again individually, in the second step of the procedure. The predictor with the lowest p-value is included to the new 'base case' model that then consists of two predictors. These steps are repeated until none of the predictors fulfill the predefined inclusion criterion (p-entry).

To illustrate the forward selection procedure, the RA-cohort [6] was used to build a prediction model for the dichotomous outcome variable development of RA within 2 years. The research question is as follows

> **?** Which variables measured at baseline can predict the development of RA within 2 years in patients with arthralgia?

A total of 283 patients were included in this analysis, after excluding all patients with a follow-up time of less than 2 years, of which 101 (36 %) developed RA within 2 years. For illustrative purposes, we used one of the imputed databases of the RA-cohort because some variables in the original database contained missing values. As this group is relatively small, we set a p-value smaller than 0.1 as inclusion criterion (i.e., p-entry $= 0.1$). We included the following variables in the selection procedure: age at baseline, gender (with male codes as one and female as two), having a first-degree relative (FDR) with RA, smoking, alcohol use, non-steroid anti-inflammatory drug (NSAID) use, duration of symptoms < 12 months ('duration'), intermittent symptoms present ('intermittent'), symmetric arthralgia ('symmetric'), arthralgia in upper and lower extremities ('extremities'), arthralgia in small joints ('smallJoints'), VAS ≥ 50 ('VAS50'), morning stiffness ≥ 1 h ('stiffness'), swollen joint(s) reported ('SJC44'), tender joint(s) reported ('TJC53'), CRP status ('CRP') and antibody status (with IgM-RF positive but aCCP negative coded as one and set as reference group, IgM-RF negative but aCCP low positive coded as two, IgM-RF negative but aCCP high positive coded as three, and IgM-RF positive and aCCP positive coded as four). For all dichotomous predictors, no or negative was coded as zero and yes or positive as one, except for alcohol use, where alcohol use was coded as zero and no alcohol use as one.

In the first step of the forward selection procedure, all potential predictors are added individually as predictors. ◻Table 7.3 shows the combined SPSS output of these univariable logistic regression models. In this case, several predictors have a p-value smaller than 0.001. Because SPSS only reports the first three decimals of the p-values, it is difficult to judge which predictor has the smallest p-value. If this would occur in the case of only non-categorical (i.e., dichotomous or continuous) predictors – so when all degrees of freedoms are 1 – the Wald statistic (under "Wald") is used to select the predictor with the smallest p-value. After all, the higher the value of the Wald statistic, the lower the p-value. In this example, a categorical predictor is included in the selection procedure and we therefore have to check the overall p-value (in the row "antibody"). Although the Wald statistic for antibody is the highest, is also has three degrees of freedoms and therefore cannot be compared to the other predictors with a p-value smaller than 0.001. So we need to check the exact p-values in SPSS, by double clicking on the output table, and double clicking on

◻ Table 7.3 Combined SPSS output for the first step in the forward selection procedure to build a prediction model for the development of RA within 2 years

	B	SE	Wald	df	Sig.	Exp(B)	95 % C.I. for EXP(B)	
							Lower	Upper
age	−.013	.011	1.371	1	.242	.987	.965	1.009
gender	.052	.290	.033	1	.857	1.054	.597	1.861
FDR	.114	.287	.158	1	.691	1.121	.639	1.966
smoking	−.444	.273	2.656	1	.103	.641	.376	1.094
alcohol	.541	.256	4.479	1	.034	1.718	1.041	2.836
NSAID	.165	.275	.360	1	.548	1.180	.688	2.023
duration	.674	.264	6.521	1	.011	1.963	1.170	3.294
intermittent	.936	.256	13.322	1	.000	2.550	1.542	4.215
symmetric	.367	.296	1.534	1	.216	1.443	.808	2.578
extremities	.550	.253	4.705	1	.030	1.732	1.054	2.846
smallJoints	−.204	.279	.534	1	.465	.816	.472	1.409
VAS50	.592	.257	5.325	1	.021	1.808	1.093	2.990
stiffness	.975	.315	9.588	1	.002	2.652	1.430	4.916
SJC44	.122	.259	18.746	1	.000	3.071	1.848	5.104
TJC53	.465	.252	3.404	1	.065	1.592	.971	2.608
CRP	.308	.418	.543	1	.461	1.361	.600	3.087
antibody			35.125	3	.000			
antibody(1)	1.013	.469	4.657	1	.031	2.753	1.097	6.906
antibody(2)	1.621	.424	14.653	1	.000	5.059	2.206	11.604
antibody(3)	2.262	.398	32.222	1	.000	9.600	4.397	20.962

the cell of the p-value. The p-value of antibody status was the lowest ($p = 0.000000114$), compared to the p-values of intermittent symptoms ($p = 0.000262$) and reported swollen joints ($p = 0.000015$). Therefore, antibody status was included first.

In the following step of the selection procedure, all remaining potential predictors were added to the logistic regression model including antibody status. The following predictors were entered into the model (in chronological order): VAS pain ($p = 0.002$), swollen joints reported ($p = 0.003$), duration of symptom ($p = 0.009$), intermittent symptoms ($p = 0.010$), morning stiffness ($p = 0.014$), smoking ($p = 0.039$), arthralgia in small joints ($p = 0.058$), and arthralgia in lower and upper extremities ($p = 0.081$). In total, 10 steps were needed to build the final prediction model. ◻Table 7.4 shows the final model, as it would be reported in a scientific paper. The regression coefficients for each predictor as well as the intercept of the model (i.e., b_0) are also reported. We need these values to compute the predicted probability that a new patient with certain characteristics will develop RA within 2 years. How this is done is explained in ▶Sect. 7.3.2.

□ Table 7.4 Final prediction model for the development of RA within 2 years

	OR	95 % CI	p-value	B
Antibody status			<0.001	
IgM-RF positive but aCCP negative	1.0			
IgM-RF negative but aCPP low positive	2.7	0.97; 7.3		0.976
IgM-RF negative but aCPP high positive	5.4	2.1; 13.7		1.686
IgM-RF and aCPP positive	9.1	3.7; 22.2		2.204
VAS pain ≥ 50	3.1	1.6; 6.0	0.001	1.140
Swollen joints reported	2.2	1.2; 4.1	0.009	0.799
Symptom duration < 12 months	2.5	1.3; 4.8	0.006	0.910
Intermittent symptoms present	2.2	1.2; 4.1	0.012	0.788
Morning stiffness ≥ 1 h	2.6	1.2; 5.4	0.013	0.943
Smoking	0.47	0.24; 0.90	0.023	−0.766
Arthralgia in small joints	0.48	0.25; 0.94	0.031	−0.735
Arthralgia in lower/upper extremities	1.7	0.93; 3.2	0.081	0.553
Intercept				−3.076

The conclusion to our research question is that the development of RA within 2 years is predicted by antibody status, VAS pain score, reported swollen joints, duration of symptoms, intermittent symptoms, morning stiffness, smoking, and arthralgia in the small joints as well as in the lower and upper extremities. All predictors, except smoking and arthralgia in small joints, increase the risk of developing RA within 2 years.

7.3   Linear Predictor (or Prediction Rule)

Since the regression model is always a linear combination of the predictors, this combination is called the linear predictor (LP) or prediction rule. For any new patient, the outcome of the prediction model is predicted with the LP. For a continuous outcome variable, the LP predicts the outcome itself. For a dichotomous outcome, the LP predicts the odds for the positive outcome. For a time to event outcome, the LP predicts the hazard function (which is translated to the survival or cumulative incidence function).

Every prediction model can be translated into an LP. The LP of a linear or logistic regression prediction model including k predictors (e.g., $x_1, x_2 \ldots x_k$) is equal to

$$\mathrm{LP} = b_0 + b_1 \times x_1 + b_2 \times x_2 + \ldots + b_k \times x_k, \qquad \text{(E7.1)}$$

where b_0 is equal to the intercept and b_i is the regression coefficient of predictor x_i. The LP of a Cox regression model is slightly different than that of a linear of logistic regression model since a Cox regression model does not have an intercept b_0 as the 'baseline' risk is given by the baseline hazard function $h_0(t)$

$$\mathrm{LP} = b_1 \times x_1 + b_2 \times x_2 + \ldots + b_k \times x_k. \qquad \text{(E7.2)}$$

7.3.1 Linear Regression Prediction Model

The LP of the linear regression prediction model to predict the DAS44 score after 52 weeks of treatment (◻Table 7.2; ▶Sect. 7.2.3) is equal to

$$\text{DAS44\_wk52} = 0.54 - 0.48 \times \text{aCCP} - 0.074 \times \text{TSJC}$$
$$+ 0.40 \times \text{DAS44\_wk0} + 0.57 \times \text{fatigue}.$$

Example 7.2

Predicted DAS44 scores after 52 weeks of treatment

Patient A: the predicted DAS44 score after 52 weeks of treatment for a new patient who is not fatigued (fatigue = 0), has a DAS44 score at baseline of 3.15, 9 swollen joints and is aCCP negative (aCCP = 0), would be

$$\text{DASS44\_wk52} = 0.54 - 0.48 \times 0 - 0.074 \times 9 + 0.40 \times 3.15 + 0.57 \times 0 \approx 1.13.$$

Patient B: the predicted DAS44 score after 52 weeks of treatment for a new patient who is fatigue, has a DAS44 score at baseline of 1.89, 12 swollen joints, and is aCCP positive, would be:

$$\text{DASS44\_wk52} = 0.54 - 0.48 \times 1 - 0.074 \times 12 + 0.40 \times 1.89 + 0.57 \times 1 \approx 0.50.$$

7.3.2 Logistic Regression Prediction Model

For a logistic regression prediction model, the probability for the outcome of interest, i.e., the 'success' outcome, is calculated from the LP. The LP looks similar as the LP of a linear regression prediction model, but the outcome of the logistic regression model is the natural logarithm (ln) of the odds instead of the actual value of the outcome variable, as is the case in a linear regression prediction model. The LP for the prediction model to predict development of RA within 2 years (◻Table 7.4; ▶Sect. 7.2.4) is equal to

$$\text{LP} = -3.08 + 0.98 \times \text{antibody}(1) + 1.69 \times \text{antibody}(2) + 2.20$$
$$\times \text{antibody}(3) + 1.14 \times \text{VAS50} + 0.80 \times \text{SJC44} + 0.91$$
$$\times \text{duration} + 0.79 \times \text{intermittent} + 0.94 \times \text{stiffness} - 0.77$$
$$\times \text{smoking} - 0.74 \times \text{smallJoints} + 0.55 \times \text{extremities}.$$

From the LP we calculate the probability that a patient with certain characteristics at baseline will develop RA within 2 years by extending ▶Eq. E4.8 (▶Sect. 4.4.1) as follows

$$P(Y = 1) = \frac{1}{1 + \exp(-\text{LP})} \tag{E7.3}$$

Example 7.3

Calculating the probability to develop RA within 2 years

Patient A: the LP for development of RA within 2 years for a new patient who is IgM-RF negative but aCPP low positive (antibody(1) = 1, antibody(2) = 0, antibody(3) = 0), has a VAS pain below 50 (VAS50 = 0), does not report having swollen joints (SJC44 = 0), has 14 months of symptom duration (duration = 1), with presence of intermittent symptoms (intermittent = 1), morning stiffness of at least one hour (stiffness = 1), who does not smoke (smoking = 0), and has arthralgia in small joints (smallJoints = 1), but not in the lower and upper extremities (extremities = 0), is equal to

$$LP = -3.08 + 0.98 \times 1 + 1.69 \times 0 + 2.20 \times 0 + 1.14 \times 0 + 0.80 \times 0 + 0.91 \times 0$$
$$+ 0.79 \times 1 + 0.94 \times 1 - 0.77 \times 0 - 0.74 \times 1 + 0.55 \times 0 \approx -1.10$$

Hence the probability to develop RA within 2 years for this patient is equal to

$$P(Y = 1) = \frac{1}{1 + \exp(-(-1.10))} \approx 0.25$$

In other words, this patient has a probability of 25 % to develop RA within 2 years.

Patient B: the LP for development of RA within 2 years for a new patient who is IgM-RF and aCPP positive (antibody(3) = 1), has a VAS pain of 50 or above (VAS50 = 1), reports having swollen joints (SJC44 = 1), has 6 months of symptom duration (duration = 0), with presence of intermittent symptoms (intermittent = 1), morning stiffness of at least one hour (stiffness = 1), who does not smoke (smoking = 0), and has arthralgia in small joints (smallJoints = 1), as well as in the lower and upper extremities (extremities = 1), is equal to

$$-3.08 + 0.98 \times 0 + 1.69 \times 0 + 2.20 \times 1 + 1.14 \times 1 + 0.80 \times 1 + 0.91$$
$$\times 1 + 0.80 \times 1 + 0.94 \times 1 - 0.77 \times 0 - 0.74 \times 1 + 0.55 \times 1 \approx 3.49$$

Hence the probability to develop RA within 2 years for this patient is equal to

$$P(Y = 1) = \frac{1}{1 + \exp(-(3.49))} \approx 0.97.$$

In other words, this patient has a probability of 97 % to develop RA within 2 years.

7.3.3 Cox Regression Prediction Model

The prediction model of van de Stadt et al. [6], predicting the time to development of RA, was built with a Cox regression model, using the backward selection procedure, with a *p*-value of 0.10 as the inclusion criteria. Of the 374 included patients, 131 developed RA after a median follow-up time of 12 months (IQR [6–23]). The final model included the following variables: having an FDR with RA, alcohol use, duration of symptoms, intermittent symptoms, arthralgia in upper and lower extremities, VAS pain, duration of morning stiffness, swollen joint(s), and antibody status classified in the four groups as used in the previous section (◻Table 7.5). The LP of the prediction model of van de Stadt et al. is equal to

◻ Table 7.5 Points assigned to each of the predictors in the prediction model of van de Stadt et al. [6]. Categories not listed were assigned zero points

Predictor (x_i)	b_i	Points
Having an FDR with RA	0.43	1
No alcohol	0.37	1
Duration of symptoms <12 months	0.54	1
Intermittent symptoms present	0.56	1
Arthralgia in upper and lower extremities	0.32	1
VAS $\geq$ 50	0.82	2
Morning stiffnes $\geq$ 1 h present	0.50	1
Swollen joint(s) reported	0.50	1
Antibody status IgM-RF positive but aCCP negative IgM-RF negative but aCCP low positive IgM-RF negative but aCCP high positive IgM-RF and aCCP positive	 0 1.00 1.58 1.94	 0 2 3 4

$$LP = 0.43 \times FDR + 0.37 \times alcohol + 0.54 \times duration + 0.55 \times intermittent$$
$$+ 0.32 \times extremities + 0.82 \times VAS50 + 0.50 \times stiffness + 0.57 \times SJC44$$
$$+ 1.00 \times antibody(1) + 1.58 \times antibody(2) + 1.94 \times antibody(3).$$

The survival function or cumulative incidence function for a new patient with certain characteristics is estimated for the LP in combination with the estimated baseline hazard function $h_0(t)$. However, in prediction models for a time to event outcome variable, this is rarely done. Instead, each predictor in the model is assigned a score (or a number of points). The regression coefficient of each predictor in the prediction model of van de Stadt et al. was rounded to half points and then multiplied by two [6]. ◻Table 7.5 shows the points assigned to each predictor in the prediction model of van de Stadt et al. The total number of points a patient could score ranged from 0 to 12. For each patient the prediction rule, based on these assigned points, is then calculated, and Kaplan-Meier curves are plotted for each number of points. When some curves lie close to each other, they could be identified as a group of patients with similar risk. In the study of van de Stadt et al. [6], patients with a score between zero and four were classified as having 'low' risk to develop RA, patients with a score of five or six points were classified as having 'intermediate' risk, and patients with a score of seven or higher were classified as having 'high' risk.

◻Figure 7.1 shows the one minus Kaplan-Meier curves for the three risk groups. From the survival table, for example, the probability that a patient with a certain risk classification will develop RA within 2 and 5 years could be obtained (◻Table 7.6).

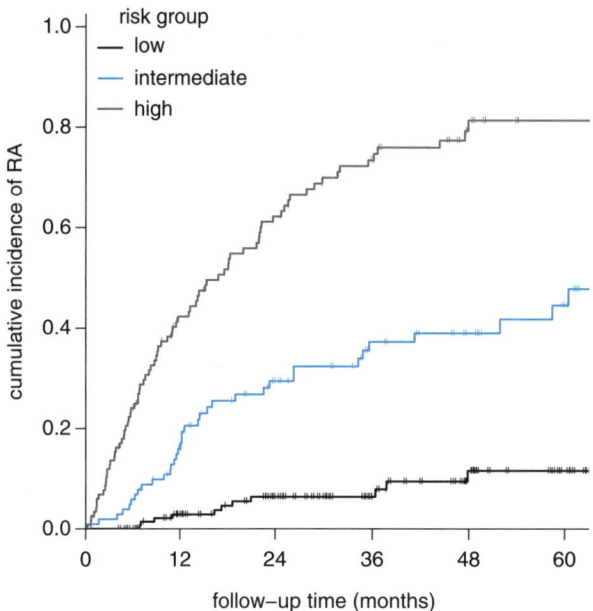

◻ Fig. 7.1 One minus Kaplan-Meier curves for the time to development of RA, stratified by risk group of the prediction model

Example 7.4

Estimating the probability to develop RA within 2 and 5 years
Patient A: the prediction rule for a new patient who has an FDR with RA, does not take alcohol, has less than 12 months of symptom duration, no intermittent symptoms present, arthralgia in the upper and lower extremities, a VAS pain below 50, morning stiffness for less than 1 hour, reported having swollen joints and is IgM-RF positive but aCPP negative, is equal to

$$1 \times 1 + 1 \times 1 + 1 \times 1 + 1 \times 0 + 1 \times 1$$
$$+ 2 \times 0 + 1 \times 0 + 1 \times 1 + 0 \times 1 = 5.$$

This patients has an intermediate risk to develop RA, and the probability that he/she will develop RA within 2 or 5 years is $1 - 0.706 = 0.294$ and $1 - 0.554 = 0.446$, i.e., 29 % and 45 %, respectively.
Patient B: the prediction rule for a new patient who has an FDR with RA, takes alcohol, has less than 12 months of symptom duration, intermittent symptoms present, arthralgia in the upper and lower extremities, a VAS pain of at least 50, morning stiffness for at least 1 hour, reported not having swollen joints and is IgM-RF positive and aCPP positive, is equal to

$$1 \times 1 + 1 \times 1 + 1 \times 1 + 1 \times 1 + 1 \times 1$$
$$+ 2 \times 1 + 1 \times 1 + 1 \times 0 + 4 \times 1 = 12.$$

This patient has a high risk to develop RA, and the probability that he/she will develop RA within 2 or 5 years is $1 - 0.378 = 0.622$ and $1 - 0.187 = 0.813$, i.e., 62 % and 81 %, respectively.

□ Table 7.6 Part of SPSS output of the survival table, stratified by risk group of the prediction model

Survival Table

Risk group	Time		Status	Cumulative Proportion Surviving at the Time		N of Cumulative Events	N of Remaining Cases
				Estimate	Std. Error		
low	1	4.140	no arthritis	.	.	0	153
	20	11.039	arthritis	.972	.014	4	134
	43	16.361	arthritis	.963	.016	5	111
	49	20.994	arthritis	.937	.022	8	105
	92	36.370	arthritis	.922	.026	9	62
	114	47.836	arthritis	.884	.036	11	40
	152	72.444	arthritis	.589	.242	12	2
intermediate	1	.624	arthritis	.990	.010	1	101
	22	11.729	arthritis	.840	.037	16	80
	28	12.025	arthritis	.829	.038	17	74
	49	23.261	arthritis	.706	.048	27	53
	56	26.218	arthritis	.676	.051	29	46
	82	58.382	arthritis	.554	.063	35	20
	86	60.386	arthritis	.521	.067	36	16
high	1	.230	arthritis	.992	.008	1	117
	62	11.729	arthritis	.577	.047	47	56
	63	13.109	arthritis	.567	.048	48	55
	82	23.688	arthritis	.378	.048	66	36
	84	24.706	arthritis	.368	.048	67	34
	109	47.836	arthritis	.187	.044	81	9
	116	64.854	arthritis	.125	.059	82	2

7.4 Quality of Multiple Regression Prediction Models

If all predictors have a p-value below the inclusion criterion, it only indicates that the predictors (independent of each other) influence the outcome variable. However, it does not provide any indication on the quality of the model. It is important to know how well the model predicts the outcome, and also to quantify how much of the variation between patients is explained by the predictors included in the prediction model. There are several measures to quantify the quality of the prediction model (called goodness-of-fit measures); for different multiple regression prediction models (i.e., linear, logistic and

Cox) different measures exist. These goodness-of-fit measures could also be computed to quantify the quality of an association regression model either a simple or a multiple association regression model, although this is not adviced.

7.4.1 Linear Regression Prediction Model

The quality of a linear regression prediction model is measured by the amount of explained variance, the R^2 (or R-square), which is equal to

$$R^2 = \frac{\text{explained variation}}{\text{total variation}} \qquad \text{(E7.4)}$$

The total variation is the squared standard deviation (SD) of the outcome variable in the study population. The explained variation is the variation explained by the multiple linear regression prediction model. In mathematical equations, the total and explained variation are equal to

$$\text{total variation} = \sum (Y_i - \text{mean}(Y_i))^2, \qquad \text{(E7.5)}$$

$$\text{explained variation} = \sum \left(\widehat{Y}_i - \text{mean}(Y_i) \right)^2, \qquad \text{(E7.6)}$$

where, for patient i, Y_i is the observed value, $\widehat{Y}_i$ is the (model) predicted value of the outcome variable, and mean(Y_i) is the study population mean of the outcome variable. The better the model, the more of the total variation in the study population is explained by the model. Put differently, the closer the value R^2 lies to 1 (or to 100 %), the better the model.

The R^2 of a linear regression prediction model is default part of the SPSS output of a linear regression model. ◘Table 7.7 shows the SPSS model summary output of the linear regression prediction model predicting the DAS44 score after 52 weeks of treatment, build with the backward selection procedure in ▶ Sect. 7.2.3. The value of R^2 is reported under "R square", the value of R (i.e., the square root of R^2) is reported under "R". The more predictors added to the model, the higher the R^2. The adjusted R^2 (under "Adjusted R Square") corrects for the number of predictors in the model as follows

$$\text{adjusted } R^2 = 1 - \left(1 - R^2 \right) \times \frac{n-1}{n-k-1}, \qquad \text{(E7.7)}$$

where k is the number of predictors in the model. Note that each dummy variable of a categorical predictor counts as one predictor for this formula. Under "Std. Error of the Estimate", the SD of the error variable ε in linear regression model is reported. From ◘Table 7.7, we conclude that 23 % (i.e., $R^2 = 0.229$) of the variation in the DAS44 score after 52 weeks of treatment is explained by differences in gender, DAS44 at baseline, total swollen joint count and aCCP status.

◻ **Table 7.7** SPSS output of the prediction model summary, including the R^2, predicting the DAS44 after 52 weeks of treatment

Model summary				
Model	R	R Square	Adjusted R Square	Std Error of the Estimate
1	.479[a]	.229	.208	.8718

[a]Predictors: (Constant), aCPP, gender, DAS44_wk0, SJC

7.4.2 Logistic Regression Prediction Model

There are several measures to assess the quality of logistic regression prediction models: with Nagelkerke's R^2, by calibration with the calibration curve and the Hosmer and Lemeshow test, and through discrimination with a receiver operating characteristic (ROC) curve and its corresponding area under the curve (AUC).

Nagelkerke's R^2

In a logistic regression prediction model, the ln(odds) for a dichotomous outcome variable is modelled. Although the ln (odds) can take any value, the outcome itself can take only two values: 'success' or 'failure'. It is therefore not possible to compute the total variation of the outcome variable itself, and the variation explained by the model as was the case for a continuous outcome variable. However, it is possible to compute a goodness-of-fit measure in a logistic regression prediction model with the same interpretation as the explained variance R^2: the Nagelkerke's R^2. SPSS reports a model summary for every logistic regression model as default output. ◻Table 7.8 shows the SPSS output of the final prediction model for the development of RA within 2 years, obtained with the forward selection procedure in ▶ Sect. 7.2.4 (◻Table 7.4). Nagelkerke's R^2 is reported under "Nagelkerke R Square". SPSS also reports the Cox & Snell R^2 (under "Cox & Snell R Square"), on which Nagelkerke's R^2 is based. However, the maximum value of the Cox & Snell R^2 is 0.75, while Nagelkerke's R^2 can take any value between zero and one. Consequently, Nagelkerke's R^2 is more comparable to the R^2 of a linear regression prediction model, and is therefore preferred as goodness-of-fit measure over the Cox & Snell R^2. Finally, the model summary output table also contains the value of $-2\ln(\text{likelihood})$ (under "-2 Log likelihood"). The likelihood (of the observations) is defined as the product of all the individual predicted probabilities for each patient, based on the prediction model. The value of $-2\ln(\text{likelihood})$ is used to compare two nested models (▶ Sect. 7.6.2). In ◻Table 7.8, we see that Nagelkerke's R^2 is equal to 0.38, hence we conclude that approximately 38 % of the variation in the development of RA within 2 years is explained by differences in the predictors included in the final prediction model.

▣ Table 7.8 SPSS output of the model summary, with Nagelkerke's R^2, predicting development of RA within 2 years

Model Summary			
Step	−2 Log likelihood	Cox & Snell R Square	Nagelkerke R Square
1	276.496[a]	.278	.382

[a]Estimation terminated at iteration number 5 because parameter estimates changed by less than .001

Calibration and Discrimination

The goodness-of-fit of a logistic regression prediction model is usually assessed by calibration and discrimination. Calibration refers to the agreement between the predicted outcome and the observed outcome, whilst discrimination refers to the ability of the model to distinguish between the patients with a positive outcome and patients with a negative outcome. Discrimination and calibration are related to each other: a model with high discrimination has lower calibration, and vice versa. Especially large prediction models provide a better discrimination, but are more difficult to fit and thus have a poorer calibration.

There are several methods to measure calibration of a logistic regression prediction model. We only describe two methods: (1) the calibration curve, and (2) the Hosmer-Lemeshow test. For other goodness-of-fit measures for calibration, we refer to the further readings (►Sect. 7.8). The first step in both methods of calibration is to determine the predicted probabilities for a positive outcome, for each patient individually, using the LP (►Eq. E7.3, ►Sect. 7.3.2). The predicted probabilities can be saved in SPSS as an additional option (Supplementary Information A.5.2). ▣Table 7.9 shows the predicted probabilities to develop RA within 2 years for several patients, based on the prediction model developed in ►Sect. 7.2.4. When the predicted probabilities are saved, descriptive statistics of the predicted probabilities can be obtained. ▣Table 7.10 shows some descriptive statistics: the minimum and maximum predicted probability (under "Minimum" and "Maximum", respectively) and the mean and SD (under "Mean" and "Std. Deviation", respectively). Also the number of patients for whom the predicted probability could be computed is reported (under "N").

Calibration Curve

With a calibration curve, the predicted probabilities are plotted against the observed probabilities. However, because the outcome variable is dichotomous, the observed probabilities cannot be computed for each individual patient separately. Instead, the predicted probabilities are grouped in deciles, i.e., ten groups of approximately the same size (the lowest 10 % of the probabilities are grouped together, the next 10 % are grouped together in the next group, etc.). For each group, the mean of the observed outcomes (i.e., the number of patients with a positive outcome divided by the total number of patients in that group) is computed as well as the mean of the predicted probabilities

◻ **Table 7.9** Predicted probabilities for development of RA within 2 years for the first ten and very last patient in the study population

ID	RA within 2 years	Predicted Probability
1	1	.60909
2	0	.43288
3	1	.61617
4	0	.33440
5	0	.24069
6	0	.78594
7	0	.56844
8	0	.10908
9	1	.58535
10	0	.41413
283	1	.45188

◻ **Table 7.10** SPSS output with some descriptive statistics on the predicted probabilities for all patients

Descriptive Statistics

	N	Minimum	Maximum	Mean	Std. Deviation
Predicted probability	283	.01017	.97139	.3568905	.26105496
Valid N (listwise)	283				

(◻Table 7.11). In the calibration curve, the mean predicted probabilities are then plotted on the x-axis, and the mean observed outcomes on the y-axis (◻Fig. 7.2). If these points lie more or less on the straight line $y = x$, the observed and predicted probabilities match with each other, indicating that the model fits the data well.

Whether the observed and predicted probabilities match, can also be tested statistically. To that end, a logistic regression model for the outcome variable is estimated with the LP as determinant

$$\ln(\text{odds}) = b_0 + b_1 \times \text{LP}. \tag{M7.1}$$

The predicted probabilities agree with the observed outcomes if the intercept b_0 is equal to zero, and the slope b_1 is equal to one. ◻Table 7.12 shows the SPSS output of this logistic regression model. Not surprisingly, the regression coefficients are indeed estimated to be zero (under "B", in the row "Constant") and one (under "B", in the row "LP"). This is because the model is now calibrated in the same study population as the model was built in. Ideally, the LP is calibrated in an external study population (▶ Sect. 7.5.2)

■ **Table 7.11**   Observed and predicted probabilities for the calibration curve

Percentile group	Mean observed outcome	Mean predicted probabilities
1	0.03	0.0319961
2	0.11	0.0706865
3	0.10	0.1173001
4	0.14	0.1804591
5	0.29	0.2613014
6	0.31	0.3650523
7	0.48	0.4708057
8	0.52	0.5505649
9	0.79	0.6810986
10	0.79	0.8348597

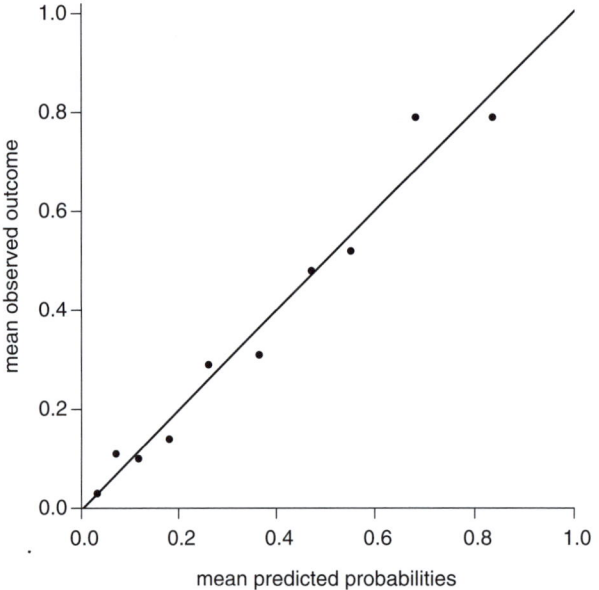

■ **Fig. 7.2**   Calibration curve of the predicted probabilities versus mean observed outcomes of the logistic prediction model for the development of RA within 2 years

Hosmer-Lemeshow Test

Another method to test whether the observed and predicted probabilities match, is with the Hosmer-Lemeshow test. The Hosmer-Lemeshow test compares the observed number of patients with a positive outcome in each decile group of the predicted probabilities

◻ **Table 7.12** SPSS output of the logistic regression model relating the development of RA within 2 years to the LP of the final prediction model

Variables in the Equation

		B	SE	Wald	df	Sig.	Exp(B)
Step 1[a]	LP	1.000	.131	58.332	1	.000	2.718
	Constant	.000	.156	.000	1	1.000	1.000

[a]Variable(s) entered on step 1: LP

◻ **Table 7.13** SPSS output of the contingency table with the number of observed and predicted patients without and with RA after 2 years

Contingency Table for Hosmer and Lemeshow Test

		arthritis within 2 years = no		arthritis within 2 years = yes		Total
		Observed	Expected	Observed	Expected	
Step 1	1	28	28.072	1	.928	29
	2	25	25.999	3	2.001	28
	3	25	24.690	3	3.310	28
	4	24	22.947	4	5.053	28
	5	20	20.684	8	7.316	28
	6	20	17.828	8	10.172	28
	7	14	14.837	14	13.127	28
	8	14	12.656	14	15.344	28
	9	5	9.105	23	18.895	28
	10	7	5.145	23	24.855	30

to the predicted number of patients with a positive outcome in that group. Because the outcome can take only two values, comparing the observed and expected number of patients with a positive outcome is equivalent to comparing the observed and expected number of patients with a negative outcome. SPSS calculates the expected number of patients from the mean predicted probability in that group. The predicted number of patients with a positive outcome is equal to the mean predicted probability in that group times the number of patients in that group. The predicted number of patients with a negative outcome is the total number of patients in that group minus the predicted number of patients with a positive outcome. ◻Table 7.13 shows the SPSS output of the observed and predicted number of patients, which is obtained as additional output of

□ **Table 7.14**   SPSS output of the Hosmer-Lemeshow test

Hosmer and Lemeshow Test			
Step	Chi-square	df	Sig.
1	5.579	8	.694

a logistic regression model (Supplementary Information A.5.2). For each decile group (in the rows "1" to "10"), the observed and expected number of patients who developed RA within 2 years are reported (under "arthritis within 2 years = yes", in "Observed" and "Expected" respectively). The observed and expected number of patients who did not developed RA within 2 years are reported under "arthritis within 2 years = no", in "Observed" and "Expected" respectively. The total number of patients in each decile group is also reported (under "Total"). The Hosmer-Lemeshow test is equal to a chi-square test (for one group), with the following null and alternative hypothesis

H0: the observed and predicted number of patients are equal;
H1: the observed and predicted number of patients are unequal.

□Table 7.14 shows the SPSS output of the Hosmer-Lemeshow test. The value of the chi-square test statistic is reported under "Chi-square", the number of degrees of freedom under "df", and the p-value under "Sig.". From this output, we conclude that there is no evidence to reject the null hypothesis ($p = 0.69$). In other words: this model is well calibrated, or, consequently, has a high goodness-of-fit.

ROC Curve and AUC

The discriminating ability of a logistic regression prediction model is investigated graphically with an ROC curve, in which the predicted probabilities are selected as test variable (▶Sect. 4.6.2). From the ROC curve, the AUC is estimated. The AUC is a measure of concordance: among patients with a low predicted probability only a few should have a positive outcome, while among patients with a high predicted probability only a few should have a negative outcome. □Figure 7.3 shows the ROC curve for the predicted probabilities of the prediction model predicting the development of RA within 2 years build in ▶Sect. 7.2.4. Instead of using the predicted probabilities, the LP (▶Sect. 7.3.2) could be used as well, and the ROC curves will be the same. □Table 7.15 shows the SPSS output with the AUC of this ROC curve. Based on the AUC, we conclude that the prediction model is of high quality, with an AUC of 0.82 (95 % CI [0.77; 0.87]). In other words, the prediction model is considered 'good' at discriminating between patients who will develop RA within 2 years and patients who will not [7].

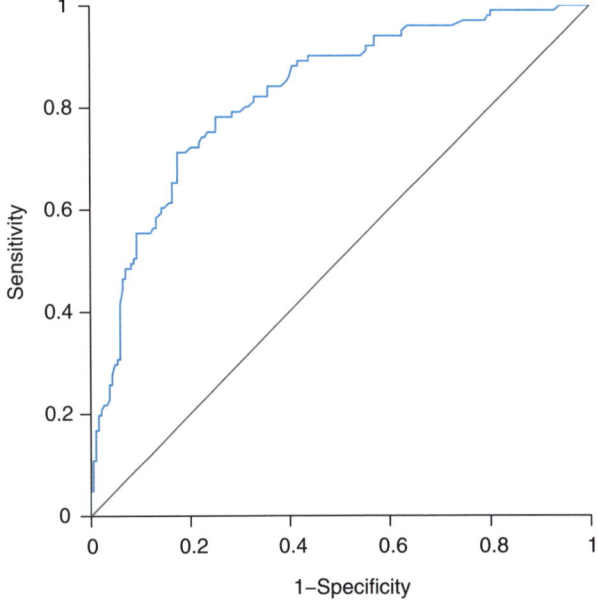

☐ **Fig. 7.3**　ROC curve for predicting the probability to develop RA within 2 years

☐ **Table 7.15**　SPSS output of the AUC for prediction the probability to develop RA within 2 years

Area under the Curve				
Test Result Variable(s): Predicted probability				
Area	**Std.Error[a]**	**Asymptotic Sig.[b]**	**Asymptotic 95 % Confidence Interval**	
			Lower Bound	**Upper Bound**
.825	.026	.000	.775	.875

The test result variable(s): Predicted probability has at least one tie between the positive actual state group and the negative actual state group
Statistics may be biased
[a]Under the nonparametric assumption
[b]Null hypothesis: true are = 0.5

7.4.3　Cox Regression Prediction Model

Harrell's C Index

Since the outcome of a Cox regression model is a function over time, the goodness-of-fit measure needs to take the time into account. There are several measures available, none of them could be computed directly in SPSS, but they could be computed in R or Stata.

We only highlight the Harrell's C index (or Harrell's C statistic), which is a concordance statistic such as the AUC of the ROC. For other goodness-of-fit measures of a Cox regression prediction model, we refer to the further readings (▶ Sect. 7.8).

In general, higher values of the LP of the Cox regression prediction model indicate a higher risk of the event. In other words, in a good prediction model, patients with higher values of the LP should have a shorter time to event. The Harrell's C index compares the time to event and the LP for all pairs of patients. The index is equal to the number of concordant pairs divided by the total number of pairs. Because the index is a ratio, its values ranges from zero to one, with higher values indicating higher concordance, and consequently a better goodness-of-fit. The Harrell's C index has one important disadvantage: pairs that cannot be compared because of censoring are discarded from the comparisons, i.e., a patient with a shorter follow-up time and a censored event cannot be compared to a patient with a longer follow-up time and an observed event. Because the Harrell's C index is a generalization of the AUC, a Harrell's C index between 0.5 and 0.6 indicates very poor concordance (or goodness-of-fit), between 0.6 and 0.7 poor, between 0.7 and 0.8 fair, between 0.8 and 0.9 good, and between 0.9 and 1.0 excellent [7].

The prediction model of van de Stadt et al., predicting the time to development of RA, had a Harrell's C index of 0.79 (95 % CI [0.74; 0.84]), and the simpler prediction rule classifying patients as low, moderate and high risk to develop RA had a Harrell's C index of 0.78 (95 % CI [0.73; 0.84]). Based on these values, the researchers concluded that both the model and the simpler prediction rule are of fair quality to predict the time to development of RA within to and 5 years.

7.5   Validation of Multiple Regression Prediction Models

Once the quality of a prediction model is deemed good enough for clinical practice, validity of the model needs to be investigated before the prediction model is implemented. Validity of a model refers to the generalizability of the model. There are two types of validation: internal and external validation.

7.5.1   Internal Validation

Internal validation is determined on the same study population that was used to build the model. There are several methods for internal validation; we only highlight two commonly used methods: the bootstrap procedure and cross-validation.

Bootstrap Procedure

With the bootstrap procedure, the predictive performance of the model is investigated by (repeatedly) creating new (random) samples from the original study population. The bootstrap procedure follows four distinctive steps.
1. Take a random sample, of the same size (with replacement) of the patients of the original study population. This new sample is called the bootstrap sample.

2. Estimate the regression coefficients of the model in the bootstrap sample, as well as the goodness-of-fit measure (e.g., the R^2 for a linear regression prediction model, the AUC for a logistic regression prediction model and Harrell's C statistic for a Cox regression prediction model).
3. Repeat steps 1 and 2 a large number of times (at least 250 times, but most commonly advised is at least 1,000 samples).
4. Compute the median and the 2.5th and 97.5th percentile of the estimated regression coefficient (per coefficient) and the goodness-of-fit measure. This results in the bootstrapped estimated regression coefficients, and the bootstrapped estimated goodness-of-fit.

Important to note in step 1 is that no new predictors are selected, only the predictors that are validated are included in the model. In this way, only the regression coefficients of the predictors are estimated in this test set. Some macros exists for the bootstrap procedure in SPSS, but generally other statistical software is used, such as Stata and R. However, this is a rather complex procedure, so when performing bootstrap, we advise to consult a statistician.

Cross-Validation

With cross-validation the predictive performance of the model is investigated by predicting the outcome in a new patient or a population of patients that was not used to build the model. There are different ways of cross-validation, such as leave-one-out cross-validation, leave-p-out cross-validation, and k-fold cross-validation. All cross-validation methods consist of several steps. In leave-one-out cross-validation the following five steps are taken.

1. Exclude patient 1 from the database, this new database is called the test set, and estimate the model.
2. Predict the outcome for patient 1 based on this new model.
3. Compute the difference between the predicted outcome and the observed outcome.
4. Repeat steps 1 to 3 for all other patients.
5. Compute the mean of the square of these differences over all patients.

The smaller the mean squared difference computed in step 5, the better the prediction model. Again, no new predictors are selected in step 1.

How to predict the outcome for each patient based on the new model in step 2 depends on the type of outcome variable. For a continuous outcome variable, the predicted outcome is directly computed from the LP of the prediction model. For a dichotomous outcome variable, the predicted outcome is based on a cut-off value for the predicted probability classifying this patient as either positive or negative, for example with the ROC curve (▶ Sect. 4.6.2). For a time to event outcome variable, the predicted outcome is based on the likelihood of the observation, which we will not elaborate on as it lies beyond the scope of this quick guide.

With leave-p-out cross-validation, a total of p patients are excluded from the test-set, and the outcome of these p patients are then predicted in step 2. This is repeated for all possible samples of p patients, which makes it rather time consuming for large samples. Instead, with k-fold cross-validation, the sample is divided in k mutually exclusive subsamples. Each of these subsamples is left out once, so that the test set consists of all other subsamples.

■ **Table 7.16**   SPSS output of the AUC for the test and the validation set to illustrate external validation

Area Under the Curve[a,d]

Test Result Variable(s): LP

Set	Area	Std. Error[b]	Asymptotic Sig.[c]	Asymptotic 95 % Confidence Interval	
				Lower Bound	Upper Bound
test	.880	.030	.000	.822	.939
validation	.717	.044	.000	.630	.804

[a]For split file set = test, the test result variable(s): LP has at least one tie between the positive actual state group and the negative actual state group. Statistics may be biased
[b]Under the nonparametric assumption
[c]Null hypothesis: true area = 0.5
[d]For split file set = validation, the test result variable(s): LP has at least one tie between the positive actual state group and the negative actual state group. Statistics may be biased

Cross-validation cannot be performed in SPSS, but it is possible in R and Stata. However, this is again rather complex, so when performing cross-validation, we advise to consult a statistician.

7.5.2 External Validation

With external validation, the goodness-of-fit measures are determined in an external (new) study population. To that end, the LP of the model to be validated is computed for all patients in the external study population. From the LP, the R^2 (in case of a continuous outcome variable), the AUC (for dichotomous outcome variable) or Harrell's C (for a time to event outcome variable) is computed, which is then compared to the goodness-of-fit of the original study population.

To illustrate external validation, let us reconsider the prediction model for the development of RA within 2 years. Unfortunately, we do not have an external sample. Therefore, the original study population was split in two datasets: a test and a validation set. We estimated the regression coefficients of the model build in ▶ Sect. 7.2.4 in one set, which we refer to as the test set. Then, we computed the LP for the patients in the other set, which we refer to as the validation set. Note that this actually is the first step of a 2-fold (internal) cross-validation. ■Table 7.16 shows the SPSS output of the AUC for both sets separately. The AUC of the original study population (test set) is much higher (0.88, 95 % CI [0.82; 0.94]) than the AUC of the external study population (validation set: 0.72, 95 % CI [0.63; 0.80]). This indicates that the model might not be valid in external samples, despite the high discrimination in the original study population. This is, however, probably due to overfitting: we included all predictors selected with the forward selection procedure in ▶ Sect. 7.2.4, while the test set and the validation set are much smaller (with 136 and 147 patients, respectively, of whom 49 and 52 patients

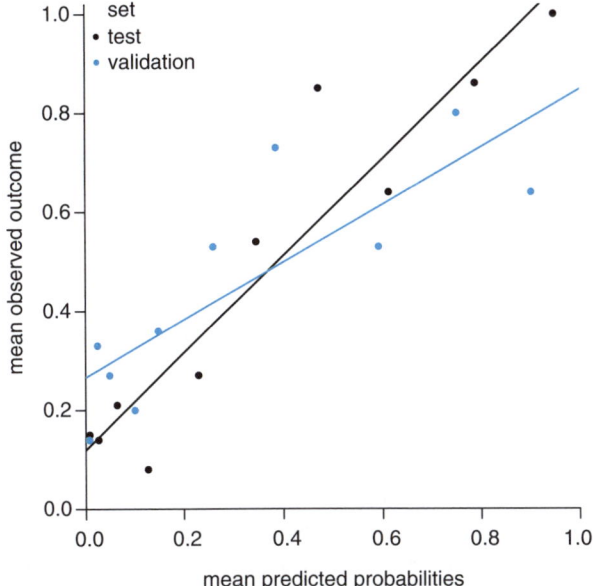

■ **Fig. 7.4**   Calibration curves for the test set and validation set

developed RA within 2 years). In other words, the number of predictors in the model is too high according to the rule of thumb. In other statistical software packages it is possible to formally test whether the AUC's differ, but this is not possible in SPSS.

Calibration-in-the-Large

For a logistic regression prediction model, external validation of the model is also possible with the calibration curve. This is called calibration-in-the-large. The predicted probabilities are computed for all patients in the external study population, using their values of the LP. These predicted probabilities are again grouped in deciles, and for each group the mean of the observed outcomes and the mean of the predicted probabilities are computed. ■Figure 7.4 shows the calibration curves of the test set and the validation set. The slope of the line through the calibration points of the validation set seems to be less steep (and smaller than one) than that of the line through the points of the test set. This could indicate optimism of the predictions, meaning that the predictions are too extreme: the predicted probabilities are too low (compared to what is actually observed) for low predicted probabilities and too high (compared to what is actually observed) for high predicted probabilities. If the slope were larger than one, this could indicate that the predictions are not sufficiently extreme. This can be tested statistically with a logistic regression model.

■Table 7.17 shows the SPSS output of a logistic regression model, with the LP as the only determinant, for each of the sets separately. The results are in line with the calibration curves: the regression coefficient in the test set is estimated to be zero (intercept) and one (slope), but that is because the model was built in this set. The intercept in the validation model does not differ significantly from zero, but the slope does differ

▣ Table 7.17   SPSS output of the logistic regression model relating the development of RA within 2 years to the LP of the final prediction model, for the test and validation set separately

Variables in the Equation

Set			B	SE	Wald	df	Sig.	Exp(B)
test	Step 1[a]	LP	1.000	.179	31.100	1	.000	2.718
		Constant	.000	.245	.000	1	.999	1.000
validation	Step 1[a]	LP	.382	.094	16.506	1	.000	1.465
		Constant	−.177	.203	.761	1	.383	.838

[a]Variable(s) entered on step 1: LP

significantly from one. This cannot be concluded from the p-value in the output as this tests whether or not the slope is equal to zero, but has to be checked with the 95 % CI for the slope (which can be computed using the standard form of a 95 % CI, ▶Eq. E2.2, ▶Sect. 2.3.3):

$$[0.382 - 1.96 \times 0.094; 0.382 + 1.96 \times 0.094] \approx [0.198; 0.566].$$

Because the value one is not contained in the 95 % CI for the slope, we conclude that the prediction model is too optimistic. Again, this is probably the result of overfitting.

7.6   Comparing Nested Multiple Regression Prediction Models

Different prediction models can be compared to each other by comparing their goodness-of-fit measures when assessed in the same study population. The (validated) model with the highest quality is then selected for use in clinical practice. However, sometimes new techniques become available which could be used to improve an existing prediction model. Then, the question rises whether this new technique, or biomarker or whatever other variable is discovered, is of added value to the existing prediction model. This can be tested statistically, with a research question and a hypothesis. The research question of interest is always of the following form

? Is (or are) the potential predictor(s) x (or $x_1, x_2, ..., x_k$) of added value in predicting outcome variable Y?

The corresponding null and alternative hypothesis of this research questions are always

H0: the predictors are not of added value;
H1: the predictors are of added value.

The models that are compared will always be nested. This means that one model is extended to the other model by adding one or more additional preditctors. Both models should include the same set of predictors, except for the newly added potential predictors. If some predictors are only included in one model and not in the other, and other predictors are not included in the first model but are included in the second model, the models are not nested. Non-nested models can never be compared with the statistical tests described below.

We explain how to analyze nested models, by using examples from ►Chap. 6, in which multiple regression prediction models were analyzed and interpreted. For illustrative purposes, these models will be considered prediction models in the following sections. However, these analyses could also be used to compare to nested association regression models.

7.6.1 Linear Regression Prediction Models

To illustrate the concept of nested models and how they are compared, let us reconsider the linear regression prediction model for the prediction of DAS44 after 52 weeks by treatment arm, erythrocyte sedimentation rate (ESR) and aCPP status of ►Sect. 6.5.1

$$\text{mean DAS44\_wk52} = b_0 + b_1 \times \text{treatment} + b_2 \times \text{DASS44\_wk0} \tag{M7.2}$$
$$+ b_3 \times \text{ESR\_wk0} + b_4 \times \text{aCCP}.$$

Assume we want to investigate the following research question

? Are the potential predictors being fatigue at baseline and being IgM-RF positive of added value to the prediction model consisting of received treatment, DAS44 at baseline, ESR at baseline and being aCCP positive to predict the DAS44 after 52 weeks of treatment?

►Model M7.2 is then compared to a linear regression prediction model in which being fatigue at baseline ('fatigue') and IgM-RF status are added

$$\text{mean DAS44\_wk52} = b_0 + b_1 \times \text{treatment} + b_2 \times \text{DAS44\_wk0} + b_3$$
$$\times \text{ESR\_wk0} + b_4 \times \text{aCCP} + b_5 \times \text{fatigue} \tag{M7.3}$$
$$+ b_6 \times \text{IgM\_RF}.$$

Since all variables of ►Model M7.2 are also included in ►Model M7.3, the models are nested. Whether the two potential predictors fatigue and IgM_RF are of added value, is investigated with the F-test. This test compares the R^2 of ►Model M7.3 to that of ►Model M7.2. The R^2 always increases when more predictors are added to the model. The F-test assesses whether this increase is statistically significant. Keep in mind that a statistically significant improvement of the R^2 does not necessarily mean that this improvement is also clinically relevant.

To create two nested models in SPSS, the 'Next' button in the linear regression model query needs to be used (Supplementary Information A.4.3): all variables in ►Model M7.2 are entered in the first block, all variables added in ►Model M7.3 are entered in the second block. ◻Table 7.18 shows the SPSS output of the F-test. The table consists of two rows: one for ►Model M7.2 and one for ►Model M7.3. The first four columns (under "R", "R Square", "Adjusted R Square", and "Std. Error of the Estimate", respectively) report the model summary for both models and is similar to the model summary output for one model

□ **Table 7.18**   SPSS output of the *F*-test, investigating the added value of the potential predictors being fatigue at baseline and being IgM-RF positive at baseline to better predict the DAS44 after 52 weeks of treatment

Model Summary

Model	R	R Square	Adjusted R Square	Std. Error of the Estimate	Change Statistics				
					R Square Change	F Change	df1	df2	Sig. F Change
1	.331[a]	.110	.077	.9679	.110	3.302	4	107	.014
2	.418[b]	.174	.127	.9410	.064	4.100	2	105	.019

[a]Predictors: (Constant), treatment, DAS44 (at baseline), ESR (at baseline), aCCP
[b]Predictors: (Constant), treatment, DAS44 (at baseline), ESR (at baseline), aCCP, fatigue (at baseline), IgM-RF

(i.e., □Table 7.7, ▶Sect. 7.4.1). The important measures for the *F*-test are found in the part "Change Statistics" of the table. The *p*-value of the first row (under "Sig. F Change") actually tests whether the predictors in ▶Model M7.2 are of added value to the null model, in which the outcome variable is assumed to be constant across all patients. To answer the research question, we need to look at the second row. The value of the test statistic of the *F*-test ("F Change") is reported, with the corresponding degrees of freedom ("df1" and "df2"). The change in R^2 is reported too ("R Square Change"). Bases on this output, we conclude that the predictors being fatigue at baseline and being IgM-RF positive at baseline are of added value to predict the DAS44 after 52 weeks of treatment (R^2 0.17, R^2 change 0.064, $p = 0.019$).

7.6.2 Logistic Regression Prediction Models

To illustrate how to compare two nested logistic regression prediction models, we reconsider the dichotomous outcome variable as assessed in ▶Sect. 6.5.2, i.e., the development of RA within 2 years, again modeled by

$$\ln(\text{odds for RA within 2 years}) = b_0 + b_1 \times \text{age} + b_2 \times \text{FDR} + b_3 \times \text{stiffness}. \tag{M7.4}$$

Let us investigate whether antibody status is of added value to this model:

❓ Is the potential predictor antibody status of added value to a prediction model consisting of age, having an FDR with RA and duration of morning stiffness to predict the chance to develop RA within 2 years?

The extended model is equal to

$$\ln(\text{odds for RA within 2 years}) = b_0 + b_1 \times \text{age} + b_2 \times \text{FDR} + b_3 \times \text{stiffness} + b_4 \times \text{antibody}(1) + b_5 \times \text{antibody}(2) + b_6 \times \text{antibody}(3). \tag{M7.5}$$

◻ Table 7.19 SPSS table with the dummy coding for antibody status in a logistic regression model

Categorical Variable Codings[a]

		Frequency	(1)	(2)	(3)
antibody[b]	1=IgM-RF +, aCCP −	82	0	0	0
	2=IgM-RF −, aCCP low +	47	1	0	0
	3=IgM-RF −, aCCP high +	63	0	1	0
	4=IgM-RF +, aCCP +	91	0	0	1

[a]Category variable: antibody
[b]Indicator Parameter Coding

In this model, the variables antibody(1), antibody(2) and antibody(3) refer to the three dummy variables for the categorical determinant antibody status. ◻Table 7.19 shows the coding of the dummy variables in ►Model M7.5.

With the estimated regression coefficients of ►Models M7.4 and M7.5, the probability to develop RA within 2 years can be predicted. The likelihood of the observations is defined as the product of all these individual probabilities. Two nested logistic regression prediction models are then compared by comparing the values of −2 ln(likelihood). Adding more variables to a model will always decrease the −2 ln(likelihood). The likelihood-ratio (LR)-test tests whether the decrease in −2 ln(likelihood) is statistically significant.

To create two nested logistic regression prediction models in SPSS, the 'Next' button in the logistic regression model query needs to be used (Supplementary Information A.5.2), similar as for a linear regression model. The LR-test is default output in SPSS. Instead of reporting the results of the two models in one table, like for two nested linear regression models, SPSS reports the two models in two different blocks. The LR-test comparing ►Model M7.4 to ►Model M7.5 is found in the second block (◻Table 7.20). The table consists of three rows: one labeled "step", one labeled "block" and one labeled "model". The values of the chi-square test statistic (under "Chi-Square") and degrees of freedom (under "df") of the first two rows are equal in this case. In the third row, ►Model M7.5 is compared to the null model, i.e., a model without any predictors included. Based on the second row of the LR-test we conclude that antibody status is of added value to predict the development of RA within 2 years ($p < 0.001$).

A remark concerning the output of the LR-test has to be made. In ◻Table 7.20 the results in rows one and two are equal. However, if a selection procedure is performed within the second block of the SPSS query, for example when one wants to correct a priori for gender and age, multiple steps are taken in the second block and the results in the first two rows will not be equal. Therefore, we advise to always use the results in the second row labeled "block".

◻ **Table 7.20**   SPSS output of the LR-test of a logistic regression prediction model, investigating the added value of antibody status to a model to a better prediction of the ln(odds) for development of RA within 2 years

Omnibus Tests of Model Coefficients

		Chi-square	df	Sig.
Step 1	Step	41.567	3	.000
	Block	41.567	3	.000
	Model	52.563	6	.000

7.6.3 Cox Regression Prediction Models

Comparing two nested Cox regression prediction models is also done with de LR-test, although the likelihood of the observations is more complex to compute in a Cox regression model and not further described here; it is not needed for interpretation and beyond the scope of this quick guide. We explain how to compared nested Cox regression models with the following research question

? Is the potential predictor antibody status of added value to a prediction model consisting of age, having an FDR with RA and duration of morning stiffness to predict the time to development of RA?

The base model (as considered in ▸ Sect. 6.5.2) is equal to

$$\ln(h(t)) = \ln(h_0(t)) + b_1 \times \text{age} + b_2 \times \text{FDR} + b_3 \times \text{stiffness}, \tag{M7.6}$$

and the extended model is then equal to

$$\ln(h(t)) = \ln(h_0(t)) + b_1 \times \text{age} + b_2 \times \text{FDR} + b_3 \times \text{stiffness} + b_4$$
$$\times \text{antibody}(1) + b_5 \times \text{antibody}(2) + b_6 \times \text{antibody}(3). \tag{M7.7}$$

The coding of the dummy variables in the Cox regression model are equal to that in the logistic regression model (◻ Table 7.19, ▸ Sect. 7.6.2, though with different frequencies because all patients were included in this analysis opposed to only patients with at least 2 years of follow-up). Two nested Cox regression prediction models are created in SPSS with the 'Next' procedure in a Cox regression query (Supplementary Information A.6.2). The results of the two models are reported in two different blocks by SPSS. The LR-test comparing Model M7.6 to Model M7.7 is found in the second block. ◻ Table 7.21 shows the SPSS output of this test. The table consists of three parts: "Overall (score)", "Change From Previous Step" and "Change From Previous Block". The first part compares Model M7.7 to the null model, and the results of the last two parts are the same (similarly as for comparing two nested logistic regression prediction models). From the last part of this table we conclude that antibody status is of added value to predict time to development of RA ($p < 0.001$).

◻ **Table 7.21** SPSS output of the LR-test of a Cox regression prediction model, investigating the added value of antibody status to the model to predict the time to development of RA

Omnibus Tests of Model Coefficients[a]

−2 Log Likelihood	Overall (score)			Change From Previous Step			Change From Previous Block		
	Chi-square	df	Sig.	Chi-square	df	Sig.	Chi-square	df	Sig.
1322.190	86.908	6	.000	73.002	3	.000	73.002	3	.000

[a]Beginning Block Number 2. Method = Enter

7.7 Pitfalls and Other Things to Consider in Prediction Models

7.7.1 Interaction Terms

Similar as in the analyses of an association model, (an) interaction term(s) could also be added to a prediction model. Contrary to an association model, where only two-way interactions are considered with the central determinant, many interactions are possible in a prediction model. This depends on the number of included predictors, for example, for a model with 20 predictors, two-way, three-way, four-way, up to 20-way interactions are possible. It is not feasible to build a prediction model that is as complete as possible with respect to all possible interactions. There are two practical solutions to this problem: (1) include only biologically plausible interactions in the model, and (2) stratify a priori before building the models. In the first solution, only those predictors with a possible cause-and-effect relation to the outcome variable are interacted with each other. For example, a three-way interaction between antibody status, the presence of RA in FDRs, and having many tender joints to predict the development of RA within 2 years. Or a three-way interaction between smoking behavior, alcohol intake and atrial stiffness to predict the occurrence of myocardial infarctions. Bear in mind that a prediction model should always be simple and easy to apply in daily practice; adding interactions is not always beneficial.

7.7.2 Collinearity

Predictors in a prediction model could be related to each other, in which case collinearity might be present. Collinearity between two predictors mathematically means that there is a linear relation between the two predictors. Loosely speaking, this means that the two predictors are highly correlated to each other. Note that collinearity can also be present in association models. Multicollinearity mathematically means that two or more predictors in a prediction model are highly linearly related, i.e., they are all highly correlated to each other. Due to collinearity, less 'information' is present in the prediction model. If two predictors are not correlated, every patient in the study population provides information on the influence of predictor 1 on the outcome as well as on the influence of predictor 2 on the outcome variable. If two predictors are correlated, information on the influence of predictor 1 on the outcome also provides some information on the influence of predictor 2 on the outcome since they are correlated, i.e., providing less 'information'. Consequently, the regression coefficients are estimated less accurately, with larger standard errors (SEs), making it more difficult to detect a significant influence of the predictor: the larger the SE, the smaller the value of the test statistic and hence the larger the p-value.

Collinearity can be detected in several ways. The easiest way is to look at changes in the regression coefficients when a predictor is added or deleted. If the coefficients change enormously, or the signs of the regression coefficient change (i.e., from positive to negative or vice versa, also known as the reverse sign phenomenon) collinearity might be present. However, sometimes the changes are minimal, but collinearity is still present. Hence, another way to detect collinearity is by determining the variance inflation factor (VIF) for each of the predictors:

$$\mathrm{VIF} = \frac{1}{\text{tolerance}}, \ \text{tolerance} = 1 - R_j^2,$$

where R_j^2 is the explained variation in a regression model with predictor x_j as outcome variable and all other predictors as determinants (so leaving out the outcome variable of interest) [8, 9]. The VIF expresses how much the variance of that predictor increases due to collinearity. The VIF ranges from one to infinity: a VIF of one indicates no collinearity, between one and five indicates moderate collinearity, and of five or higher indicates high collinearity. The VIF is an additional option in the linear regression model query of SPSS (Supplementary Information A.4.3). ◻Table 7.22 shows the SPSS output of the final prediction model of ▶Sect. 7.2.3. The tolerance and the VIF are reported in the last two columns (under "Collinearity Statisics"). In the prediction model to predict the DAS44 after 52 weeks of treatment, we conclude that moderate collinearity is present for the total SJC and the DAS44 at baseline: with an VIF of 1.7 and 1.6, respectively.

A third method to detect collinearity is to construct a correlation matrix among all pairs of predictors. This provides an indication of the likelihood that any given pair of predictors could create (multi)collinearity problems. Correlations of 0.4 or higher are considered indicators of a (multi)collinearity problem. A disadvantage of the correlation matrix is that the correlation cannot be computed with categorical predictors.

There is no preferred method to detect collinearity, but eye-balling, in other words, just looking at the changes in the model when adding a predictor, is the easiest to perform. By doing so, at least predictors that strongly correlate are noticed, and can be acted on. And when collinearity is encountered, actions need to be taken. There are several options to eliminate collinearity in a prediction model, below we explain three options that are simple to perform. First, if a categorical predictor is included in a linear regression prediction model, check whether one category is set as the reference category and whether the reference category itself was not included as a separate dummy variable. That is, if a categorical predictor with k categories is included, make sure that only $k - 1$ dummy variables are included in the model. Secondly, if a categorical predictor was

◨ **Table 7.22** SPSS output of the prediction model for the DAS44 after 52 weeks of treatment, with collinearity statistics

Coefficients[a]

Model		Unstandardized Coefficients		Standardized Coefficients	t	Sig.	Collinearity Statistics	
		B	Std. Error	Beta			Tolerance	VIF
1	(Constant)	.537	.491		1.093	.277		
	aCCP	−.482	.183	−.232	−2.635	.010	.911	1.097
	SJC	−.074	.020	−.395	−3.595	.000	.586	1.707
	DAS44_wk0	.574	.140	.438	4.093	.000	.617	1.621
	fatigue	.404	.189	.184	2.140	.035	.956	1.046

[a]Dependent Variable: DAS44 (after 52 weeks)

computed from a continuous predictor e.g., because of violation of the linearity assumption, make sure that not both the categorical predictor and the continuous predictor for the same measure are included in the model, as this will always result in high collinearity. A last simple option is to drop one of the predictors that causes collinearity. However, this will lead to loss of information. For example, the DAS44 score is a composite score, based on the ESR, the total tender and swollen joint count and the VAS general well-being. Including these individual predictors as well as the DAS44 leads to multicollinearity. We refer to the further readings (►Sect. 7.8) for references on more sophisticated techniques to deal with collinearity.

7.7.3 Selection Procedures in SPSS

In the examples of the backward and forward procedure in ►Sects. 7.2.3 and 7.2.4, the selection procedures were performed manually. An advantage of making a prediction model by hand is that in-depth knowledge of the data is obtained. A disadvantage is that it is time consuming, especially when many predictors are included in the selection procedure of a forward selection process. After all, in the first step of the procedure, each possible predictor is added to the null model. Then, in the second step, only one model less has to be checked, etc. If many potential predictors are included in the dataset, a forward procedure might be needed to fulfill the rule of thumb for the number of predictors to be included.

SPSS can also perform the selection procedures automatically. SPSS has several different options to build a prediction model. ◨Figure 7.5 shows screenshots of the linear and the logistic regression query in SPSS with different options. In this figure, a drop down menu is shown which drops down after clicking on the arrow at the right side of

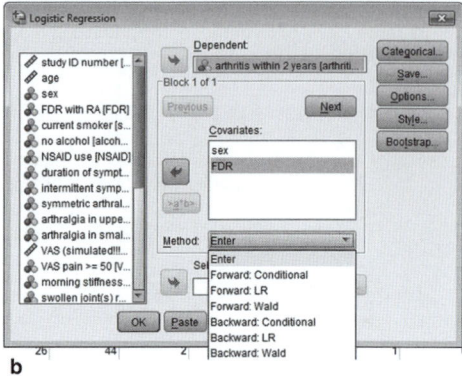

Fig. 7.5 Screenshot of a linear regression query (**a**) and a logistic regression query (**b**) in SPSS

"Enter". The default setting in SPSS is "Enter", in which case all predictors listed in the box "Independent(s)" or "Covariates", are included in the model. From the dropdown menu, different procedures could be selected.

For the linear regression model (◻Fig. 7.5a) there are four selection procedures: "stepwise", "remove", "backward" and "forward". The backward and forward procedures are as explained and illustrated in ▶Sects. 7.2.3 and 7.2.4. The "remove" procedure is the opposite of the "enter" procedure, and is only used to remove all listed predictors at once in a new block. This is not of interest when building a prediction model. With the "stepwise" procedure, SPSS starts with the first step of a forward selection procedure: the strongest predictor is added. It continues with a forward selection procedure until one or more variables do not fulfill the inclusion criterion any more (i.e., its/their p-value(s) is/ are larger than p-entry). Then, SPSS performs one or more backward selection steps. At each step, SPSS checks whether another predictor has to be removed from or added to the current model, until none of the remaining (not included) potential predictors fulfill the inclusion criterion (i.e., no p-values larger than p-entry or -removal) and all of the included predictors do.

For the logistic regression model (◻Fig. 7.5b) there is only a forward or a backward selection procedure, each with three different options to choose from: "conditional", "LR" (likelihood ratio) and "Wald". With "conditional", the predictors are entered (forward) or removed (backward) based on their p-values (of the Wald statistic) in the model. With "LR" the decision to enter or remove a predictor is based on the change in the LR-test between a model with all predictors and a model excluding the specific predictor. With "Wald", again two models (one with all predictors and one without that specific predictor) are compared, now using the Wald statistic instead of the LR-test.

It must be said that with the automatic selection procedure in SPSS, the final prediction model could be different from the one developed by hand. There are several reasons for that. SPSS keeps adding predictors that have been removed previously to the model to assess if these predictors in the new model do fulfill the inclusion criterion (backward procedure), or removing predictors that were added before from the model, to asses if

▢ **Table 7.23** Part of the SPSS output for the final prediction model (step "16") of the DAS44 after 52 weeks of treatment developed by the automatic selection procedure in SPSS

Variables in the Equation[a]

Step		Unstandardized Coefficients		Standardized Coefficients	t	Sig.	95.0 % Confidence Interval for B	
		B	Std. Error	Beta			Lower Bound	Upper Bound
16	(Constant)	.440	.505		.873	.385	−.561	1.442
	aCCP	−.485	.188	−.232	−2.576	.011	−.859	−.111
	SJC	−.080	.022	−.416	−3.601	.000	−.124	−.036
	DAS44_wk0	.620	.149	.473	4.158	.000	.324	.916
	Fatigue	.448	.197	.201	2.271	.025	.057	.840

[a]Dependent Variable: DAS44 (after 52 weeks)

these predictors in the new model still fulfill the inclusion criterion (forward procedure). Moreover, SPSS only includes data from patients in the study population with complete data on all predictors included in the selection procedure, i.e., patients with missing values on one or more predictors are excluded from the selection procedure, decreasing the number of patients included for building the prediction model. For example, if we would have built the prediction model for predicting DAS44 after 52 weeks of treatment (▶ Sect. 7.2.3) with the automatic backward selection procedure in SPSS, a different final prediction model would have been obtained, as can be seen in ▢Table 7.23. The same variables are included, but the regression coefficients differ (▢Table 7.2, ▶ Sect. 7.2.3). The difference is mainly driven by missing data: this model was built on data from 103 patients, instead of 154 patients. Therefore, if predictors have (many) missing data, building a prediction model manually is the preferred method.

Finally, for a linear regression prediction model with categorical predictors, the automatic selection procedure cannot be used, because the dummy variables for each category compared to the reference category have to be created by hand. SPSS then considers these dummy variables as separate predictors, while in fact they have to be kept together for the correct comparison of all groups. Hence, it could be that one dummy variable is removed by SPSS, while others are left in. Because SPSS creates dummy variables for categorical variables in a logistic or Cox regression automatically, when a categorical variable is defined as 'categorical' in the logistic or Cox regression query, this is not a problem for a dichotomous and time to event outcome variable.

A last thing to keep in mind when building a prediction model, is that both selection procedures can lead to different models. This is mostly due to the fact that with a backward selection procedure, the starting point is the complete model including all possible predictors, and therefore accounts for the influence of the predictors on each other. This has an effect on the regression coefficients and their SE, and consequently influences the *p*-values. With the forward selection procedure, the starting point is the null model to which, one by one, predictors are added, limiting the influence of several predictors on each other. Therefore, in the first few steps of a forward selection procedure, a predictor could fulfill the inclusion criterion, while adding more predictors to the model increases its *p*-value to above *p*-entry. In a linear regression model with a backward or forward procedure, SPSS does not add these predictors to the model or does not remove them, whereas with a "stepwise" procedure, they are removed. In a logistic or Cox regression model with a backward or forward procedure, SPSS does add or remove the predictors to or from the model. Therefore, always check which predictors were entered to or removed from the model in each step, and do not just look at the last step of the automatic procedure (the final block of rows in the output table).

7.8   Further Readings

Steyerberg wrote a book, and co-authored a paper covering all aspects of prediction models: selection of the predictors, and the quality and validity of the models [10, 11]. Multivariable Cox regression models are also described in the tutorials on survival analysis in the British Journal of Cancer: part II is an introduction to multivariable model, parts III and IV discuss the goodness-of-fit of prediction models, including other goodness-of-fit measures for Cox regression models [12–14]. Some information on the *F*-test and LR-test to compare nested models can be found in the book written by Armitage et al. [8]. The concept of collinearity is described in the books written by Armitage et al. and by Belsey et al. [8, 9]. Another way to deal with collinearity is by using partial least squares regression. This technique is described, for example, by Wold et al. and by Helland [15, 16]. Another more sophisticated technique to deal with collinearity is principal components analysis, which Jackson and Jolliffe have both written on [17, 18].

References

1. Kannel WB, McGee D, Gordon T. A general cardiovascular risk profile: the Framingham study. Am J cardiol. 1976;38(1):46–51.
2. Anderson KM, Wilson PW, Odell PM, Kannel WB. An updated coronary risk profile. A statement for health professionals. Circulation 1991;83(1):356–62.
3. Engels MA, Twisk JW, Blankenstein MA, van Vugt JM. Age independent first trimester screening for Down syndrome: improvement in test performance. Prenat Diagn. 2013;33(9):884–8. ► https://doi.org/10.1002/pd.4153.
4. Engels MA, Bhola SL, Twisk JW, Blankenstein MA, van Vugt JM. Evaluation of the introduction of the national Down syndrome screening program in the Netherlands: age-related uptake of prenatal screening and invasive diagnostic testing. Eur J Obstet Gynecol Reprod Biol. 2014;174:59–63. ► https://doi.org/10.1016/j.ejogrb.2013.12.009.
5. ter Wee MM, den Uyl D, Boers M, Kerstens P, Nurmohamed M, van Schaardenburg D, et al. Intensive combination treatment regimens, including prednisolone, are effective in treating patients with early rheumatoid arthritis regardless of additional etanercept: 1-year results of the COBRA-light open-label, randomised, non-inferiority trial. Ann Rheum Dis. 2015;74(6):1233–40. ► https://doi.org/10.1136/annrheumdis-2013-205143.

6. van de Stadt LA, Witte BI, Bos WH, van Schaardenburg D. A prediction rule for the development of arthritis in seropositive arthralgia patients. Ann Rheum Dis. 2013;72(12):1920–6. ▶https://doi.org/10.1136/annrheumdis-2012-202127.

7. Šimundić A-M. Measures of diagnostic accuracy: basic definitions. EJIFCC 2009;19(4):203–11.

8. Armitage P, Berry G, Matthews JNS. Statistical methods in medical research. Oxford: Blackwell Science Ltd; 2002.

9. Belsey DA, Kuh D, Welsch RE. Regression diagnostics. New York: John Wiley; 1980.

10. Steyerberg EW. Clinical prediction models. New York: Springer; 2009.

11. Steyerberg EW, Vickers AJ, Cook NR, Gerds T, Gonen M, Obuchowski N, et al. Assessing the performance of prediction models: a framework for traditional and novel measures. Epidemiology 2010;21(1):128–38. ▶https://doi.org/10.1097/ede.0b013e3181c30fb2.

12. Bradburn MJ, Clark TG, Love SB, Altman DG. Survival analysis part II: multivariate data analysis – an introduction to concepts and methods. Br J Cancer. 2003;89(3):431–6. ▶https://doi.org/10.1038/sj.bjc.6601119.

13. Bradburn MJ, Clark TG, Love SB, Altman DG. Survival analysis part III: multivariate data analysis – choosing a model and assessing its adequacy and fit. Br J Cancer. 2003;89(4):506–11. ▶https://doi.org/10.1038/sj.bjc.6601120.

14. Clark TG, Bradburn MJ, Love SB, Altman DG. Survival analysis part IV: further concepts and methods in survival analysis. Br J Cancer. 2003;89(5):781–6. ▶https://doi.org/10.1038/sj.bjc.6601117.

15. Wold S, Martens H, Wold H. The multivariate calibration problem in chemistry solved by the PLS method. In: Kågström B, Ruhe A, editors. Matrix Pencils. Lecture Notes in Mathematics, vol 973. Heidelber: Springer; 1983. pp. 286–93.

16. Helland IS. Some theoretical aspects of partial least squares regression. Chemometr Intell Lab Syst. 2001;58(2):97–107. ▶https://doi.org/10.1016/s0169-7439(01)00154-x.

17. Jackson JE. A user's guide to principal components. New York: John Wiley & Sons, Inc; 1991.

18. Jolliffe IT. Principal component analysis. 2nd ed. New York: Springer-Verlag; 2002.

Missing data

Abstract
Ideally, all data in the database is complete and no information is missing for any patient. However, in medical research, data is often missing, for example due to the fact that patients might not fill out certain questions or that patients are lost to follow up. For the correct statistical inference, missing data needs to be dealt with properly. In this chapter we explore different mechanisms behind missing data and provide several methods on how to deal with missing data.

© Bohn Stafleu van Loghum is een imprint van Springer Media B.V., onderdeel van Springer Nature 2019
M. M. ter Wee and B. I. Lissenberg-Witte, *A Quick Guide on How to Conduct Medical Research*,
https://doi.org/10.1007/978-90-368-2248-0_8

8.1   Mechanisms of Missingness

There are several reasons for data to be missing, for example due to nonresponse of the patient, non-applicability of a certain question, drop-out of the patient, technical failure of the measurement instrument, etc. Nonresponse of a patient occurs if a patient overlooks or is not willing to answer an item on a questionnaire, or a researcher forgets to measure a certain variable during the patients study visit. An example of a non-applicable question is the age of menopause which is not applicable for pre-menopausal women or men in general. Data that is missing due to drop-out occurs if, for example, the patient decided to discontinue a new treatment in a randomized controlled trial (RCT) because of serious side effects. When entering data into a database, it is important to keep track of these different types of missingness, i.e., code not applicable differently from nonresponse. Whenever we speak about missing data in this chapter, we mean data missing due to nonresponse, drop-out or a technical failure; inapplicability of a variable is just a fact and is not truly missing for that patient. Missing data could be present in data on the outcome variable, on the determinant, potential confounders and effect modifiers, and on predictors.

Before analyzing the data, the amount of missing data in the study population has to be investigated, to acquire insight on the potential impact of data that is missing. The first step is a univariable description of the missing data of the outcome variable and the determinant, which is obtained by the missing values analysis query in SPSS (Supplementary Information A.7). ◻Table 8.1 summarizes the missing data for several variables measured in the rheumatoid arthritis (RA)-cohort [1]. The included variables were age, gender, having a first-degree relative (FDR) with RA, smoking, alcohol use, non-steroid anti-inflammatory drug (NSAID) use, duration of symptoms <12 months ('duration'), intermittent symptoms present ('intermittent'), symmetric arthralgia ('symmetric'), arthralgia in upper and lower extremities ('extremities'), arthralgia in small joints ('smallJoints'), VAS pain $\geq$ 50 ('VAS50'), morning stiffness $\geq$ 1h ('stiffness'), swollen joint(s) reported ('SJC44'), tender joint(s) reported ('TJC53'), CRP status ('CRP') and antibody status ('antibody', based on the values of rheumatoid factor type immunoglobulin M (IgM-RF) and anticyclic citrullinated peptide (aCCP)). For each variable, SPSS reports the number of patients with a missing value and the percentage (under "Count" and under "Percent", respectively). For continuous variables, SPSS also reports the mean (under "Mean") and standard deviation (SD; under "Std. Deviation") as well as the number of patients with extremely low values or extremely high values (i.e., below/above the 25th/75th percentile minus/plus 1.5 times the interquartile range (IQR), under "Low" and under "High", respectively). From ◻Table 8.1, we conclude that the total amount of missing values is considerably low, ranging from 0 % to 3.7 %. In total, however, 59 patients of the 374 included (16 %) had at least one missing value.

Missing data needs to be dealt with properly in the analyses, otherwise incorrect conclusions could be drawn from the data. To decide on the appropriate method to handle missing data, the underlying mechanisms that causes data to be missing, needs to be investigated first. We consider three missing data mechanisms:

⬛ **Table 8.1** SPSS output of the missing value analysis, summarizing the amount of missing data in the important variables of the study population

Univariate Statistics

	N	Mean	Std. Deviation	Missing		No. of Extremes[a]	
				Count	Percent	Low	High
age	374	48.77	11.495	0	.0	0	0
gender	374			0	.0		
FDR	374			0	.0		
smoking	372			2	.5		
alcohol	361			13	3.5		
NSAID	374			0	.0		
duration	368			6	1.6		
intermittent	360			14	3.7		
symmetric	369			5	1.3		
extremities	367			7	1.9		
smallJoints	368			6	1.6		
VAS50	374			0	.0		
stiffness	374			0	.0		
SJC44	374			0	.0		
TJC53	374			0	.0		
CRP	367			7	1.9		
antibody	374			0	.0		

[a]Number of cases outside the range (Q1 − 1.5 * IQR, Q3 + 1.5 * IQR)

1. Missing completely at random (MCAR): this mechanism assumes that there is no relation between the missingness of the data and any other variables, observed or missing. That is, missing data points are a random subset of the data, and there is no pattern visible by which some data is more likely to be missing than other.
2. Missing at random (MAR): this mechanism assumes that there is a systematic relation between the propensity of a value to be missing and other variables, but that this has nothing to do with the missing value itself. For example, if women are less likely to report their weight than men, weight is MAR.
3. Missing not at random (MNAR): this mechanism assumes that there is a relation between the propensity of a value to be missing and other variables, which has to do with the missing value itself. This is the case when patients who were already very frail at the start of the study are also more likely to drop out of the study.

▶ Table 8.2   *P*-values for the comparison of patients with and without any missing data in the RA-cohort

variable	p-value	tested with
age	0.75	independent samples *t*-test
gender	0.50	chi-square test
FDR with RA	0.25	chi-square test
current smoker	0.47	chi-square test
no alcohol	0.48	chi-square test
NSAID use	0.77	chi-square test
duration of symptoms <12 months	0.52	chi-square test
intermittent symptoms present	1.00	chi-square test
symmetric arthralgia	0.55	chi-square test
arthralgia in upper and lower extremities	0.85	chi-square test
arthralgia in small joints	0.78	chi-square test
VAS pain $\geq$ 50	0.064	chi-square test
morning stiffness $\geq$ 1 hour	0.53	chi-square test
swollen joint(s) reported	0.39	chi-square test
tender joint(s) reported	0.48	chi-square test
CRP	0.20	Fisher's exact test
shared epitope	0.22	chi-square test
antibody status	0.62	chi-square test

To distinguish MAR from MCAR in the (outcome) variable, a dichotomous variable can be computed that indicates, for each patient, whether or not one or more variables are missing. Differences in characteristics between patients with and without missing data are statistically tested with an independent samples *t*-test or a chi-square test, depending on the type of variable, i.e., continuous or dichotomous. This holds for both the outcome variable as well as determinants and predictors. If there are no differences between these two groups, the data is probably MCAR. The missing data in the RA-cohort seemed to be MCAR based on the above described analysis: ▶Table 8.2 shows the *p*-values comparing all important variables in the RA-cohort between patients with missing data ($n = 59$) and patients without missing data ($n = 315$). There was no evidence for any differences between the groups for any of the variables ($p \geq 0.064$).

The only way to distinguish between MNAR and M(C)AR is to actually measure some of the missing data, and then compare the missing values with observed values. If the missing values differ significantly from the observed values, the data is probably MNAR. However, measuring missing data is a big challenge or even impossible. For example, in a longitudinal study regarding the quality of life amongst first time cardiac infarct patients during the first year after their cardiac infarct, patients may have died during the follow-up period. It might be argued that their quality of life is the worst

□ **Table 8.3** Part of the database of the RA-cohort to illustrate the different methods for handling missing data

patient ID	smoking	alcohol	duration	intermittent	antibody
1	no	yes	no	no	IgM-RF −, aCCP low +
7		no	yes	yes	IgM-RF +, aCCP +
48	no	no	no		IgM-RF +, aCCP −
64	yes	no	yes	yes	IgM-RF −, aCCP low +
70	no				IgM-RF +, aCCP +

possible, but if their death is not the result of a cardiac infarct, this does not reflect their quality of life properly. Unfortunately, we can never be 100 % sure whether missing data is at random, or whether the missingness depends on unobserved variables or even on the missing data itself.

8.2 Handling Missing Data

There are several ways to deal with missing data, which we illustrate with data of the RA-cohort. We evaluate the effect of these methods with the following Cox regression model for the time to development of RA

$$\ln(h(t)) = \ln(h_0(t)) + b_1 \times \text{smoking} + b_2 \times \text{alcohol} + b_3$$
$$\times \text{duration} + b_4 \times \text{intermittent} + b_5 \times \text{antibody}(1) \qquad \text{(M8.1)}$$
$$+ b_6 \times \text{antibody}(2) + b_7 \times \text{antidbody}(3).$$

For the determinants smoking, duration, and intermittent, no was coded as zero and yes as one, while alcohol use was coded as zero and no alcohol use as one. For the categorical determinant antibody being IgM-RF positive but aCCP negative was coded as one and set as the reference group; being IgM-RF negative but aCCP low positive was coded as two ('antibody(1)'); IgM-RF negative but aCCP high positive coded as three ('antibody(2)') and IgM-RF positive and aCCP positive coded as four ('antibody(3)'). □Table 8.3 shows part of the database for some of the patients, some of whom have missing data for one or more variables.

8.2.1 Complete Case Analysis

The most rigid method to deal with missing data is to exclude subjects with missing data (on all variables in the analyses) completely. This is called a complete case analysis. □Table 8.4 shows the SPSS output of ▶model M8.1 for the complete case analysis. We know some patients had missing values for one or more variables in the model, based on

□ **Table 8.4**   SPSS output of the Cox regression model for the time to development of RA for a complete case analysis

Variables in the Equation

	B	SE	Wald	df	Sig.	Exp(B)	95.0 % CI for Exp(B)	
							Lower	Upper
smoking	−.073	.200	.132	1	.716	.930	.628	1.376
alcohol	.477	.190	6.313	1	.012	1.612	1.111	2.339
duration	.476	.198	5.778	1	.016	1.610	1.092	2.374
intermittent	.588	.188	9.762	1	.002	1.801	1.245	2.605
antibody			38.522	3	.000			
antibody(1)	1.058	.385	7.549	1	.006	2.880	1.354	6.125
antibody(2)	1.547	.356	18.909	1	.000	4.697	2.339	9.431
antibody(3)	1.952	.336	33.839	1	.000	7.041	3.648	13.591

□ **Table 8.5**   SPSS output of the case processing summary for the Cox regression model for the time to development of RA

Case Processing Summary

		N	Percent
Cases available in analysis	Event[a]	121	32.4 %
	Censored	224	59.9 %
	Total	345	92.2 %
Cases dropped	Cases with missing values	29	7.8 %
	Cases with negative time	0	0.0 %
	Censored cases before the earliest event in a stratum	0	0.0 %
	Total	29	7.8 %
Total		374	100.0 %

[a]Dependent Variable: follow-up time (months)

□Table 8.1. SPSS reports how much data is missing exactly in the output "Case Processing Summary" (□Table 8.5). SPSS always produces such a summary output table with a description of the used cases. The number (under "N") and percentage (under "Percent") of patients included in the analysis are reported in the rows "Cases available in analysis". The total number of patients is reported in the row "Total", the number of patients who developed RA during the total follow-up period in the row "Event" and the number of patients who did not develop RA during the follow-up (i.e., are censored) in the row

"Censored". The number and percentage of patients not included in the analysis, with specification for reason of exclusion, are reported in the rows "Cases dropped". The total number of excluded patients is reported in the row "Total", and the number of patients excluded due to missing data in the row "Cases with missing values". Other reasons for exclusion are a negative follow-up time (in the row "Cases with negative time") and a censored time to event before the first observed event time (in the row "Censored cases before the earliest event in a stratum"). The total number of patients, the included and excluded, are reported in the last row of the table (in "Total"). From ◻Table 8.5, we see that 345 of the 374 patients (92 %) were included in the analysis, of which 121 (32 %) developed RA, and that the remaining 29 patients had a missing value for at least one of the variables in the model.

Complete case analysis is only used when the data is missing completely at random. If data is missing at random or missing not at random, systematic differences between complete and incomplete cases could introduce a bias in the results. Moreover, if there are many variables included in the analyses, for example when building a prediction model, there might be only a few complete cases left for the analysis. Therefore, we advise to use this approach only as part of a sensitivity analysis. A sensitivity analysis is an analysis in which different methods to handle missing data are applied and compared to each other. The conclusion of the research question is strengthened if these different methods yield comparable results as the main result in which missing data was dealt with.

A more strict complete case analysis in a randomized controlled trial (RCT) is the per-protocol analysis. In such analysis, patients are excluded in case of large protocol deviations due to, for example, intake of concomitant medication or non-sufficient exposure or non-availability of measurement of the primary endpoint. This analysis is also part of the sensitivity analysis. The main analysis is usually the intention-to-treat analysis, in which all randomized patients, ignoring missing data, are included in the analysis.

The missing values of patients with missing data can also be imputed, instead of removing these patients from the analyses. There are different ways to impute data, some are based on deterministic methods (without any random variation), others are based on more complex stochastic methods (with random variation).

8.2.2 Deterministic Imputation

Mean Imputation

The easiest way to impute a single value of a variable is by imputing the missing value with the mean (mean imputation). With mean imputation, each missing value is replaced by their mean of the observed values. For example, two patients in the RA-cohort had a missing value for their smoking status, and 113 of the remaining 372 patients (30 %) currently smoked. The mean imputed value for smoking of the patient with ID 7, would then be equal to 0.30. However, smoking is a dichotomous determinant, hence the mean has to be dichotomized as well. To do so, values smaller than 0.5 are rounded to zero and values larger than 0.5 to one. The mean values for alcohol,

▪ Table 8.6 Part of the dataset of the RA-cohort in which missing values are replaced by the mean values and then rounded to zero or one

patient ID	smoking	alcohol	duration	intermittent	antibody
1	no	no	no	no	IgM-RF −, aCCP low +
7	no	yes	yes	yes	IgM-RF +, aCCP +
48	no	yes	no	no	IgM-RF +, aCCP −
64	yes	yes	yes	yes	IgM-RF −, aCCP low +
70	no	yes	no	no	IgM-RF +, aCCP +

▪ Table 8.7 SPSS output of the Cox regression model for the time to development of RA, where missing values were imputed with mean imputation

Variables in the Equation

	B	SE	Wald	df	Sig.	Exp(B)	95.0 % CI for Exp(B)	
							Lower	Upper
smoking	.028	.189	.022	1	.882	1.029	.709	1.491
alcohol	.525	.183	8.259	1	.004	1.690	1.182	2.417
duration	.419	.191	4.817	1	.028	1.520	1.046	2.209
intermittent	.452	.181	6.235	1	.013	1.571	1.102	2.240
antibody			43.924	3	.000			
antibody(1)	1.082	.371	8.496	1	.004	2.950	1.425	6.106
antibody(2)	1.539	.342	20.254	1	.000	4.661	2.384	9.112
antibody(3)	2.009	.323	38.743	1	.000	7.458	3.961	14.041

duration and intermittent were 0.37, 0.32 and 0.36. Therefore, all missing values are imputed with the value zero. ▪Table 8.6 shows the result of this imputation method for the patients in ▪Table 8.3.

▪Table 8.7 shows the SPSS output of the Cox regression model (with all 374 patients included). The results differ slightly from the results of the complete case analysis (▪Table 8.4, ▶Sect. 8.2.1). The p-value of smoking increased from $p = 0.72$ to $p = 0.88$. The influence of the duration of symptoms (hazard ratio (HR) 1.6, 95 % confidence interval (CI) [1.1; 2.4], $p = 0.016$ versus HR 1.5, 95 % CI [1.05; 2.2], $p = 0.028$) and the presence of intermittent symptoms (HR 1.8, 95 % CI [1.2; 2.6], $p = 0.002$ versus HR 1.6, 95 % CI [1.1, 2.2], $p = 0.013$) became slightly weaker. Only the association between antibody status and the time to development of RA became slightly stronger.

Although this method is easy to implement, it also has its disadvantages. It underestimates the standard deviation (SD) of the variable, leading to underestimation of the standard error (SE). Consequently, the p-values will be too small. Moreover, the relation with other variables is completely ignored. In other words, the imputed values are not related to any of the other variables, which lead to a bias of the association.

Last Observation Carried Forward

Another deterministic way of handling missing data in longitudinal studies with repeated measurements of the outcome variable, such as the COmbinatie Behandeling Reumatoïde Artritis (COBRA)-light trial [2], is the last observation carried forward method. With this method, the missing value of a measurement is imputed with the value of the last observed measurement. We cannot illustrate this method in the RA-cohort, because the Cox regression prediction model only contains predictors that are measured once, at baseline, and not repeatedly over time. Therefore, let us consider a patient in the COBRA-light trial with a missing value of the disease activity score in 44 joints (DAS44) after 26 weeks of treatment. Assume that this patient had a DAS44 of 5.4 at baseline and a DAS44 of 4.5 after 13 weeks of treatment. Then, the last observation carried forward imputed value of the DAS44 after 26 weeks is 4.5. However, because of regression to the mean, low values after 13 weeks are more likely to result in higher values after 26 weeks, whereas high values are more likely to result in lower values after 26 weeks. Therefore, this method is not advised to use when handling missing data.

8.2.3 Stochastic Imputation

Regression Imputation

The methods described in ▶Sects. 8.2.2 and 8.2.3, do not take into account that missing values could be related to other variables, or are more present in specific groups of patients (as is the case in MAR missing data). With a linear or logistic regression model, the missing value is predicted to account for dependencies with and differences between other variables. This method is called regression imputation. This can be augmented by adding a residual term to the prediction (single stochastic regression imputation), to preserve the same variability in the imputed data as is present in the observed data.

To impute the missing values of smoking in the RA-cohort, a logistic regression model was estimated, with smoking as dichotomous outcome variable and all other patient characteristics and disease related characteristics as determinants. For two patients, smoking status was imputed using the predicted probability of this model (◻Table 8.8). The procedure was repeated for all other variables with at least one missing variables. With this imputation method, the missing values for 'alcohol' and 'intermittent' of the patient with ID 70 were now imputed by the values 'no' and 'yes', respectively. The other missing values in ◻Table 8.3 (▶Sect. 8.2) were imputed with the same value as in ◻Table 8.6 (▶Sect. 8.2.2).

◻Table 8.9 shows the SPSS output of the Cox regression model based on this imputed database. The results differ slightly from the results of the complete case analysis (◻Table 8.4, ▶Sect. 8.2.1) and the mean imputed method (◻Table 8.7, ▶Sect. 8.2.2), as expected.

◾ **Table 8.8**   Part of the dataset of the RA-cohort, missing values are imputed with single stochastic regression imputation

patient ID	smoking	alcohol	duration	intermittent	antibody
1	no	no	no	no	IgM-RF −, aCCP low +
7	no	yes	yes	yes	IgM-RF +, aCCP +
48	no	yes	no	no	IgM-RF +, aCCP −
64	yes	yes	yes	yes	IgM-RF −, aCCP low +
70	no	no	no	yes	IgM-RF +, aCCP +

◾ **Table 8.9**   SPSS output of the Cox regression model for the time to development of RA, where missing values were imputed with single stochastic regression imputation

Variables in the Equation

	B	SE	Wald	df	Sig.	Exp(B)	95.0 % CI for Exp(B)	
							Lower	Upper
smoking	.041	.190	.046	1	.830	1.042	.718	1.510
alcohol	.565	.182	9.633	1	.002	1.760	1.232	2.514
duration	.424	.191	4.936	1	.026	1.528	1.051	2.220
intermittent	.514	.182	8.026	1	.005	1.673	1.172	2.388
antibody			43.128	3	.000			
antibody(1)	1.079	.371	8.457	1	.004	2.943	1.422	6.091
antibody(2)	1.540	.342	20.242	1	.000	4.667	2.385	9.130
antibody(3)	1.992	.323	38.152	1	.000	7.331	3.896	13.795

Multiple Imputation

The disadvantage of single stochastic regression imputation is that the SE of the effect sizes are too small and consequently the p-values are too small. Multiple imputation method deals with this limitation, and consists of three steps:

1. create m datasets of imputations for the missing values, using a stochastic regression imputation method for each set;
2. analyze each of the m complete datasets separately (due to the stochastic component of each data set, each estimated effect will differ);
3. pool the results by taking the average over the different effect sizes.

◻ **Table 8.10** Part of the dataset of the RA-cohort, missing values are imputed with multiple imputation (m = 3)

Imp_[a]	patient ID	smoking	alcohol	duration	intermittent	antibody
1	1	no	no	no	no	IgM-RF −, aCCP low +
1	7	**no**	yes	yes	yes	IgM-RF +, aCCP +
1	48	no	yes	no	**no**	IgM-RF +, aCCP −
1	64	yes	yes	yes	yes	IgM-RF −, aCCP low +
1	70	no	**no**	**no**	yes	IgM-RF +, aCCP +
2	1	no	no	no	no	IgM-RF −, aCCP low +
2	7	**no**	yes	yes	yes	IgM-RF +, aCCP +
2	48	no	yes	no	**no**	IgM-RF +, aCCP −
2	64	yes	yes	yes	yes	IgM-RF −, aCCP low +
2	70	no	**yes**	**no**	**no**	IgM-RF +, aCCP +
3	1	no	no	no	no	IgM-RF −, aCCP low +
3	7	**no**	yes	yes	yes	IgM-RF +, aCCP +
3	48	no	yes	no	**no**	IgM-RF +, aCCP −
3	64	yes	yes	yes	yes	IgM-RF −, aCCP low +
3	70	no	**no**	**no**	**no**	IgM-RF +, aCCP +

[a]Imp_ is imputation set

Depending on the percentage of missing data, 5 to 10 different datasets are enough to pool the estimates properly. In SPSS it is possible to create these m sets automatically, with the Multiple Imputation query (see Supplementary Information A.7). Van de Stadt et al. used this procedure to create $m = 5$ imputation sets. SPSS automatically adds a new variable to the database "Imputation_", in the first column of the database. ◻Table 8.10 shows the imputed values for some patients with missing values, for three imputed databases.

◻Table 8.11 shows the SPSS output of the Cox regression model for these three imputed databases. SPSS recognizes that the database is a multiple imputation database because of the first variable in the database "Imputation_". The Cox regression model is estimated for the original dataset (i.e., the complete case analysis, in the rows in "Original data" under "Imputation Number") and each imputed dataset separately (in the rows "1", "2" and "3" under "Imputation Number"). SPSS also pools these results automatically (in the rows "Pooled" under "Imputation Number"). This is not the case for all statistical analyses in SPSS, but it is for all analyses described in this quick guide. The output of the pooled results is basically the same as the output of a Cox regression model based on a non-imputed database: the estimated regression coefficients for the different variables

▣ Table 8.11 SPSS output of the Cox regression model for the time to development of RA, applying the multiple imputation method

| Variables in the Equation | | | | | | | 95.0 % CI for Exp(B) | | | | |
Imputation Number	B	SE	Wald	df	Sig.	Exp(B)	Lower	Upper	Fraction Missing Info.	Relative Increase Variance	Relative Efficiency
Original data											
smoking	−.073	.200	.132	1	.716	.930	.628	1.376			
alcohol	.477	.190	6.313	1	.012	1.612	1.111	2.339			
duration	.476	.198	5.778	1	.016	1.610	1.092	2.374			
intermittent	.588	.188	9.762	1	.002	1.801	1.245	2.605			
antibody			38.522	3	.000						
antibody(1)	1.058	.385	7.549	1	.006	2.880	1.354	6.125			
antibody(2)	1.547	.356	18.909	1	.000	4.697	2.339	9.431			
antibody(3)	1.952	.336	33.839	1	.000	7.041	3.648	13.591			
1											
smoking	.041	.190	.046	1	.830	1.042	.718	1.510			
alcohol	.565	.182	9.633	1	.002	1.760	1.232	2.514			
duration	.424	.191	4.936	1	.026	1.528	1.051	2.220			
intermittent	.514	.182	8.026	1	.005	1.673	1.172	2.388			
antibody			43.128	3	.000						
antibody(1)	1.079	.371	8.457	1	.004	2.943	1.422	6.091			
antibody(2)	1.540	.342	20.242	1	.000	4.667	2.385	9.130			
antibody(3)	1.992	.323	38.152	1	.000	7.331	3.896	13.795			

■ **Table 8.11** SPSS output of the Cox regression model for the time to development of RA, applying the multiple imputation method (continued)

Variables in the Equation

Imputation Number		B	SE	Wald	df	Sig.	Exp(B)	95.0 % CI for Exp(B)		Fraction Missing Info.	Relative Increase Variance	Relative Efficiency
								Lower	Upper			
2	smoking	.029	.189	.023	1	.878	1.029	.710	1.492			
	alcohol	.576	.182	9.998	1	.002	1.778	1.245	2.541			
	duration	.454	.190	5.718	1	.017	1.574	1.085	2.284			
	intermittent	.514	.181	8.093	1	.004	1.673	1.174	2.384			
	antibody			44.339	3	.000						
	antibody(1)	1.107	.371	8.924	1	.003	3.025	1.463	6.253			
	antibody(2)	1.564	.342	20.904	1	.000	4.779	2.444	9.345			
	antibody(3)	2.018	.321	39.452	1	.000	7.523	4.008	14.121			
3	smoking	.032	.190	.028	1	.866	1.033	.712	1.497			
	alcohol	.543	.182	8.922	1	.003	1.720	1.205	2.456			
	duration	.445	.192	5.388	1	.020	1.561	1.072	2.273			
	intermittent	.483	.182	7.054	1	.008	1.621	1.135	2.315			
	antibody			43.055	3	.000						
	antibody(1)	1.069	.372	8.281	1	.004	2.913	1.406	6.035			
	antibody(2)	1.513	.342	19.538	1	.000	4.541	2.321	8.881			
	antibody(3)	1.991	.323	37.909	1	.000	7.325	3.886	13.808			

□ **Table 8.11**   SPSS output of the Cox regression model for the time to development of RA, applying the multiple imputation method (continued)

Variables in the Equation

Imputation Number		B	SE	Wald	df	Sig.	Exp(B)	95.0 % CI for Exp(B)		Fraction Missing Info.	Relative Increase Variance	Relative Efficiency
								Lower	Upper			
Pooled	smoking	.034	.190			.858	1.034	.713	1.500	.001	.002	1.000
	alcohol	.561	.183			.002	1.753	1.224	2.509	.012	.012	.996
	duration	.441	.192			.021	1.554	1.068	2.262	.009	.009	.997
	intermittent	.504	.183			.006	1.655	1.157	2.368	.013	.013	.996
	antibody(1)	1.085	.372			.004	2.960	1.428	6.134	.004	.004	.999
	antibody(2)	1.539	.344			.000	4.661	2.377	9.140	.007	.007	.998
	antibody(3)	2.000	.323			.000	7.393	3.926	13.920	.003	.003	.999

in model ►M8.1 are reported, with the corresponding SEs, the exponential (exp) of the regression coefficients, i.e., the hazard ratios (HRs) and the 95 % CIs. SPSS adds three more columns to the table to provide information on the pooled analyses. The fraction of missing information (under "Fraction Missing Info") is an estimate of the proportion of patients with a missing value for that variable based on the relative increase variance. The relative increase in variance (under "Relative Increase Variance") is the ratio of the between-imputation and the mean within-imputation variance of the regression coefficients. The relative efficiency (under "Relative Efficiency") is equal to the ratio of missing information and relative increase in variance. The closer the relative efficiency values lie to one, the closer the pooled estimate (for each parameter) is to an estimate based on an infinite number of imputations. If the relative efficiency is not close to one, more imputations are needed for more accurate estimates of the effects.

Only the results of the complete case analysis (i.e., Imputation Number = Original data) and the pooled results (i.e., Imputation Number = Pooled) of the Cox regression model are reported in a paper. The results for each of the imputation datasets are not reported. ◻Table 8.12 shows an example of how the results are reported in a scientific paper. Based on ◻Table 8.12, we conclude that the pooled results are very similar to the results of the complete case analysis. This is because only a small proportion of patients had missing values for one or more variables in the model (8 %), if this proportion would have been higher, the results would differ more.

The multiple imputation method requires the data to be at least MAR (possible even MCAR, but definitely not MNAR). Moreover, the imputation model that is used to impute the missing data needs to be well specified and valid. Large differences between the complete case analysis and the pooled results for a dataset with a low proportion of missing data, could indicate a poorly specified imputation model.

One last remark has to be made regarding the multiple imputation method. Because the missing values are imputed with stochastic models, different imputation sets are obtained when the procedure is repeated on the same dataset. Therefore, the new dataset has to be saved, once the multiple imputation model is final and missing values are imputed. If an imputed database is opened again, SPSS will always generate a warning message in the output file (►Warning 8.1).

❗ Warning 8.1

Note # 5268. Command name: GET FILE
This appears to be a Multiple Imputation dataset. In addition to the original data, a multiple imputation dataset contains multiple copies of the data in which missing values have been replaced with imputed values. If you want this dataset to be treated as a multiple imputation dataset, use the SPLIT FILE command to define the Imputation_ variable as a SPLIT FILE variable before performing analyses.

In other words, if the Split File query is used, SPSS will automatically provide the estimated effects for the original data, each of the imputation datasets and the pooled results. If forgotten, analyses are performed on a database in which all imputation

■ **Table 8.12** Estimated effects on the time to development of the different determinants in the Cox regression model, for the original data (complete case analysis) and the pooled results of multiple imputation (with three datasets)

	original data (n = 345)			pooled results (n = 374)		
	HR	95 % CI	p-value	HR	95 % CI	p-value
Current smoker	0.93	0.63; 1.4	0.72	1.03	0.71; 1.5	0.86
No alcohol	1.6	1.1; 2.3	0.012	1.7	1.2; 2.5	0.002
Symptom duration < 12 months	1.6	1.1; 2.4	0.016	1.6	1.1; 2.3	0.021
Intermittent symptoms present	1.8	1.2; 2.6	0.002	1.7	1.2; 2.4	0.006
Antibody status			<0.001			
IgM-RF positive but aCCP negative	1			1		
IgM-RF negative but aCPP low positive	2.9	1.4; 6.1		3.0	1.4; 6.1	
IgM-RF negative but aCPP high positive	4.7	2.3; 9.4		4.6	2.4; 9.1	
IgM-RF positive and aCPP positive	7.0	3.6; 13.6		7.4	3.9; 13.9	

datasets as well as the original dataset are considered as one large dataset. As a consequence, the SEs of the effects will be too small and the p-value to low, possibly leading to an incorrect conclusion.

8.3 Further Readings

Rubin has written an excellent paper and co-authored a great book on missing data and multiple imputation [3, 4].

References

1. Stadt LA van de, Witte BI, Bos WH, Schaardenburg D van. A prediction rule for the development of arthritis in seropositive arthralgia patients. Ann Rheum Dis. 2013;72(12):1920–6. ▶ https://doi.org/10.1136/annrheumdis-2012-202127.
2. Uyl D den, Wee MM ter, Boers M, Kerstens P, Voskuyl A, Nurmohamed M, et al. A non-inferiority trial of an attenuated combination strategy ('COBRA-light') compared to the original COBRA strategy: clinical results after 26 weeks. Ann Rheum Dis. 2014;73(6):1071–8. ▶ https://doi.org/10.1136/annrheumdis-2012-202818.
3. Rubin DB. Multiple imputation after 18+ years. J Am Stat Assoc. 1996;91:473–89. ▶ https://doi.org/10.1080/01621459.1996.10476908.
4. Little RJA, Rubin DB. Statistical Analysis with Missing Data. 2nd ed. New York: John Wiley & Sons; 2002.

Writing and Critically Appraising a Scientific Paper

Abstract

After setting up a medical research, and collecting and analyzing the data, a scientific paper is written. Writing a scientific paper is not the easiest task. Therefore, in the first part of this chapter, we provide general tips for writing a scientific paper as well as tips what to include in the specific parts of a paper. In the second part of this chapter, we focus on how to critically appraise existing literature. After all, a publication in a journal with a high impact factor does not necessarily indicate that the scientific paper is of good quality. Therefore it is necessary to know what to check when reading existing literature.

© Bohn Stafleu van Loghum is een imprint van Springer Media B.V., onderdeel van Springer Nature 2019
M. M. ter Wee and B. I. Lissenberg-Witte, *A Quick Guide on How to Conduct Medical Research*,
https://doi.org/10.1007/978-90-368-2248-0_9

9.1   Writing a Scientific Paper

Medical research aims to provide the world with new discoveries and insights. The results of the research becomes available to the greater public through scientific papers in journals. Most journals are peer-reviewed, which means that peers or experts on the topic evaluate the manuscript. These peers provide the editor of the journal with a recommendation to publish, revise or reject the paper. The process of writing, submitting and revising is often a discouraging process, which takes time and patience. With the following tips, this process might be shortened, which hopefully leads to acceptance of the paper for publication.

Try to write the paper in a quite formal and passive style, not referring to 'we', or 'you', but as if a third person has watched all the steps that were performed in the research, and has to write the paper. For example use 'the authors found…'. However, some journals do prefer the use of a more personal and active style, so always check the guidelines for authors of the journal of interest, before starting to write. Keep the main message of the paper in mind, and explain all aspects of the research in such a way that a lay-person knows what was done. Read many papers to see how others describe certain scientific aspects. Also ask for input from more experienced writers or a native English speaker for comments on style, grammar and spelling of the paper. A poor writing style or bad grammar are common reasons to reject a manuscript.

A scientific paper usually follows a fixed format: abstract, introduction, patients and methods, results, discussion and conclusion. Below, we provide some tips and tricks for writing these different parts of the manuscript. We start, however, with an overview of general guidelines for different types of research designs that are advised to be followed when writing a scientific paper.

9.1.1   General Guidelines

Each journal has its own guideline for the writing style (active or passive) as well as for the word limit and reference style which a scientific paper should convey. For medical research, more general guidelines have been developed for different research designs, and journals require that these guidelines are followed as well when submitting a scientific paper. To make sure no time is wasted on rewriting a paper that is ready for submission to a journal, the appropriate guidelines should always be checked before beginning to write. They help to improve the quality of the scientific paper and increase the chance of getting the paper published. The following guidelines have been developed:

- The STrengthening the Reporting of OBservational studies in Epidemiology (STROBE) statement is a guideline to report the results of cohort studies, case-control studies or cross-sectional studies [1, 2]. This statement provides guidelines on how to write and critically appraise observational studies and can be found at ▶ http://www.strobe-statement.org [3].

- The REporting of studies Conducted using Observational Routinely collected health Data (RECORD) statement is a guideline to report the results of observational studies with routinely collected health data, for example through hospital records [4, 5]. This statement can be found at ▶ http://www.record-statement.org [6].
- The CONsolidated Standards Of Reporting Trials (CONSORT) statement is a guideline to report the results of experimental studies, such as randomized controlled trials (RCTs) [7, 8]. The CONSORT statement has several extensions for non-inferiority and equivalence trials, clustered trials, parallel group trials, pragmatic trials, N-of-1 trials, pilot and feasibility trials, and within person trials. This statement, and the extensions, can be found at ▶ http://www.consort-statement.org [9].
- The Preferred Reporting Items for Systematic reviews and Meta-Analyses (PRISMA) statement is a guideline to report the results of systematic reviews and meta-analyses [10, 11]. It can be found at ▶ http://www.prisma-statement.org [12].
- The Transparent Reporting of a multivariable prediction model for Individual Prognosis Or Diagnosis (TRIPOD) statement is a guideline to describe the results of prediction modelling studies [13]. This statement can be found at ▶ http://www. tripod-statement.org [14].
- The STAndards for Reporting of Diagnostic accuracy (STARD) statement is a guideline to report the results of studies on diagnostic accuracy [15, 16]. This statement can be found at ▶ http://www.equator-network.org/reporting-guidelines/stard/ [17].
- The Transparent Reporting of Evaluations with Nonrandomized Designs (TREND) statement is a guideline to report the results of nonrandomized controlled trials [18]. This statement can be found at ▶ https://www.cdc.gov/trendstatement/index.html [19].
- The Consolidated Health Economic Evaluation Reporting Standards (CHEERS) statement [20, 21] as well as the recommendations of the Panel on Cost-Effectiveness in Health and Medicine [22–25] can be used to report the results of economic evaluations or cost-effectiveness analyses (CEAs).
- The Meta-analyses Of Observational Studies in Epidemiology (MOOSE) guideline can be used to report the results of systematic reviews and meta-analyses of observational studies [26]. This guideline can also be used to review results of meta-analyses.
- The COnsolidated criteria for Reporting Qualitative research (COREQ) guideline needs to be used to report the results of qualitative studies [27].
- The COnsensus-based Standards for selection of health Measurement Instruments (COSMIN) standard is a checklist that can be used to define and determine the psychometric properties of Health-Related Patient-Reported Outcome Measures (HR-PROMs). This standard can also be used to develop a new PROM [28–30]. The checklist can be found at ▶ http://www.cosmin.nl [31].

9.1.2 The Abstract

The abstract is a summary of the scientific paper and is the first thing read by the target audience. The reader will decide whether the paper is interesting enough to read in more detail based on the abstract. In addition, the journal editor decides whether the paper is relevant to their journal based on the abstract. It should therefore be attractive on the one hand, but also brief and concise on the other. Moreover, it should highlight the most important results and the final conclusion.

The abstract can be either structured or unstructured. A structured abstract has a similar format as the paper itself: background/objective, methods, results and conclusion. Most structured abstracts are between 250 and 300 words. An unstructured abstract contains the same information as the structured abstract, but is written as one single paragraph, often used in systematic reviews. An unstructured abstract is usually shorter than a structured abstract: between 100 and 250 words. The type of abstract, and the word limit of the abstract, depends on the journal guidelines.

Another type of abstract is the conference abstract. This is an abstract which is submitted to a conference organization, and published in conference books if accepted for an oral presentation or a poster (presentation). Conference abstracts can be longer, sometimes up to 500 words, because they stand alone.

Some authors decide to write the abstract after completing the paper. However, writing the abstract in advance, will help to keep a focus on the important messages of the paper.

9.1.3 The Introduction

In ▶ Chap. 1, we introduced the hourglass template (◘ Fig. 1.1, ▶ Sect. 1.3) that can be used to write the scientific background of the research for the research proposal. It can also be used to write the introduction of the paper. Writing the introduction is often underestimated.

The introduction starts with the importance of the topic, for example with the impact of the disease. This is followed by a description of the research gap. What information is missing in the existing literature and why is it important to narrow this gap? This leads to the research question or aim. The research aim usually starts with 'The purpose/aim of this study/review/case report is to …'. The research question or aim is translated to the null and alternative hypothesis, in the research proposal (▶ Sect. 1.4), but these hypotheses are rarely stated in the introduction of the scientific paper. ◘ Figure 9.1 shows these different aspects of the introduction of the published scientific paper of van de Stadt et al. [32].

9.1.4 The Patients and Methods

The best written papers are the ones that make it possible to reproduce the research. That is why the methods section has to be written objectively. Use sub-headers to clearly outline the different aspects: study population, laboratory tests, questionnaires, statistical analyses, etc. The methods section cannot contain any results.

The first paragraph of the methods section provides a description of the research population. The in- and exclusion criteria are summarized, allowing the reader to judge if selection bias might be present. If applicable, a statement on approval by the Medical Ethical Review Board (MERB) is added as well a description of the informed consent procedure.

INTRODUCTION

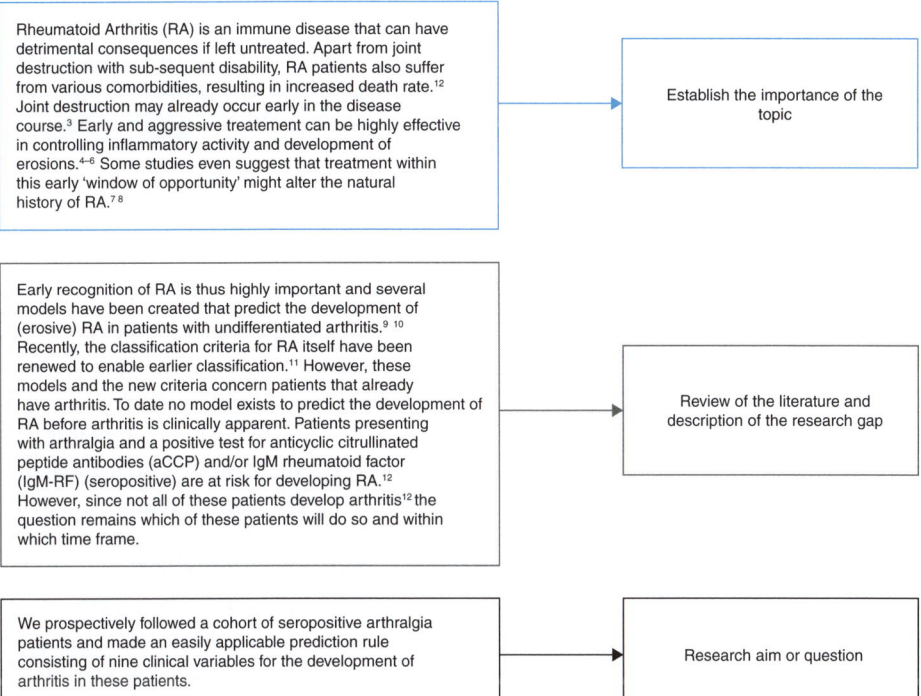

Fig. 9.1 Example of the different aspects of an introduction (Taken from van de Stadt et al. [32]. © BMJ and EULAR 2018)

The second paragraph lists the data collection methods. Which data is collected, how is it collected/measured and how often? If questionnaires are used, preferably through validated questionnaires, provide results on their reliability and validity. If medication is used, provide information on the daily dosage used and the treatment protocol. Do not provide a rationale or justification for the used questionnaires or test measures, this should be addressed in the discussion.

The last paragraph of the methods sections is devoted to the statistical analyses. The analysis plan, developed for the research proposal (▶ Sect. 1.5.3), forms the basis of the statistical analyses paragraph. Start this paragraph with a description of the descriptive statistics (▶ Chap. 2). Continue with a description of the statistical tests (inferential statistics) and/or which kind of regression models are estimated (▶ Chap. 3–5). Do not forget to report how the assumptions of these tests and/or models are checked. Provide this information for the primary objective, as well as for the secondary and tertiary objectives. If the focus lies on analyzing an association between the outcome variable and a central determinant, describe how confounding and effect modification is investigated and corrected for (▶ Chap. 6). If the primary objective of the study is to build a prediction model, describe the selection procedure, the inclusion criterion and goodness-of-fit measures to assess the quality of the final model (▶ Chap. 7). It is also important to describe how missing data is handled (if applicable), whether the primary analysis is based on intention-to-treat or per-protocol and whether sensitivity analyses are performed (▶Chap. 8). Finally, the significance level of the statistical tests, whether this is one-sided or two-sided, and the statistical software used, need to be reported. For example, all analyses in this book were conducted in SPSS (IBM Corp., Armonk, NY, USA, version 22) and in all tests a two-sided significance level α of 0.05 was used, unless specified otherwise.

9.1.5 The Results

Most parts of the introduction and the methods section of the paper could be written before the research has even started, using parts of the research proposal. This is not the case for the results section. All results of the study are reported in the results section of the paper. Provide information on the study population in the first paragraph of this section. Describe how many patients were screened and how many were actually included in the study. For every screened but not included patient, provide the reason for exclusion. This contributes to a better judgement on whether selection bias is present or not. Also state the number of patients that dropped out, with a specification of the reasons for drop-out, and the number of patients that were lost to follow-up. The best way to visualize the flow of number of patients included in the study, from screening to the final analyses, is with a flowchart (◘Fig. 1.3, ▶Sect. 1.5.1). The flowchart is shown for each group separately, when two or more groups are compared. Also ellaborate shortly in the text on the numbers mentioned in the flowchart. ◘Figure 9.2 shows the flowchart of the COmbinatie Behandeling Reumatoïde Artritis (COBRA)-light trial [33]. Subsequently, in the published paper on the results of 26 weeks of treatment in the COBRA-light trial, the flowchart was described as follows: *Of all patients screened (n=246), 33% were not included because they did not meet the entry criteria or declined participation. The predominant reason to decline was the intensity of the study rather than the treatment. Two patients did not initiate treatment and dropped out immediately after randomisation. These patients were excluded from the ITT analyses.*© BMJ and EULAR 2018 [40]. In the first paragraph, also descriptive statistics, including missing data of the patients in the study population, are reported (◘Table 2.4 and 2.5, ▶Sect. 2.2.5).

In the second paragraph of the results section, the results of the primary analysis, corresponding to the primary objective, are reported. Use the appropriate effect size with the 95 % confidence interval (CI) and exact p-value of the statistical test. Only report the objective results: the interpretation of the results should be postponed to the discussion section. Results of the secondary/tertiary analyses and sensitivity analyses – if performed – follow in the subsequent paragraphs.

Use clear figures to support the main message. Tables should be readable as standalone, without forcing the reader to read the scientific paper in detail. Remember that every journal has guidelines, which include the maximum number of tables and figures that can be included in the scientific paper, and in what format and quality the figures should be uploaded to the submission system.

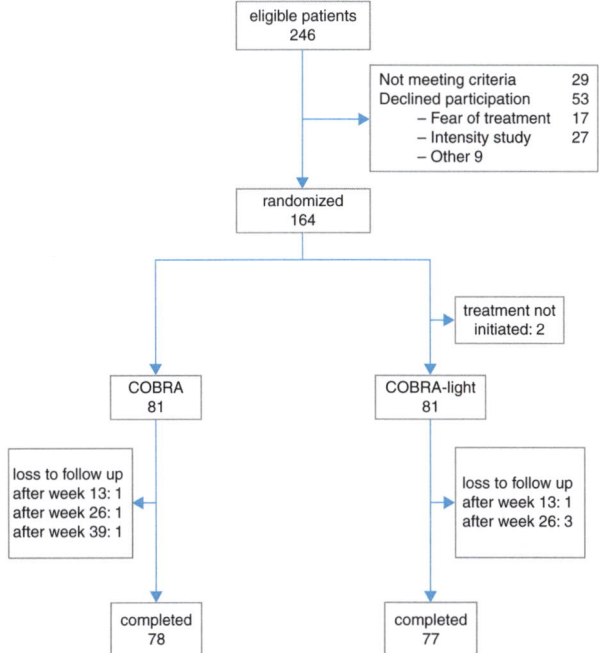

eligible patients
246

Not meeting criteria   29
Declined participation   53
– Fear of treatment   17
– Intensity study   27
– Other 9

randomized
164

treatment not
initiated: 2

COBRA
81

COBRA-light
81

loss to follow up
after week 13: 1
after week 26: 1
after week 39: 1

loss to follow up
after week 13: 1
after week 26: 3

completed
78

completed
77

Fig. 9.2 Flowchart of the COBRA-light trial for 52 weeks of treatment [33] © BMJ and EULAR (2018)

9.1.6 The Discussion and Conclusion

The results of the research are reported in the results section, while they are interpreted in the discussion section. A good discussion often follows a certain structure as well. It starts with a short summary of the most important results. Make sure that no new results are reported in the discussion. Then, the results are interpreted and compared to existing literature. How do the findings differ from other studies or why are they similar. After that, elaborate on the strengths and limitations of the performed study. The discussions ends with a short, firm conclusion. The conclusion should answer the research question and state implications of the results for clinical practice. The hourglass template (◘ Fig. 1.1, ▶ Sect. 1.3) can also be used to help write the discussion.

9.1.7 Research Integrity

Research integrity is an important aspect of (medical) research. It means that a researcher is honest, adheres to rules, regulations and guidelines, such as the Good Clinical Practice (GCP) guidelines, and follows specific research codes and norms. Research integrity should be propagated in all steps of research. Be truthful, honor commitments, be precise, avoid errors and report all results. This includes also reporting the negative results. Reporting negative results reduces publication bias, a type of bias that occurs if the outcome of a research influences the decision to publish (in case of a positive result) or not (in case of a negative result). It must be said that positive results have a much higher chance of being published compared to negative findings. This automatically results in publication bias. When performing a systematic review, try to include negative results, or if they cannot be found, make sure a statement is made on this in the discussion section.

Another important aspect of research integrity is the author contribution. The International Committee of Medical Journal Editors (ICMJE) has developed recommendations for criteria that define authorship. These recommendations can be found at ► www.icmje. org [34]. Finally, potential conflict of interest for (some of) the authors should always be reported.

9.1.8 Submission Process to a Journal

After the paper has been written, the paper is send to all coauthors. They will read the paper and provide comments and suggestions for changes. This process can be time consuming. However, approval of all authors is needed to submit the paper to the selected journal.

Submission of a scientific paper should be accompanied with a submission letter. This letter contains a short description of the research with the most important conclusion and implications for daily practice. The editor of the journal will first read this letter as well as the title and abstract of the paper. Therefore, the title should be catchy and the abstract clear, with a firm but solid conclusion. Based on the submission letter and the abstract, the editor decides whether or not the paper is interesting for the journal and its readers. If deemed interesting, the paper is sent to peer reviewers for review. Otherwise, the corresponding author receives an email stating that the paper has not been considered for publication.

The review process might take quite some time: depending on the journal, up to two or three months, and sometimes even longer. The reviewers provide the editor with feedback on the importance and scientific quality of the paper. Depending on the journal, one of the reviewers could be a statistician, who reviews the statistical analyses section of the paper, and checks whether the results are obtained and interpreted correctly. The editor then decides what to do, using the feedback of the reviewers: reject the paper, ask for major revisions of the paper or accept it provisionally with minor revisions.

In case of (major or minor) revisions, the author needs to reply to each of the issues raised by the reviewers. However, one does not always have to agree with the reviewers. Make sure that the issues are replied to with solid arguments. Always write the reply in a respectful manner, and thank the reviewers for their time. The revised version of the paper (usually two documents, one in which the changes to the previous version are highlighted and one clean version) as well as the reply to the reviewers are then submitted to the journal again. Sometimes, the editor sends the revised version with replies back to the reviewers for a second review process. Otherwise, the editor decides him-/ herself to accept the paper, or to reject the paper completely.

If the paper is accepted for publication, the journal will edit the paper to match the journal's style and the corresponding author receives a proof. Take the time to read the proof and check all results, figures and tables as errors occur quite often. After the proof is submitted, the paper is finished and usually appears as an online-publication at the journal's website first. This allows other researchers to use the results for their own new research as quickly as possible. Congratulations, the research is now finished. On to the next!

9.2   Critical Appraisal of Existing Literature

Although the pile of published scientific papers is enormous, selecting those papers that are of the best quality is quite difficult. Many researchers have the opinion that if a paper is published in a journal with a high impact factor, it has to be of good quality. Sadly enough, this is not necessarily true. Therefore, every paper that is read or used as a reference, should be critically appraised.

Of course, all the mentioned statements and guidelines in ▶Sect. 9.1.1 are a good starting point to judge the quality of published papers. Common sense, together with the methods described in the previous chapters, also allows for a solid appraisal. Critical appraisal starts with determining the main research question and the secondary aims. Formulate the corresponding null and alternative hypothesis (if not provided in the paper). Review the method section to determine if the research design is appropriate to answer the research question. Also check for potential selection bias in the description of how the study population was selected.

The statistical analyses paragraph is also an important part of the paper for critical appraisal. Establish the outcome variable: is it a continuous, a dichotomous or a time to event variable? Decide on the main focus: is it an association model or a prediction model? Is the association model corrected for confounding and/or effect modification? What selection procedure is used to build the prediction model, and what was the selection criterion? Use ◻Table 9.1 to investigate whether the statistical tests and models are applied correctly. Also check if the corresponding assumptions are tested. When more complex statistical methods are used, check the further readings sections at the end of ▶Chaps. 3–5 (▶Sects. 3.6, 4.7 and 5.6) for references to these methods, or seek help of a statistician. Check if the provided results are reported in the correct way. Could the results provide an answer to the question, and secondary aims?

At last, read the discussion. Are there no new results reported? Are the interpretations of the results correct? Are the results (correctly) compared to existing literature? Are all strengths and limitations of the study acknowledged? And most importantly, does the final conclusion give an answer to the research question?

When performing a systematic review, critical appraisal of the selected papers is done through a risk of bias assessment. This can be done through risk of bias tools such as the Cochrane risk of bias [35], or the Newcastle-Ottawa Scale (NOS) tool [36]. The Cochrane risk of bias tool is an assessment of RCTs, and consists of the following topics: allocation sequence and concealment, precautionary measures to ensure blinding, blinding of outcome assessment, incomplete outcome data, selective reporting and

▢ Table 9.1 Overview of the important statistical methods, with the effects size to report and the assumptions to check, for the analyses described in ▸ Chaps. 3–7

		Outcome variable			
		Continuous - normally distributed	Continuous - non-normally distributed	Dichotomous	Time to event
Dichotomous determinant	Statistical test	Independent samples t-test	Mann-Whitney U test	Chi-square test	Log-rank test; Cox regression model
	Effect size	Mean difference	None	OR/RR/RD	Kaplan-Meier curve/cumulative incidence; HR
	Assumptions	Normally distributed in each group separately	None	Expected count ≥ 5 in all cells	None; Proportionality
Categorical determinant	Statistical test	ANOVA	Kruskal-Wallis	Chi-square test	Log-rank test; Cox regression model
	Effect size (one group set as reference)	Mean difference	None	OR/RR/RD	Kaplan-Meier curve/cumulative incidence; HR
	Assumptions	Normally distributed in each group	None	Expected count ≥ 5 in all cells	None; Proportionality
Continuous determinant	Statistical model	Linear regression model		Logistic regression model	Cox regression model
	Effect size (per increase of 1 unit)	Regression coefficient (mean difference)		Exponential of regression coefficient (OR)	Exponential of regression coefficient (HR)
	Assumptions	Linearity; Normality residuals; Homoscedasticity		Linearity	Linearity; Proportionality

◻ **Table 9.1** Overview of the important statistical methods, with the effects size to report and the assumptions to check, for the analyses described in ▸ Chaps. 3–7 (continued)

		Outcome variable			
		Continuous – normally distributed	Continuous – non-normally distributed	Dichotomous	Time to event
Paired data	Statistical test	Paired sample *t*-test	Wilcoxon signed rank test	McNemar test	
	Effect size	Mean difference	None	Percentage positive outcomes	
	Assumptions	Normally distributed at both measurements	None	None	
Multiple regression/ prediction model	Statistical model	Linear regression model		Logistic regression model	Cox regression model
	Assumptions	Linearity for each continuous predictor		Linearity for each continuous predictor	Linearity for each continuous predictor
		Normality residuals			Proportionality for each predictor
		Homoscedasticity			
	Number of patients per predictor	10 patients		10 patients with event and 10 without event	10 patients with event and 10 without event
	SPSS remarks	Dummy variables manually		Dummy variables automatic	Dummy variables automatic
		Interaction between two variables manually		Interaction between two variables automatic	Interaction between two variables automatic
	Quality of the model	R^2		AUC under ROC	Harrell's C
				calibration curve	
				Hosmer-Lemeshow test	
	Comparing nested models	*F*-test		LR-test	LR-test

other sources of bias. The NOS tool is a risk of bias tool for nonrandomized studies and assesses the following topics: representativeness, definition of exposure, assessment of outcome, non-response rate and sufficient follow-up. Each tool focuses on certain topics. Therefore, a combination of tools is advised.

9.3   Further Readings

Many books and papers have been written on how to write a scientific paper, such as the one written by Hoogenboom & Manske or by Wallwork et al. [37, 38]. Hoogenboom also co-authored a commentary, in which the peer review process is visualized [39].

References

1. Elm E von, Altman DG, Egger M, Pocock SJ, Gotzsche PC, vandenbroucke JP, et al. The strengthening the reporting of observational studies in epidemiology (STROBE) statement: guidelines for reporting observational studies. Ann Intern Med. 2007;147(8):573–7. ►https://doi.org/10.7326/0003-4819-147-8-200710160-00010.
2. Vandenbroucke JP, von Elm E, Altman DG, Gotzsche PC, Mulrow CD, Pocock SJ, et al. Strengthening the Reporting of Observational Studies in Epidemiology (STROBE): explanation and elaboration. Ann Intern Med. 2007;147(8):W163–94. ►https://doi.org/10.7326/0003-4819-147-8-200710160-00010-w1.
3. STROBE Initiative. STROBE Statement. 2009. ►http://www.strobe-statement.org. Accessed 9 Oct 2009.
4. Benchimol EI, Smeeth L, Guttmann A, Harron K, Moher D, Petersen I, et al. The REporting of studies Conducted using Observational Routinely-collected health Data (RECORD) statement. PLoS Med. 2015;12(10):e1001885. ►https://doi.org/10.1371/journal.pmed.1001885.
5. Langan SM, Benchimol EI, Guttmann A, Moher D, Petersen I, Smeeth L, et al. Setting the RECORD straight: developing a guideline for the REporting of studies Conducted using Observational Routinely collected Data. Clin Epidemiol. 2013;5:29–31. ►https://doi.org/10.2147/clep.s36885.
6. RECORD Group. RECORD Reporting Guidelines. 2017. ►http://www.record-statement.org. Accessed 9 Oct 2018.
7. Schulz KF, Altman DG, Moher D, for the CONSORT Group. CONSORT 2010 statement: updated guidelines for reporting parallel group randomised trials. BMJ. 2010;340(9609):c332. ►https://doi.org/10.1136/bmj.c332.
8. Moher D, Hopewell S, Schulz KF, Montori V, Gøtzsche PC, Devereaux PJ, et al. CONSORT 2010 explanation and elaboration: updated guidelines for reporting parallel group randomised trials. BMJ. 2010;340:c869. ►https://doi.org/10.1136/bmj.c869.
9. CONSORT Group. CONSORT Website. 2010. ►http://www.consort-statement.org. Accessed 9 Oct 2018.
10. Moher D, Liberati A, Tetzlaff J, Altman DG, PRISMA Group. Preferred reporting items for systematic reviews and meta-analyses: the PRISMA Statement. Ann Intern Med. 2009;151(4):264–9. ►https://doi.org/10.7326/0003-4819-151-4-200908180-00135.
11. Shamseer L, Moher D, Clarke M, Ghersi D, Liberati A, Petticrew M, et al. Preferred reporting items for systematic review and meta-analysis protocols (PRISMA-P) 2015: elaboration and explanation. BMJ. 2015;350:g7647. ►https://doi.org/10.1136/bmj.g7647.
12. PRISMA Group. PRISMA Statement. 2015. ►http://www.prisma-statement.org. Accessed 9 Oct 2018.
13. Moons KG, Altman DG, Reitsma JB, Ioannidis JP, Macaskill P, Steyerberg EW, et al. Transparent Reporting of a multivariable prediction model for Individual Prognosis or Diagnosis (TRIPOD): explanation and elaboration. Ann Intern Med. 2015;162(1):55–63. ►https://doi.org/10.7326/m14-0698.
14. TRIPOD Group. TRIPOD Statement. 2018. ►http://www.tripod-statement.org. Accessed 9 Oct 2018.
15. Bossuyt PM, Reitsma JB, Bruns DE, Gatsonis CA, Glasziou PP, Irwig L, et al. STARD 2015: an updated list of essential items for reporting diagnostic accuracy studies. BMJ. 2015;351:h5527. ►https://doi.org/10.1136/bmj.h5527.

16. Cohen JF, Korevaar DA, Altman DG, Bruns DE, Gatsonis CA, Hooft L, et al. STARD 2015 guidelines for reporting diagnostic accuracy studies: explanation and elaboration. BMJ Open. 2016;6(11):e012799. ▶ https://doi.org/10.1136/bmjopen-2016-012799.

17. EQUATOR Network. STARD 2015: an updated list of essential items for reporting diagnostic accuracy studies. 2017. ▶ http://www.equator-network.org/reporting-guidelines/stard/. Accessed 9 Oct 2018.

18. Jarlais DC des, Lyles C, Crepaz N, Trend Group. Improving the reporting quality of nonrandomized evaluations of behavioral and public health interventions: the TREND statement. Am J Public Health. 2004;94(3):361–6. ▶ https://doi.org/10.2105/ajph.94.3.361.

19. Centers for Disease Control and Prevention. TREND Statement. 2018. ▶ https://www.cdc.gov/trendstatement/index.html. Accessed 9 Oct 2018.

20. Husereau D, Drummond M, Petrou S, Carswell C, Moher D, Greenberg D, et al. Consolidated Health Economic Evaluation Reporting Standards (CHEERS) statement. Int J Technol Assess Health Care. 2013;29(2):117–22. ▶ https://doi.org/10.1017/s0266462313000160.

21. Husereau D, Drummond M, Petrou S, Greenberg D, Mauskopf J, Augustovski F, et al. Reply to Roberts et al.: CHEERS is sufficient for reporting cost-benefit analysis, but may require further elaboration. Pharmacoeconomics. 2015;33(5):535–6. ▶ https://doi.org/10.1007/s40273-015-0277-8.

22. Mandelblatt JS, Fryback DG, Weinstein MC, Russell LB, Gold MR. Assessing the effectiveness of health interventions for cost-effectiveness analysis. Panel on Cost-Effectiveness in Health and Medicine. J Gen Intern Med. 1997;12(9):551–8. PMC: 1497158.

23. Siegel JE, Torrance GW, Russell LB, Luce BR, Weinstein MC, Gold MR. Guidelines for pharmacoeconomic studies. Pharmacoeconomics. 1997;11(2):159–68. ▶ https://doi.org/10.2165/00019053-199711020-00005.

24. Siegel JE, Weinstein MC, Russell LB, Gold MR. Recommendations for reporting cost-effectiveness analyses. Panel on cost-effectiveness in health and medicine. JAMA. 1996;276(16):1339–41. ▶ https://doi.org/10.1001/jama.1996.03540160061034.

25. Weinstein MC, Siegel JE, Gold MR, Kamlet MS, Russell LB. Recommendations of the panel on cost-effectiveness in health and medicine. JAMA. 1996;276(15):1253–8. ▶ https://doi.org/10.1001/jama.1996.03540150055031.

26. Stroup DF, Berlin JA, Morton SC, Olkin I, Williamson GD, Rennie D, et al. Meta-analysis of observational studies in epidemiology: a proposal for reporting. Meta-analysis Of Observational Studies in Epidemiology (MOOSE) group. JAMA. 2000;283(15):2008–12. ▶ https://doi.org/10.1001/jama.283.15.2008.

27. Tong A, Sainsbury P, Craig J. Consolidated criteria for reporting qualitative research (COREQ): a 32-item checklist for interviews and focus groups. Int J Qual Health Care. 2007;19(6):349–57. ▶ https://doi.org/10.1093/intqhc/mzm042.

28. Mokkink LB, Prinsen CA, Bouter LM, de Vet HCW, Terwee CB. The COnsensus-based Standards for the selection of health Measurement INstruments (COSMIN) and how to select an outcome measurement instrument. Braz J Phys Ther. 2016;20(2):105–13. ▶ https://doi.org/10.1590/bjpt-rbf.2014.0143.

29. Mokkink LB, Terwee CB, Knol DL, Stratford PW, Alonso J, Patrick DL, et al. Protocol of the COSMIN study: COnsensus-based Standards for the selection of health Measurement INstruments. BMC Med Res Methodol. 2006;6:2. ▶ https://doi.org/10.1186/1471-2288-6-2.

30. Mokkink LB, Terwee CB, Knol DL, Stratford PW, Alonso J, Patrick DL, et al. The COSMIN checklist for evaluating the methodological quality of studies on measurement properties: a clarification of its content. BMC Med Res Methodol. 2010;10:22. ▶ https://doi.org/10.1186/1471-2288-10-22.

31. COSMIN initiative. Checklists for assessing study qualities. 2005. ▶ https://www.cosmin.nl/tools/checklists-assessing-methodological-study-qualities/. Accessed 9 Oct 2018.

32. van de Stadt LA, Witte BI, Bos WH, van Schaardenburg D. A prediction rule for the development of arthritis in seropositive arthralgia patients. Ann Rheum Dis. 2013;72(12):1920–6. ▶ https://doi.org/10.1136/annrheumdis-2012-202127.

33. ter Wee MM, den Uyl D, Boers M, Kerstens P, Nurmohamed M, van Schaardenburg D, et al. Intensive combination treatment regimens, including prednisolone, are effective in treating patients with early rheumatoid arthritis regardless of additional etanercept: 1-year results of the COBRA-light open-label, randomised, non-inferiority trial. Ann Rheum Dis. 2015;74(6):1233–40. ▶ https://doi.org/10.1136/annrheumdis-2013-205143.

34. International Committee of Medical Journal Editors. ICMJE recommendations. 2017. ▶ http://www.icmje.org/recommendations/. Accessed 9 Oct 2018.

35. Higgins JPT, Green S, editors. Cochrane handbook for systematic reviews of interventions version 5.1.0 [updated March 2011]. The Cochrane Collaboration; 2011. Available from ► http://handbook.cochrane.org.
36. Wells GA, Shea B, O'Connel D, Peterson J, Welch V, Losos M, et al. The Newcastle-Ottawa Scale (NOS) for assessing the quality of nonrandomised studies in meta-analyses. 2013. ► http://www.ohri.ca/programs/clinical_epidemiology/oxford.asp. Accessed 9 Sept 2018.
37. Hoogenboom BJ, Manske RC. How to write a scientific article. Int J Sports Phys Ther. 2012;7(5):512–7. PMC: 3474301.
38. Wallwork A. English for writing research papers. New York: Springer; 2011.
39. Voight ML, Hoogenboom BJ. Publishing your work in a journal: understanding the peer review process. Int J Sports Phys Ther. 2012;7(5):452–60. PMC: 3474310.
40. Uyl D den, Wee MM ter, Boers M, Kerstens P, Voskuyl A, Nurmohamed M, et al. A non-inferiority trial of an attenuated combination strategy ('COBRA-light') compared to the original COBRA strategy: clinical results after 26 weeks. Ann Rheum Dis. 2014;73(6):1071–8. ► https://doi.org/10.1136/annrheumdis-2012-202818

9

Supplementary Information

© Bohn Stafleu van Loghum is een imprint van Springer Media B.V., onderdeel van Springer Nature 2019
M. M. ter Wee and B. I. Lissenberg-Witte, *A Quick Guide on How to Conduct Medical Research*,
https://doi.org/10.1007/978-90-368-2248-0

SPSS Quick Guide

A.1 Introduction to SPSS

SPSS is a statistical program to analyze a database (with extension .sav). The data can be viewed by using two different 'Views':

1. **Data View**

    The database is seen as a table. The first column contains the row-numbers, the following columns contain the data. The first row contains the variable names. Data can be entered by typing in the values.

2. **Variable View**

    Contains information about each variable:

    a. Name: name of the variable

    b. Label: short description of the variable

    c. Values: short description of the values of the variable, in case the variable is binary or categorical. To add values or change/remove current values, select the cell, click on the appearing '...' and add/change/remove the values.

    d. Missing: value(s) that represent a missing value for that variable, for example if that variable was not measured (i.e., unknown) or is not applicable for a patient.

    e. Measure: type of the variable. Scale = continuous variable; ordinal = ordered dichotomous or categorical variable; nominal = unordered dichotomous or categorical variable.

The results of the statistical analysis appear in an output-file (with extension .spv). These results could be exported as a word-document (figures and tables), an excel-file (tables) or a power-point presentation (figures and tables). To do so, select the object(s) of interest for export, right-click with the computer mouse and choose 'Export...'. The output-file also contains the 'commands' (called syntax) SPSS executed to obtain the results. The syntax ("Log") could be copied to an SPSS-syntax file (with extension .sps), and used to rerun the analysis more quickly. Moreover, by using the syntax, a log of all analyses is kept.

This command-code could also be pasted into a syntax-file directly by clicking on 'Paste' instead of 'OK' in the final steps below. If this option is chosen, SPSS will NOT run the command. To run the syntax, select the part to run, and use CTRL + R (or click on ▶).

This SPSS quick guide takes you through all the necessary and optional steps to perform the analyses discussed in ▶Chap. 2 to 8. Each instruction follows a specific style:

- **Type of analysis**

Menu to be selected from the menu bar $\Rightarrow$ submenu $\Rightarrow$ analysis…

1. Steps that NEED to be followed are numbered 1., 2., etc.
   a. Steps that could be followed to obtain results that are not printed by default are numbered a., b., etc.
   b. This also holds for some additional options.
2. The last step is always to Click on 'OK'. This can be replaced by 'Paste' to obtain the syntax printed in the syntax-file.

A.2 Getting Started

- **Export output object(s)**

FIRST select the object(s) to be exported: File $\Rightarrow$ Export…

1. Select the type of document the object(s) are exported to.
2. Make sure that the check-box 'Selected' is checked to export only a selection of the output and not the whole output-file.
3. Click on 'Browse…' to select the location to export the object(s) to.
4. Change the filename to the desired name.
5. Click on 'OK'.

- **Select cases (for analyses in a specific group of patients)**

Data $\Rightarrow$ Select Cases…

1. Select 'If condition is satisfied' and click on 'If…'.
2. Select the variable in the left column and finish the expression in the white area (right top).
3. Click on 'Continue'.
   a. To copy the selected cases to a new dataset, select 'Copy selected cases to a new dataset' and type a name for this new dataset.
   b. To delete unselected cases from the current dataset, select 'Delete unselected cases'.
4. Click on 'OK'.

NOTE: to analyze all cases after a selection, select 'All cases' in step 1.

- **Stratify analyses [split file] (to compare groups of patients)**

Data $\Rightarrow$ Split file…

1. Select 'Compare groups'.
2. Select the splitting variable(s) in the left column and click on the arrow.
3. Click on 'OK'.

NOTE: to remove the split, select 'Analyze all cases, do not create groups' in step 1.

- ### Compute a new variable

Transform $\Rightarrow$ Compute variable…

1. Type the name of the new variable in the field below 'Target Variable:'.
   a. Click on 'Type & Label' to add a description of the variable (i.e., add a variable label).
   b. Type the description of the variable after 'Label:'.
   c. Click on 'Continue'.
2. Type the equation in the field below 'Numeric Expression:'. Select variables from the database in the left column and click on the arrow. Specific functions can be searched below 'Function group:'.
3. Click on 'OK'.

- ### Divide a continuous variable into groups of equal size

Transform $\Rightarrow$ Rank Cases…

1. Select the variable to categorize from the left column and click on the first arrow.
2. Click on 'Rank Types…'.
3. Select 'Ntiles', and type the number of categories (i.e., 4 for quartiles).
4. Unselect 'Rank' and click on 'Continue'.
5. Click on 'OK'.

NOTE: the new categorical variable can be found in the last column(s) of the database, and the name(s) of this variable starts with 'N'.

- ### Recode a categorical or continuous variable into a new variable

Transform $\Rightarrow$ Recode into Different Variables…

1. Select the variable to recode from the left column and click on the arrow.
2. Type the name and label (optional) of the new variable in the field(s) below 'Name:' under Output Variable. Click on 'Change'.
3. Click on the button 'Old and New Values…'.
4. Select the (range of) old value(s) to recode on the left side below 'Old Value'.
   a. 'Value:' and type the value to recode.
   b. 'Range:' and type the lower and upper values of the old variable.
   c. 'Range, LOWEST through value:' and type the upper value of the category of the old variable.
   d. 'Range, value through HIGHEST:' and type the lower value of the category of the old variable.
5. Select the option for the new value at the right side below 'New Value'.
   a. 'Value:' and type the new value.
   b. 'Copy old value(s)' to copy value(s) of the old variable.
6. Click 'Add'.
7. Repeat steps 4. – 6. until all categories are defined.
8. Click on 'Continue' and then 'OK'.

A.3 Descriptive Statistics

- **Frequency tables**

Analyze $\Rightarrow$ Descriptive Statistics $\Rightarrow$ Frequencies…

1. Select the variable(s) in the left column and click on the arrow.
2. Click on 'OK'.

- **Descriptive statistics**

Analyze $\Rightarrow$ Descriptive Statistics $\Rightarrow$ Frequencies…

1. Select the variable(s) in the left column and click on the arrow.
2. Click on 'Statistics…'.
3. Select the statistics and click on 'Continue'.
   a. For the IQR select 'Quartiles'.
4. Unselect 'Display frequency tables'.
5. Click on 'OK'.

NOTE: via Analyze $\Rightarrow$ Descriptive Statistics $\Rightarrow$ Descriptives… also some basic descriptive statistics can be obtained, but only the mean, standard deviation, minimum and maximum

- **Correlation coefficients**

Analyze $\Rightarrow$ Correlate $\Rightarrow$ Bivariate…

1. Select the variables in the left column and click on the arrow.
   a. 'Pearson' is the predefined setting in SPSS.
   b. For Spearman rank correlation, select 'Spearman' and unselect 'Pearson'.
2. Click on 'OK'.

- **Histogram**

Graphs $\Rightarrow$ Legacy Dialogs $\Rightarrow$ Histogram…

1. Select the variable from the left column and click on the first arrow.
   a. To obtain the histograms of different groups plotted under each other (without splitting the output), select the grouping variable from the left column and click on the second arrow.
   b. To obtain the histograms of different groups plotted next to each other (without splitting the output), select the grouping variable from the left column and click on the third arrow.
2. Click on 'OK'.
3. Double-click on the figure to change the style of the figure.

- **Boxplot**

Graphs $\Rightarrow$ Legacy Dialogs $\Rightarrow$ Boxplot…

1. Select 'Simple' and 'Summaries for groups of cases' and click on 'Define'.
2. Select the variable from the left column and click on the first arrow.
   a. Select the grouping variable from the left column and click on the second arrow for separate boxplots for different groups.
3. Click on 'OK'.
4. Double-click on the figure to change the style of the figure.

- **QQ-plot**

Analyze $\Rightarrow$ Descriptive Statistics $\Rightarrow$ Q-Q Plots…

1. Select the variable in the left column and click on the arrow.
2. Click on 'OK'.

- **Scatter plot**

Graphs $\Rightarrow$ Legacy Dialogs $\Rightarrow$ Scatter/Dot…

1. Select 'Simple Scatter' and click on 'Define'.
2. Select the variable for the y-axis from the left column and click on the first arrow.
3. Select the variable for the x-axis from the left column and click on the second arrow.
4. Click on 'OK'.
5. Double-click on the figure to change the style of the figure or add items.

A.4 Analyzing Continuous Outcome Variables

A.4.1 Comparing Two Groups

- **Independent samples t-test**

Analyze $\Rightarrow$ Compare Means $\Rightarrow$ Independent-Samples T Test…

1. Select the outcome variable in the left column, and click on the first arrow.
2. Select the dichotomous determinant in the left column, and click on the second arrow.
3. Click on 'Define Groups…'.
4. Enter the two values of the grouping variable and click on 'Continue'.
5. Click on 'OK'.

- **Nonparametric Mann-Whitney test**

Analyze $\Rightarrow$ Nonparametric Tests $\Rightarrow$ Legacy Dialogs $\Rightarrow$ 2 Independent Samples

1. Select the outcome variable in the left column, and click on the first arrow.
2. Select the dichotomous determinant in the left column, and click on the second arrow.
3. Click on 'Define Groups…'.
4. Enter the two values of the grouping variable and click on 'Continue'.
5. Click on 'OK'.

A.4.2 Comparing More Than Two Groups

- **ANOVA**

Analyze $\Rightarrow$ Compare Means $\Rightarrow$ One-Way ANOVA…

1. Select the outcome variable in the left column, and click on the first arrow.
2. Select the categorical determinant in the left column, and click on the second arrow.
   a. To obtain descriptive statistics of the different groups, click on 'Options…', select 'Descriptives' and click on 'Continue'.
   b. To obtain the test of homogeneity for equal variances, click on 'Options…', select 'Homogeneity of variance test' and click on 'Continue'.
   c. To obtain the results of the Welch's ANOVA or the Brown-Forsythe ANOVA, click on 'Options…', select 'Welch' or 'Brown-Forsythe' and click on 'Continue'.
   d. To obtain the post hoc comparison of each factor to all other factors click on 'Post Hoc…', select the correction-type you want to use (i.e., Bonferroni, Scheffe, Tukey, etc.) and click on 'Continue'.
3. Click on 'OK'.

- **Nonparametric Kruskal-Wallis test**

Analyze $\Rightarrow$ Nonparametric Tests $\Rightarrow$ Legacy Dialogs $\Rightarrow$ K Independent Samples

1. Select the outcome variable in the left column, and click on the first arrow.
2. Select the categorical determinant in the left column, and click on the second arrow.
3. Click on 'Define Range…'.
4. Enter the lowest and highest values of the grouping variable and click on 'Continue'.
5. Click on 'OK'.

NOTE: automatic post hoc analysis is not possible with this test.

A.4.3 Association with a Continuous Determinant

- **Linear regression**

Analyze $\Rightarrow$ Regression $\Rightarrow$ Linear...

1. Select the outcome variable in the left column and click on the first arrow.
2. Select the variable(s) to be included the model from the left column and click on the second arrow.
   a. To obtain the confidence intervals for the coefficients, select 'Statistics...', select 'Confidence intervals' and click on 'Continue'.
   b. To investigate collinearity between the variables, click on 'Statistics...', select 'Collinearity diagnostics' and click on 'Continue'.
   c. To save the predicted values or the residuals, click on 'Save' and select the check-box(es) of the values to be saved in the database.
3. Select the variable-selection method from the drop-down menu right of 'Method' (enter = all variables in the model [default]; Remove = remove all variables in that block at once; Step-wise = combined forward and backward selection procedure; Forward = forward selection procedure; Backward = backward selection procedure) .
   a. To define a new block with new variables, for example to compare two nested models or to check for confounding, click on 'Next' right above the area for the independent variables. Select the new variable(s) and possibly the selection-method from the drop-down menu.
   b. To compare to nested models, using the F-statistic, click on 'Statistics...', select 'R squared change' and click on 'Continue'.
   c. To change the p-value of the inclusion criterion, click on 'Options...', change the entry and/or removal probability and click on 'Continue'.
4. Click on 'OK'.

NOTE: interaction-terms and dummy-variables should be computed by hand first, by computing a new variable!

- **Linear regression with quadratic term**

Analyze $\Rightarrow$ Regression $\Rightarrow$ Curve Estimation...

1. Select the outcome variable in the left column and click on the first arrow.
2. Select the determinant in the left column and click on the second arrow.
3. Select the check-box 'Quadratic' in the different models.
4. Select the check-box 'Display ANOVA table' to obtain the SPSS ANOVA output.
   a. Unselect the check-box 'Plot models' if you do not want to obtain a scatter plot with the fitted regression lines.
   b. Unselect the check-box 'Linear' if you do not want to obtain a simple linear regression model with only the determinant, and not its square, included.

   c. Select the check-box 'Cubic' to obtain a linear regression model with the determinant, its square and cubic included.
5. Click on 'OK'.

A.4.4 Comparing Paired Data

- **Paired sample *t*-test**

Analyze $\Rightarrow$ Compare Means $\Rightarrow$ Paired-Samples T Test…

1. Select both measurements in the left column and click on the arrow.
2. Click on 'OK'.

- **Nonparametric Wilcoxon signed rank test**

Analyze $\Rightarrow$ Nonparametric Tests $\Rightarrow$ Legacy Dialogs $\Rightarrow$ 2 Related Samples

1. Select both measurements in the left column, and click on the arrow.
2. Click on 'OK'.

A.5 Analyzing Dichotomous Outcome Variables

A.5.1 Comparing Two or More Groups, or Paired Data

- **Contingency tables**

Analyze $\Rightarrow$ Descriptive Statistics $\Rightarrow$ Crosstabs

1. Select the row-variable (usually determinant) from the left column and click on the first arrow.
2. Select the column-variable (usually outcome variable) from the left column and click on the second arrow.
   a. To obtain the percentages per row or per column, click on 'Cells…', select either 'Row' or 'Column' or both.
   b. To obtain the results of the chi-square test, click on 'Statictics…', select 'Chi-square' and click on 'Continue'.
   c. To obtain the results of the McNemar test, click on 'Statictics…', select 'McNemar' and click on 'Continue'.
   d. To obtain the Odds Ratio, click on 'Statictics…', select 'Risk' and click on 'Continue'.

e. To obtain a 3-way table, select the next grouping variable in the left column and click on the third arrow. To obtain a 4-way table, click on 'Next', select the next grouping variable in the left column and click on the third arrow. For each next layer, repeat this step.

f. To obtain the Mantel-Haenszel pooled OR, click on 'Statistics...', select 'Cochran's and Mantel-Haenszel statistics' and click on 'Continue'.

3. Click on 'OK'.

A.5.2 Association with a Continuous Determinant

- **Logistic regression**

Analyze ⇒ Regression ⇒ Binary Logistic...

1. Select the outcome variable in the left column and click on the first arrow.
2. Select the determinant/predictor(s) to be included in (the selection procedure for) the model and click on the second arrow.
   a. If (one of) the variable(s) is categorical, click on 'Categorical...', select that (those) variable(s) in the left column, click on the arrow, select 'First' instead of 'Last', click on 'Change' and then on 'Continue'.
   b. To add an interaction term between two variables, select both variables at the same time and click on '≥a*b>'.
   c. To obtain the confidence intervals for the odds ratio(s), click on 'Options...', select 'CI for exp(B)' and click on 'Continue'.
   d. To obtain the results of the Hosmer-Lemeshow test, click on 'Options...', select 'Hosmer-Lemeshow goodness-of-fit' and click on 'Continue'.
   e. To save the estimated probabilities $P(Y = 1)$ obtained by the (final) model, click on 'Save...', select 'Probabilities' and click on 'Continue'. The predicted probabilities for each patient can be found in the database, the name of the new variable starts with 'PRE_'.
3. Select the variable-selection method from the drop-down menu right of 'Method' (enter = all variables in the model [default]; Forward: Conditional/LR/Wald = forward selection procedures; Backward: Conditional/LR/Wald = backward selection procedures).
   a. To define a new block with new variables, for example to compare two nested models or to check for confounding, click on 'Next' right above the area for the independent variables. Select the new variable(s) and possibly the selection-method from the drop-down menu.
   b. To change the p-value of the inclusion criterion, click on 'Options...', change the entry and/or removal probability in 'Probability for Stepwise' and click on 'Continue'.
4. Click on 'OK'.

- **ROC curve**

Analyze ⇒ ROC curve…

1. Select the test variable in the left column and click on the first arrow.
2. Select the outcome variable (state variable) and click on the second arrow.
   a. To obtain the diagonal reference line, select the check-box 'With diagonal reference line'
   b. To obtain the standard error and confidence interval for the AUC under the ROC, select the check-box 'Standard error and confidence interval'.
   c. To obtain a table with the coordinate points of the ROC curve, select the check-box 'Coordinate points of the ROC Curve'.
   d. If smaller values of the test variable are indicative of a successful outcome, click on 'Options…', select the check-box 'Smaller test result indicates more positive test' and click on 'Continue'.
3. Click on 'OK'.

A.6 Analyzing Time to Event Outcome Variables

A.6.1 Comparing Two or More Groups

- **Kaplan-Meier curves**

Analyze ⇒ Survival ⇒ Kaplan-Meier…

1. Select the time-variable in the left column and click on the first arrow.
2. Select the status-variable in the left column and click on the second arrow.
3. Click on 'Define Events…', enter the value which codes the event (usually 1) and click on 'Continue'.
   a. To obtain separate curves for different groups, select the grouping variable in the left column and click on the third arrow (left of 'Factor:').
4. Click on 'Options…', and select 'Survival' and click on 'Continue'.
   a. If you do not want to obtain the survival table, unselect 'Survival table(s)' before clicking on 'Continue'.
   b. If you do not want to obtain the mean and median survival times printed in the Output, unselect 'Mean and median survival' before clicking on 'Continue'.
5. Click on 'OK'.

- **Log-rank test**

Analyze ⇒ Survival ⇒ Kaplan-Meier…

1. Select the time-variable in the left column and click on the first arrow.
2. Select the status-variable in the left column and click on the second arrow.
3. Click on 'Define Events…', enter the value which codes the event (usually 1) and click on 'Continue'.

4. Select the grouping variable in the left column and click on the third arrow (left of 'Factor:').
5. Click on 'Compare Factor…', select 'Log rank' and click on 'Continue'.
    a. To obtain the p-values (not corrected for multiple testing) for all pairwise comparisons, select 'Pairwise over strata'.
    b. To obtain the p-value for the overall comparison, select 'Pooled over strata'.
6. Click on 'OK'.

A.6.2 Cox Regression Model

- **Cox regression model**

Analyze $\Rightarrow$ Survival $\Rightarrow$ Cox Regression…

1. Select the time-variable in the left column and click on the first arrow.
2. Select the status-variable with the status in the left column and click on the second arrow.
3. Click on 'Define Events…', enter the value which codes the event (usually 1) and click on 'Continue'.
4. Select the determinant/predictor(s) to be included in (the selection procedure for) the model and click on the third arrow.
    a. If (one of) the variable(s) is categorical, click on 'Categorical…', select that(those) variable(s) in the left column, click on the arrow, select 'First' instead of 'Last', click on 'Change' and then on 'Continue'.
    b. To add an interaction term between two variables, select both variables at the same time and click on '$\geq$a*b>'.
    c. To obtain the confidence intervals for the hazard ratios, click on 'Options…' and select 'CI for exp(B):' and click on 'Continue'.
    d. To obtain the estimated survival functions, click on 'Plots…', select 'Survival', select the grouping variable(s) for the separate lines from the list, click on the arrow and then on 'Continue'. Note that grouping variables (also dichotomous) have to be declared categorical as described in step 4a.
    e. To save the estimated cumulative hazard of each patient to compute the Martingale residuals from, click on 'Save…', select 'Hazard function' and click on 'Continue'. The estimated cumulative hazard for each patient can be found in the database, the name of the new variable starts with 'HAZ_'. Note that the Martingale residuals have to be computed manually from these estimated cumulative hazards.
    f. To save the Schoenfeld residuals for each patient with an event, click on 'Save…', select 'Partial residuals' and click on 'Continue'. The Schoenfeld residuals for each patient can be found in the database; the name of the new variable starts with 'PR'.
5. Select the variable-selection method from the drop-down menu right of 'Method' (enter = all variables in the model [default]; Forward: Conditional/LR/Wald = forward selection procedures; Backward: Conditional/LR/Wald = backward selection procedures).
    a. To define a new block with new variables, for example to compare two nested models or to check for confounding, click on 'Next' right above the area for the independent variables. Select the new variable(s) and possibly the selection-method from the drop-down menu.

b. To change the p-value of the inclusion criterion, click on 'Options...', change the entry and/or removal probability in 'Probability for Stepwise' and click on 'Continue'.
6. Click on 'OK'.

A.6.3 Testing Proportionality

- **Log-log plot**

Analyze ⟹ Survival ⟹ Kaplan-Meier...

1. Select the time-variable in the left column and click on the first arrow.
2. Select the status-variable in the left column and click on the second arrow.
3. Click on 'Define Events...', enter the value which codes the event (usually 1) and click on 'Continue'.
4. Select the grouping variable in the left column and click on the third arrow (left of 'Factor:').
5. Click on 'Save...', select 'Survival' and click on 'Continue' to save the survival probabilities. The survival probabilities for each patient can be found in the database, the name of the new variable starts with 'SUR_'.
6. Click on 'OK'.
7. Compute a new variable, with the expression '-ln(-ln(SURV_))'.

Graphs ⟹ Chart Builder...

8. Choose a 'Line' plot with multiple groups by clicking twice on the second type of plot ('Multiple Line').
9. Move the new variable (computed in step 7.) to the field 'Y-Axis?', move the time-variable to the field 'X-Axis?' and the grouping variable to the field 'Set color'.
10. Click on 'X-Axis1 (Line1)' in the second box 'Element Properties', choose 'Logarithmic' for the 'Scale Type' and click on 'Apply'.
11. Click on 'OK' in the 'Chart Builder' box.

- **Cox-regression with time-dependent covariate**

Analyze ⟹ Survival ⟹ Cox w/Time-Dep Cov ...

1. Create the equation for the time-dependency in the top-right area; use the first variable in the left column (T_) as time-variable.
   a. For the model $b_1(t) = c_0 + c_1 \times d_T(t)$ where d is zero for all $t \le T$ and d is one for all $t > T$, the equation is equal to '(T_ > T)'.
   b. For the model $b_1(t) = c_0 + c_1 \times t$, the equation is equal to 'T_'.
   c. For the model $b_1(t) = c_0 + c_1 \times \ln(t)$, the equation is equal to 'ln(T_)'.
2. Click on 'Model...', the rest of the steps are equal to the usual Cox regression, with one additional step: add the interaction between the time-dependent variable 'T_COV_' (the first variable in the left column) and the grouping variable to the model.

A.7 Missing Data Analysis

- ■ **Missing value analyses**

Analyze ⇒ Missing Values Analysis…

1. Select continuous variables in the left column and click on the first arrow.
2. Select dichotomous and categorical variables in the left column and click on the second arrow.
3. Click on 'OK'.

- ■ **Multiple imputation**

Analyze ⇒ Multiple Imputation ⇒ Impute Missing Data Values…

1. Select the variables with missing data that need to be imputed from the left column and click on the first arrow.
2. Select the variables (without missing values) used in the imputation model from the left column and click again on the first arrow.
3. Type the name of the new dataset with the imputed data SPSS will create, in the text field to the right of 'Dataset name:'
    a. To increase the number of imputation sets, click on ▲ until the desired number of imputation sets is reached.
4. Click on the tab 'Constraints'.
5. For each of the variables selected in steps 1. and 2., assign its role in the model [default = 'Impute and use as predictor']:
    a. Click on ▼ and select 'Impute only' for variables whose missing values have to be imputed, but are not used in the model to predict other missing values.
    b. Click on ▼ and select 'Use as predictor only' for variables without missing values that should only be used in the model to predict other missing values.
6. Click on 'OK'.

Mathematical Equations and Models

B.1 The Basics

In this appendix, we provide an overview of the important mathematical equations and models, that we used and defined in this book. We start with the basic equations for descriptive statistics and inferential statistics and then provide the equations for the analyses of a continuous, a dichotomous and a time to event outcome variable.

B.1.1 Descriptive Statistics

Throughout this appendix, the observed value of an outcome variable Y of patient i is denoted by Y_i. The size of the study population is denoted by n. The mean value of variable Y in the study population is equal to ($\blacktriangleright$ Sect. 2.2.1)

$$\bar{Y} = \frac{1}{n} \sum_{i=1}^{n} Y_i,$$

and the standard deviation (SD) of variable Y in the study population is equal to ($\blacktriangleright$ Sect. 2.2.1)

$$SD = \sqrt{\frac{1}{n-1} \sum_{i=1}^{n} (Y_i - \bar{Y})^2}.$$

If we compare multiple groups, the size of group g is denoted by n_g. The mean and SD in group g is denoted by $\bar{Y}_g$ and SD_g. The pooled SD of two groups is equal to ($\blacktriangleright$ Eq. E2.1, $\blacktriangleright$ Sect. 2.3.1)

$$\text{pooled SD} = \sqrt{\frac{(n_1 - 1) \times SD_1^2 + (n_2 - 1) \times SD_2^2}{n_1 + n_2 - 2}}$$

B.1.2 Inferential Statistics

The general form of a 95% confidence interval (CI) for a general effect size is equal to ($\blacktriangleright$ Eq. E2.2, $\blacktriangleright$ Sect. 2.3.3)

$$[\text{effect size} - 1.96 \times SE; \text{effect size} + 1.96 \times SE],$$

where SE is the standard error (SE) of the effect size.

B.2 A Continuous Outcome Variable

B.2.1 Independent Samples *T*-Test

The SE for the mean difference between two groups is equal to ($\blacktriangleright$ Eq. E3.1, $\blacktriangleright$ Sect. 3.2.1)

$$SE_{diff} = \sqrt{\frac{(n_1 - 1) \times SD_1^2 + (n_2 - 1) \times SD_2^2}{n_1 + n_2 - 2}} \sqrt{\frac{1}{n_1} + \frac{1}{n_2}}.$$

The test statistic of the independent samples *t*-test is equal to ($\blacktriangleright$ Eq. E3.3, $\blacktriangleright$ Sect. 3.2.1)

$$t = \frac{\text{mean diff}}{SE_{diff}},$$

and follows a *t*-distribution with $n_1 + n_2 - 2$ degrees of freedom.

B.2.2 Analyses of Variance

The total sum of squares (SS_{tot}), the sum of squares between groups ($SS_{between}$) and within groups (SS_{within}) are equal to ($\blacktriangleright$ Eqs. E3.4 to E3.6, $\blacktriangleright$ Sect. 3.3.1)

$$SS_{tot} = \sum_{g=1}^{k} \sum_{i=1}^{n_g} (Y_{i,g} - Y)^2,$$

$$SS_{between} = \sum_{g=1}^{k} n_g (\bar{Y}_g - \bar{Y})^2,$$

$$SS_{within} = \sum_{g=1}^{k} \sum_{i=1}^{n_g} (Y_{i,g} - \bar{Y}_g)^2.$$

In these equations, $Y_{i,g}$ is the value of the outcome variable for patient i in group g. The test statistic of the analysis of variance (ANOVA) is equal to ($\blacktriangleright$ Eq. E3.7, $\blacktriangleright$ Sect. 3.3.1)

$$F = \frac{SS_{between}/(k-1)}{SS_{within}/(n-k)},$$

and follows an *F*-distribution with $k - 1$ and $n - k$ degrees of freedom.

B.2.3 Linear Regression Model

- ■ **Simple linear regression model**

A simple linear regression model for outcome variable Y with a single determinant x is equal to (▶ Models M3.2 and M3.3, ▶ Sect. 3.4.2)

$$\bar{Y} = b_0 + b_1 \times x, \text{ or equivalently}$$

$$Y = b_0 + b_1 \times x + \varepsilon.$$

The interpretation of the regression coefficients b_0 and b_1 are as follows
- b_0 is the mean outcome for patients for whom their determinant is equal to zero, i.e., $x = 0$;
- b_1 is the mean difference in outcome between two patients who differ by one unit in their determinant.

A simple linear regression model for outcome variable Y with a single categorical determinant x (with k groups) is equal to

$$\bar{Y} = b_0 + b_1 \times d_1 + b_2 \times d_2 + \ldots + b_{k-1} \times d_{k-1},$$

where $d_1, d_2, \ldots, d_{k-1}$ are the $k-1$ dummy variables. If the group 1 is set as the reference group, i.e., the dummies $d_1, d_2, \ldots, d_{k-1}$ are coded as in ◻Table B.1, the interpretation of the regression coefficients $b_0, b_1, b_2, \ldots, b_{k-1}$ are as follows
- b_0 is the mean outcome for patients in group 1;
- b_i is the mean difference in outcome between group $i+1$ and group 1.

- ■ **Multiple linear regression model**

A multiple linear regression model for outcome variable Y with k determinants $x_1, x_2, \ldots, x_k$ is equal to (▶ Model M6.15, ▶ Sect. 6.5.4)

$$Y = b_0 + b_1 \times x_1 + b_2 \times x_2 + \ldots + b_k \times x_k + \varepsilon.$$

The interpretation of the regression coefficients $b_0, b_1, b_2, \ldots, b_k$ are as follows
- b_0 is the mean outcome for patients for whom all determinants are equal to zero, i.e., $x_1 = x_2 = \ldots = x_k = 0$;
- b_i is the mean difference in outcome between two patients who differ by one unit in their determinant x_i while their values of the other determinants are equal.

- ■ **Linear regression prediction model**

The linear predictor (LP) for a linear regression prediction model is equal to (▶ Eq. E6.1, ▶ Sect. 6.5.4/▶ Eq. E7.1, ▶ Sect. 7.3)

$$LP = b_0 + b_1 \times x_1 + b_2 \times x_2 + \ldots + b_k \times x_k.$$

Table B.1 Categorical dummy coding for a regression model with a categorical determinant x with k groups

Group	d_1	d_2	...	d_{k-1}
1	0	0	...	0
2	1	0	...	0
3	0	1	...	0
⋮	⋮	⋮	...	⋮
k	0	0	...	1

The explained variance R^2 of a linear regression prediction model is equal to (▶ Eqs. E7.4 to E7.6, ▶ Sect. 7.4.1)

$$R^2 = \frac{\text{explained variation}}{\text{total variation}}, \text{with}$$

$$\text{total variation} = \sum_{i=1}^{n} (Y_i - \bar{Y})^2,$$

$$\text{explained variation} = \sum \left(\widehat{Y}_i - \bar{Y}\right)^2,$$

where, for patient i, $\widehat{Y}_i$ is the predicted value of the outcome variable by the model, i.e., the value of the LP for patient i.

B.2.4 Paired Sample *T*-Test

The test statistic for the paired sample t-test is equal to (▶ Eq. E3.8, ▶ Sect. 3.5.1)

$$t = \frac{\text{mean difference}}{\text{SD}_\Delta / \sqrt{n}},$$

where SD_Δ is the SD of the delta-variable. The test statistic follows a t-distribution with $n - 1$ degrees of freedom

B.3 A Dichotomous Outcome Variable

B.3.1 Different Effect Sizes

Table B.2 shows the general form of a 2×2 crosstab. With this table, the risk difference (RD) and the relative risk (RR) are computed to compare the risk of a 'success' outcome between two groups (denoted by p_1 and p_2) as well as the odds ratio (OR) to compare the odds (i.e., $p/(1-p)$) for a 'success' outcome between two groups (▶ Sect. 2.3.2/4.2.1)

⊡ Table B.2 General form of a 2 × 2 crosstab

		Outcome		
		Event	No event	Total
group	1	a	b	$n_1 = a + b$
	2	c	d	$n_2 = c + d$
total		$a + c$	$b + d$	$n = n_1 + n_2$

$$RD = p_1 - p_2 = \frac{a}{n_1} - \frac{c}{n_2}$$

$$RR = \frac{p_1}{p_2} = \frac{a}{n_1} / \frac{c}{n_2} = \frac{a \times n_2}{n_1 \times c}$$

$$OR = \frac{p_1/(1 - p_1)}{p_2/(1 - p_2)} = \frac{a \times d}{b \times c}$$

The SE for the RD and the natural logarithm (ln) of the RR and OR are equal to (▶Eqs. E4.1, E4.4 and E4.3, ▶Sect. 4.2.1)

$$SE_{RD} = \sqrt{\frac{p_1 \times (1 - p_1)}{n_1} + \frac{p_2 \times (1 - p_2)}{n_2}},$$

$$SE_{\ln(RR)} = \sqrt{\frac{1}{a} + \frac{1}{c} - \frac{1}{n_1} - \frac{1}{n_2}},$$

$$SE_{\ln(OR)} = \sqrt{\frac{1}{a} + \frac{1}{b} + \frac{1}{c} + \frac{1}{d}}.$$

The 95 % CI for the RD, ln(RR) and ln(OR) follow from the standard form of the 95 % CI, the 95 CI for the RR or OR is obtained by taking the exponential (exp) of the 95 % CI for the ln(RR) or ln(OR).

B.3.2 Chi-Square Test for Two Groups

The test statistic of the chi-square test is equal to (▶Eq. E4.6, ▶Sect. 4.2.2)

$$X^2 = \sum_{i,j=1}^{2} \frac{(O_{i,j} - E_{i,j})^2}{E_{i,j}},$$

and follows a χ^2-distribution with 1 degree of freedom. The test statistic for comparing k groups follows a χ^2-distribution with $k - 1$ degrees of freedom.

B.3.3 Logistic Regression Model

- **Simple logistic regression model**

A simple logistic regression model for outcome variable Y with a single determinant x is equal to (▶Sect. 4.4.1)

$$\ln(\text{odds for 'success'}) = b_0 + b_1 \times x.$$

The interpretation of the regression coefficients b_0 and b_1 are as follows
- b_0 is the $\ln(\text{odds})$ for the 'success' outcome for patients for whom their determinant is equal to zero, i.e., $x = 0$;
- b_1 is the difference in $\ln(\text{odds})$ for the 'success' outcome between two patients who differ by one unit in their determinant.

This is equivalent to
- $\exp(b_0)$ is the odds for the 'success' outcome for patients for whom their determinant is equal to zero;
- $\exp(b_1)$ is the OR for the 'success' outcome between two patients who differ by one unit in their determinant.

The estimated probability for a 'success' outcome, denoted by $P(Y = 1)$, is equal to (▶Eq. E4.8, ▶Sect. 4.4.1)

$$P(Y = 1) = \frac{1}{1 + \exp(-(b_0 + b_1 \times x))}.$$

A simple logistic regression model for outcome variable Y with a single categorical determinant x (with k groups) is equal to

$$\ln(\text{odds for 'success'}) = b_0 + b_1 \times d_1 + b_2 \times d_2 + \ldots + b_{k-1} \times d_{k-1},$$

where $d_1, d_2, \ldots, d_{k-1}$ are the $k - 1$ dummy variables coded as in ◻Table B.1. The interpretation of exponential of the regression coefficients $b_0, b_1, b_2, \ldots, b_{k-1}$ are as follows
- $\exp(b_0)$ is the odds for the 'success' outcome in group 1;
- $\exp(b_i)$ is the OR for the 'success' outcome between group $i + 1$ and group 1.

- **Multiple logistic regression model**

A multiple logistic regression model for outcome variable Y with k determinants $x_1, x_2, \ldots, x_k$ is equal to (▶Sect. 6.5.2)

$$\ln(\text{odds for 'success'}) = b_0 + b_1 \times x_1 + b_2 \times x_2 + \ldots + b_k \times x_k.$$

The interpretation of the regression coefficients b_0 and b_i are as follows
- b_0 is the ln(odds) for the 'success' outcome for patients for whom all determinants are equal to zero, i.e., $x_1 = x_2 = \ldots = x_k = 0$;
- b_i is the difference in ln(odds) for the 'success' outcome between two patients who differ by one unit in their determinant x_i while their values of the other determinants are equal.

This is equivalent to
- $\exp(b_0)$ is the odds for the 'success' outcome for patients for patients for whom all determinants are equal to zero;
- $\exp(b_i)$ is the OR for the 'success' outcome between two patients who differ by one unit in their determinant x_i while their values of the other determinants are equal.

- **Logistic regression prediction model**

The LP for a logistic regression prediction model is equal to ($\blacktriangleright$ Eq. E7.1, $\blacktriangleright$ Sect. 7.3)

$$LP = b_0 + b_1 \times x_1 + b_2 \times x_2 + \ldots + b_k \times x_k.$$

The estimated probability for a 'success' outcome is equal to ($\blacktriangleright$ Eq. E7.3, $\blacktriangleright$ Sect. 7.3.2)

$$P(Y = 1) = \frac{1}{1 + \exp(-LP)}.$$

B.3.4 Measures of Diagnostic Accuracy

The diagnostic accuracy of a diagnostic test is also determined with a 2×2 crosstab. However, the rows represent the two possible outcomes of the diagnostic test (i.e., positive and negative) and the columns the true status of the subject (i.e., the gold standard test is positive or negative). $\square$ Table B.3 shows the general form of such a crosstab. The diagnostic accuracy measures are then equal to ($\blacktriangleright$ Eqs. E4.10 to E4.13, $\blacktriangleright$ Sect. 4.6.1)

$$\text{sensitivity} = \frac{a}{n_+},$$

$$\text{specificity} = \frac{d}{n_-},$$

$$\text{PPV} = \frac{a}{m_+},$$

$$\text{NPV} = \frac{d}{m_-}.$$

▣ **Table B.3**   General form of a 2 × 2 crosstab, to assess the diagnostic accuracy of a diagnostic test

| | | Gold standard test | | |
		Positive	Negative	Total
diagnostic test	positive	a	b	n_+
	negative	c	d	n_-
total		m_+	m_-	n

The SE for one proportion (of a dichotomous outcome variable, e.g., the sensitivity or specificity) is equal to (▶Eq. E4.9, ▶Sect. 4.5.1)

$$\text{SE}_p = \sqrt{\frac{p \times (1-p)}{n}}.$$

B.4 A Time to Event Outcome Variable

B.4.1 Kaplan-Meier Curve

The number of patients at risk at time t is denoted by n_t and the number of patients who experienced the event at time t by d_t. Then, the survival fraction at time t is equal to (▶Eq. E5.1, ▶Sect. 5.1)

$$\text{survival fraction}(t) = \frac{n_t - d_t}{n_t} = 1 - \frac{d_t}{n_t}.$$

The Kaplan-Meier estimator, denoted by $\widehat{S}(t_i)$, at follow-up time t_i is equal to (▶Eq. E5.2, ▶Sect. 5.1)

$$\widehat{S}(t_i) = \widehat{S}(t_{i-1}) \times \text{survival fraction}(t_i),$$

in which the previous observed event time is denoted by t_{i-1}.

B.4.2 Cox Regression Model

▪ **Simple Cox regression model**

A simple Cox regression model for the hazard function $h(t)$ of a time to event outcome variable with a single determinant x is equal to (▶Sect. 5.2.3/5.4.1)

$$\ln(h(t)) = \ln(h_0(t)) + b_1 \times x$$

The baseline hazard $h_0(t)$ is the (estimated) hazard function for the time to event for patients for whom their determinant is equal to zero, i.e., $x = 0$. The interpretation of the regression coefficient b_1 is as follows

- b_1 is the difference in $\ln(h(t))$ between two patients who differ by one unit in the determinant.

This is equivalent to

- $\exp(b_1)$ is the hazard ratio (HR) for the time to event between two patients who differ by one unit in their determinant.

A simple Cox regression model for a time to event outcome variable Y with a single categorical determinant x (with k groups) is equal to (▶ Sect. 5.3.3)

$$\ln(h(t)) = \ln(h_0(t)) + b_1 \times d_1 + b_2 \times d_2 + \ldots + b_{k-1} \times d_{k-1}$$

where $d_1, d_2, \ldots, d_{k-1}$ are the $k-1$ dummy variables coded as in ◘ Table B.1. The baseline hazard $h_0(t)$ is the (estimated) hazard function for the time to event for patients in group 1. The interpretation of exponential of the regression coefficients $b_1, b_2, \ldots, b_{k-1}$ are as follows

- $\exp(b_i)$ is the HR for the time to event between group $i+1$ and group 1.

■ **Multiple Cox regression model**

A multiple Cox regression model for the hazard function $h(t)$ of a time to event outcome variable with k determinants $x_1, x_2, \ldots, x_k$ is equal to (▶ Sect. 6.5.3)

$$\ln(h(t)) = \ln(h_0(t)) + b_1 \times x_1 + b_2 \times x_2 + \ldots + b_k \times x_k$$

The baseline hazard $h_0(t)$ is the (estimated) hazard function for the time to event for patients for whom all determinants are equal to zero, i.e., $x_1 = x_2 = \ldots = x_k = 0$. The interpretation of the regression coefficients b_i are as follows

- b_i is the difference in $\ln(h(t))$ between two patients who differ by one unit in the determinant x_i while their values of the other determinants are equal.

This is equivalent to

- $\exp(b_i)$ is the HR for the time to event between two patients who differ by one unit in the determinant x_i while their values of the other determinants are equal.

■ **Cox regression prediction model**

The LP for a Cox regression prediction model is equal to (▶ Eq. E7.2, ▶ Sect. 7.3)

$$LP = b_1 \times x_1 + b_2 \times x_2 + \ldots + b_k \times x_k.$$

References

Agresti A. An introduction to categorical data analysis. 2nd ed. Hoboken: John Wiley & Sons; 2002.

Ahrens W, Pigeot I. Handbook of epidemiology. New York: Springer; 2014.

Altman DG. Practical statistics for medical research. London: Chapman & Hall; 1991.

Anderson KM, Wilson PW, Odell PM, Kannel WB. An updated coronary risk profile. A statement for health professionals. Circulation. 1991;83(1):356–62.

Armitage P, Berry G, Matthews JNS. Statistical methods in medical research. Oxford: Blackwell Science Ltd; 2002.

Belsey DA, Kuh D, Welsch RE. Regression diagnostics. New York: John Wiley; 1980.

Benchimol EI, Smeeth L, Guttmann A, Harron K, Moher D, Petersen I, et al. The REporting of studies Conducted using Observational Routinely-collected health Data (RECORD) statement. PLoS Med. 2015;12(10):e1001885. ►https://doi.org/10.1371/journal.pmed.1001885.

Bossuyt PM, Reitsma JB, Bruns DE, Gatsonis CA, Glasziou PP, Irwig L, et al. STARD 2015: an updated list of essential items for reporting diagnostic accuracy studies. BMJ. 2015;351:h5527. ►https://doi.org/10.1136/bmj.h5527.

Bouter LM, van Dongen MJCM, Zielhuis GA. Textbook of epidemiology. Houten: Bohn Stafleu van Loghum; 2017.

Bradburn MJ, Clark TG, Love SB, Altman DG. Survival analysis part II: multivariate data analysis – an introduction to concepts and methods. Br J Cancer. 2003;89(3):431–6. ►https://doi.org/10.1038/sj.bjc.6601119.

Bradburn MJ, Clark TG, Love SB, Altman DG. Survival analysis part III: multivariate data analysis – choosing a model and assessing its adequacy and fit. Br J Cancer. 2003;89(4):506–11. ►https://doi.org/10.1038/sj.bjc.6601120.

Butt JH, Rorth R, Kragholm K, Kristensen SL, Torp-Pedersen C, Gislason GH, et al. Return to the workforce following coronary artery bypass grafting: a Danish nationwide cohort study. Int J Cardiol. 2017. ►https://doi.org/10.1016/j.ijcard.2017.10.032.

Centers for Disease Control and Prevention. TREND statement. 2018. ►https://www.cdc.gov/trendstatement/index.html. Accessed 9 Oct 2018.

Chan AW, Tetzlaff JM, Altman DG, Dickersin K, Moher D. SPIRIT 2013: new guidance for content of clinical trial protocols. Lancet. 2013;381(9861):91–2. ►https://doi.org/10.1016/S0140-6736(12)62160-6.

Chan AW, Tetzlaff JM, Altman DG, Laupacis A, Gotzsche PC, Krleza-Jeric K, et al. SPIRIT 2013 statement: defining standard protocol items for clinical trials. Ann Intern Med. 2013;158(3):200–7. ►https://doi.org/10.7326/0003-4819-158-3-201302050-00583.

Chan AW, Tetzlaff JM, Gotzsche PC, Altman DG, Mann H, Berlin JA, et al. SPIRIT 2013 explanation and elaboration: guidance for protocols of clinical trials. BMJ. 2013;346:e7586. ►https://doi.org/10.1136/bmj.e7586.

Clark TG, Bradburn MJ, Love SB, Altman DG. Survival analysis part IV: further concepts and methods in survival analysis. Br J Cancer. 2003;89(5):781–6. ►https://doi.org/10.1038/sj.bjc.6601117.

Clark TG, Bradburn MJ, Love SB, Altman DG. Survival analysis part I: basic concepts and first analyses. Br J Cancer. 2003;89(2):232–8. ►https://doi.org/10.1038/sj.bjc.6601118.

Cleophas TJ, Zwinderman AH. Modern meta-analysis. Review and update of methodologies. New York: Springer; 2017.

Cochrane. Cochrane library. ►http://www.cochranelibrary.com. Accessed 2 Oct 2018.

Cohen J. Statistical power analysis for the behavioral sciences. 2nd ed. Hilllsdale: Erlbaum Associated; 1988.

Cohen JF, Korevaar DA, Altman DG, Bruns DE, Gatsonis CA, Hooft L, et al. STARD 2015 guidelines for reporting diagnostic accuracy studies: explanation and elaboration. BMJ Open. 2016;6(11):e012799. ►https://doi.org/10.1136/bmjopen-2016-012799.

Collet D. Modelling survival data in medical research. 2nd ed. Boca Raton: Chapman & Hall/CRC; 2004.

CONSORT Group. CONSORT website. 2010. ►http://www.consort-statement.org. Accessed 9 Oct 2018.

COSMIN initiative. Checklists for assessing study qualities. 2005. ►https://www.cosmin.nl/tools/checklists-assessing-methodological-study-qualities/. Accessed 9 Oct 2018.

de Vet HCW, Terwee CB, Mokkink LB, Knol DL. Measurement in medicine. Cambridge: Cambridge University Press; 2011.

de Vries VA, Muller MCA, Sesmu Arbous M, Biemond BJ, Blijlevens NMA, Kusadasi N, et al. Time trend analysis of long term outcome of patients with haematological malignancies admitted at dutch intensive care units. Br J Haematol. 2018. ►https://doi.org/10.1111/bjh.15140.

den Uyl D, ter Wee MM, Boers M, Kerstens P, Voskuyl A, Nurmohamed M, et al. A non-inferiority trial of an attenuated combination strategy ('COBRA-light') compared to the original COBRA strategy: clinical results after 26 weeks. Ann Rheum Dis. 2014;73(6):1071–8. ►https://doi.org/10.1136/annrheumdis-2012-202818.

des Jarlais DC, Lyles C, Crepaz N, Trend group. Improving the reporting quality of nonrandomized evaluations of behavioral and public health interventions: the TREND statement. Am J Public Health. 2004;94(3):361–6. ►https://doi.org/10.2105/ajph.94.3.361.

Dragt E. How to research trends: move beyond trend watching to kick start innovation. Amsterdam: BIS Publishers; 2017.

Elashoff JD, Lemeshow S. Sample size determination in epidemiologic studies. In: Ahrens W, Pigeot I, editors. Handbook of epidemiology. New York: Springer; 2014.

Elliot P, Cuzick D, English D, Stern R. Geographical and environmental epidemiology. Methods for small-area studies. Oxford: Oxford University Press; 1996.

Engels MA, Twisk JW, Blankenstein MA, van Vugt JM. Age independent first trimester screening for Down syndrome: improvement in test performance. Prenat Diagn. 2013;33(9):884–8. ►https://doi.org/10.1002/pd.4153.

Engels MA, Bhola SL, Twisk JW, Blankenstein MA, van Vugt JM. Evaluation of the introduction of the national Down syndrome screening program in the Netherlands: age-related uptake of prenatal screening and invasive diagnostic testing. Eur J Obstet Gynecol Reprod Biol. 2014;174:59–63. ►https://doi.org/10.1016/j.ejogrb.2013.12.009.

EQUATOR Network. STARD 2015: an updated list of essential items for reporting diagnostic accuracy studies. 2017. ►http://www.equator-network.org/reporting-guidelines/stard/. Accessed 9 Oct 2018.

Fang P, Lu J, Liu YH, Deng HM, Zhang L, Zhang HQ. Benefit of an operating vehicle preventing peritonitis in peritoneal dialysis patients: a retrospective, case-controlled study. Int Urol Nephrol. 2018. ►https://doi.org/10.1007/s11255-018-1823-z.

Flick U. An introduction to qualitative research. London: Sage Publications Ltd; 2014.

Gough D, Oliver S, Thomas J. An Introduction to systematic reviews. Los Angeles: Sage Publications Ltd; 2017.

Greenland S, Senn SJ, Rothman KJ, Carlin JB, Poole C, Goodman SN, et al. Statistical tests, P values, confidence intervals, and power: a guide to misinterpretations. Eur J Epidemiol. 2016;31(4):337–50. ►https://doi.org/10.1007/s10654-016-0149-3.

Gunzler D, Chen T, Wu P, Zhang H. Introduction to mediation analysis with structural equation modeling. Shanghai Arch Psychiatry. 2013;25(6):390–4. ►https://doi.org/10.3969/j.issn.1002-0829.2013.06.009.

Helland IS. Some theoretical aspects of partial least squares regression. Chemometr Intell Lab Syst. 2001;58(2):97–107. ►https://doi.org/10.1016/S0169-7439(01)00154-X.

Higgins JPT, Green S, editors. Cochrane handbook for systematic reviews of interventions version 5.1.0 [updated March 2011]. The Cochrane Collaboration; 2011. Available from ►http://handbook.cochrane.org.

Hoogenboom BJ, Manske RC. How to write a scientific article. Int J Sports Phys Ther. 2012;7(5):512–7. PMC: 3474301.

Husereau D, Drummond M, Petrou S, Carswell C, Moher D, Greenberg D, et al. Consolidated Health Economic Evaluation Reporting Standards (CHEERS) statement. Int J Technol Assess Health Care. 2013;29(2):117–22. ►https://doi.org/10.1017/S0266462313000160.

Husereau D, Drummond M, Petrou S, Greenberg D, Mauskopf J, Augustovski F, et al. Reply to Roberts et al. Cheers is sufficient for reporting cost-benefit analysis, but may require further elaboration. Pharmacoeconomics. 2015;33(5):535–6. ►https://doi.org/10.1007/s40273-015-0277-8.

International Committee of Medical Journal Editors. ICMJE | Recommendations. 2017. ►http://www.icmje.org/recommendations/. Accessed 9 Oct 2018.

Jackson JE. A user's guide to principal components. New York: John Wiley & Sons, Inc; 1991.

Jadad AR, Enkin MW. Randomized controlled trials. Questions, answers and musings. Malden: Wiley-Blackwell; 2007.

Jolliffe IT. Principal component analysis. 2nd ed. New York: Springer-Verlag; 2002.

Kannel WB, McGee D, Gordon T. A general cardiovascular risk profile: the Framingham study. Am J Cardiol. 1976;38(1):46–51.

Kirkwood BR, Sterne JAC. Essential medical statistics. 2nd ed. Oxford: Blackwell Science Ltd; 2003.

Kleinbaum DG, Klein M. Survival analysis. New York: Springer; 2012.

Kobayashi D, Turner DR, Forbes TJ, Aggarwal S. Parental anxiety among children undergoing cardiac catheterisation. Cardiol Young. 2017:1–7. ►https://doi.org/10.1017/s1047951117002074.

Kvrgic Z, Asiedu GB, Crowson CS, Ridgeway JL, Davis JM. "Like no one is listening to me": a qualitative study of patient-provider discordance between global assessments of disease activity in rheumatoid arthritis. Hoboken: Arthritis Care Res; 2017. ►https://doi.org/10.1002/acr.23501.

Langan SM, Benchimol EI, Guttmann A, Moher D, Petersen I, Smeeth L, et al. Setting the RECORD straight: developing a guideline for the REporting of studies Conducted using Observational Routinely collected Data. Clin Epidemiol. 2013;5:29–31. ►https://doi.org/10.2147/CLEP.S36885.

Last JM, editor. A dictionary of epidemiology. New York: Oxford University Press; 2001.

Lin DL, Wu CS, Tang CH, Kuo TY, Tu TY. The safety and risk factors of revision adenoidectomy in children and adolescents: a nationwide retrospective population-based cohort study. Auris Nasus Larynx. 2018;45(6):1191–8. ►https://doi.org/10.1016/j.anl.2018.03.002.

Little RJA, Rubin DB. Statistical analysis with missing data. 2nd ed. New York: John Wiley & Sons; 2002.

MacKinnon DP, Krull JL, Lockwood CM. Equivalence of the mediation, confounding and suppression effect. Prev Sci. 2000;1(4):173–81. ►https://doi.org/10.1023/A:1026595011371.

MacKinnon DP, Lockwood CM, Hoffman JM, West SG, Sheets V. A comparison of methods to test mediation and other intervening variable effects. Psychol Methods. 2002;7(1):83–104. PMC: 2819363.

MacKinnon DP, Fairchild AJ, Fritz MS. Mediation analysis. Annu Rev Psychol. 2007;58:593–614. ►https://doi.org/10.1146/annurev.psych.58.110405.085542.

MacKinnon DP. Introduction to statistical mediation analyses. New York: Routledge; 2008.

Mahla RS. Stem cells applications in regenerative medicine and disease therapeutics. Int J Cell Biol. 2016;2016:6940283. ▶https://doi.org/10.1155/2016/6940283.

Mandelblatt JS, Fryback DG, Weinstein MC, Russell LB, Gold MR. Assessing the effectiveness of health interventions for cost-effectiveness analysis. Panel on cost-effectiveness in health and medicine. J Gen Intern Med. 1997;12(9):551–8. PMC: 1497158.

Maxwell JA. Qualitative research design: an interactive approach. Thousands Oaks: Sage Publications Ltd; 2013.

McCusker K, Gunaydin S. Research using qualitative, quantitative or mixed methods and choice based on the research. Perfusion. 2015;30(7):537–42. ▶https://doi.org/10.1177/0267659114559116.

Miller RG Jr. Simultaneous statistical inference. New York: Springer-Verlag Inc; 1981.

Moher D, Liberati A, Tetzlaff J, Altman DG, PRISMA Group. Preferred reporting items for systematic reviews and meta-analyses: the PRISMA statement. Ann Intern Med. 2009;151(4):264–9. ▶https://doi.org/10.7326/0003-4819-151-4-200908180-00135.

Moher D, Hopewell S, Schulz KF, Montori V, Gøtzsche PC, Devereaux PJ, et al. CONSORT 2010 explanation and elaboration: updated guidelines for reporting parallel group randomised trials. BMJ. 2010;340:c869. ▶https://doi.org/10.1136/bmj.c869.

Mokkink LB, Terwee CB, Knol DL, Stratford PW, Alonso J, Patrick DL, et al. Protocol of the COSMIN study: COnsensus-based Standards for the selection of health Measurement INstruments. BMC Med Res Methodol. 2006;6:2. ▶https://doi.org/10.1186/1471-2288-6-2.

Mokkink LB, Terwee CB, Knol DL, Stratford PW, Alonso J, Patrick DL, et al. The COSMIN checklist for evaluating the methodological quality of studies on measurement properties: a clarification of its content. BMC Med Res Methodol. 2010;10:22. ▶https://doi.org/10.1186/1471-2288-10-22.

Mokkink LB, Prinsen CA, Bouter LM, de Vet HCW, Terwee CB. The COnsensus-based Standards for the selection of health Measurement INstruments (COSMIN) and how to select an outcome measurement instrument. Braz J Phys Ther. 2016;20(2):105–13. ▶https://doi.org/10.1590/bjpt-rbf.2014.0143.

Moons KG, Altman DG, Reitsma JB, Ioannidis JP, Macaskill P, Steyerberg EW, et al. Transparent Reporting of a multivariable prediction model for Individual Prognosis or Diagnosis (TRIPOD): explanation and elaboration. Ann Intern Med. 2015;162(1):55–63. ▶https://doi.org/10.7326/M14-0698.

Muennig P. Cost-effectiveness analysis in health: a practical approach. 2nd ed. San Fransisco: Jossey-Bass; 2007.

Neumann PJ, Ganiats TG, Russel LB, Sanders GD, Siegel JE. Cost-effectiveness in health and medicine. New York: Oxford University Press; 2016.

PRISMA Group. PRISMA statement. 2015. ▶http://www.prisma-statement.org. Accessed 9 Oct 2018.

Putter H, Fiocco M, Geskus RB. Tutorial in biostatistics: competing risks and multi-state models. Stat in Med. 2007;26:2389–430. ▶https://doi.org/10.1002/sim.

RECORD Group. RECORD reporting guidelines. 2017. ▶http://www.record-statement.org. Accessed 9 Oct 2018.

Riffenburgh RH. Statistics in medicine. San Diego: Academic Press; 1999.

Rossello X, Huo Y, Pocock S, van de Werf F, Chin CT, Danchin N, et al. Global geographical variations in ST-segment elevation myocardial infarction management and post-discharge mortality. Int J Cardiol. 2017;245:27–34. ▶https://doi.org/10.1016/j.ijcard.2017.07.039.

Rothman KJ, Lash TL, Greenland S. Modern epidemiology. 3rd ed. Philadelphia: Lippincott-Raven; 2012.

Rubin DB. Multiple imputation after 18+ years. J Am Stat Assoc. 1996;91:473–89. ▶https://doi.org/10.1080/01621459.1996.10476908.

Schulz KF, Altman DG, Moher D, for the CONSORT Group. CONSORT 2010 statement: updated guidelines for reporting parallel group randomised trials. BMJ. 2010;340(9609):c332. ▶https://doi.org/10.1136/bmj.c332.

Shamseer L, Moher D, Clarke M, Ghersi D, Liberati A, Petticrew M, et al. Preferred reporting items for systematic review and meta-analysis protocols (PRISMA-P) 2015: elaboration and explanation. BMJ. 2015;350:g7647. ▶https://doi.org/10.1136/bmj.g7647.

Siegel JE, Weinstein MC, Russell LB, Gold MR. Recommendations for reporting cost-effectiveness analyses. Panel on cost-effectiveness in health and medicine. JAMA 1996;276(16):1339–41. ▶https://doi.org/10.1001/jama.1996.03540160061034.

Siegel JE, Torrance GW, Russell LB, Luce BR, Weinstein MC, Gold MR. Guidelines for pharmacoeconomic studies. Pharmacoeconomics. 1997;11(2):159–68. ▶https://doi.org/10.2165/00019053-199711020-00005.

Siegel JP. Equivalence and noninferiority trials. Am Heart J. 2000;139(4):S166–70. ▶https://doi.org/10.1016/S0002-8703(00)90066-8.

Šimundić A-M. Measures of diagnostic accuracy: basic definitions. EJIFCC. 2009;19(4):203–11.

Sterne JAC, Smith GD. Sifting the evidence–what's wrong with significance tests? Phys Ther. 2001;81(8):1464–9. ▶https://doi.org/10.1093/ptj/81.8.1464.

Steyerberg EW. Clinical prediction models. New York: Springer; 2009.

Steyerberg EW, Vickers AJ, Cook NR, Gerds T, Gonen M, Obuchowski N, et al. Assessing the performance of prediction models: a framework for traditional and novel measures. Epidemiology. 2010;21(1):128–38. ▶https://doi.org/10.1097/EDE.0b013e3181c30fb2.

STROBE Initiative. STROBE statement. 2009. ►http://www.strobe-statement.org. Accessed 9 Oct 2019.

Stroup DF, Berlin JA, Morton SC, Olkin I, Williamson GD, Rennie D, et al. Meta-analysis of observational studies in epidemiology: a proposal for reporting. Meta-analysis Of Observational Studies in Epidemiology (MOOSE) group. JAMA 2000;283(15):2008–2012. ►https://doi.org/10.1001/jama.283.15.2008.

ter Wee MM, den Uyl D, Boers M, Kerstens P, Nurmohamed M, van Schaardenburg D, et al. Intensive combination treatment regimens, including prednisolone, are effective in treating patients with early rheumatoid arthritis regardless of additional etanercept: 1-year results of the COBRA-light open-label, randomised, non-inferiority trial. Ann Rheum Dis. 2015;74(6):1233–40. ►https://doi.org/10.1136/annrheumdis-2013-205143.

ter Wee MM, van Tuyl LH, Blomjous BS, Lems WF, Boers M, Terwee CB. Content validity of the Dutch Rheumatoid Arthritis Impact of Disease (RAID) score: results of focus group discussions in established rheumatoid arthritis patients and comparison with the international classification of functioning, disability and health core set for rheumatoid arthritis. Arthritis Res Ther. 2016;18:22. ►https://doi.org/10.1186/s13075-015-0911-z.

Tong A, Sainsbury P, Craig J. Consolidated criteria for reporting qualitative research (COREQ): a 32-item checklist for interviews and focus groups. Int J Qual Health Care. 2007;19(6):349–57. ►https://doi.org/10.1093/intqhc/mzm042.

TRIPOD Group. TRIPOD statement. 2018. ►http://www.tripod-statement.org. Accessed 9 Oct 2018.

Twisk JWR. Applied longitudinal data analysis for epidemiology. New York: Cambridge University Press; 2003.

van de Stadt LA, Witte BI, Bos WH, van Schaardenburg D. A prediction rule for the development of arthritis in seropositive arthralgia patients. Ann Rheum Dis. 2013;72(12):1920–6. ►https://doi.org/10.1136/annrheumdis-2012-202127.

Vandenbroucke JP, von Elm E, Altman DG, Gotzsche PC, Mulrow CD, Pocock SJ, et al. Strengthening the Reporting of Observational Studies in Epidemiology (STROBE): explanation and elaboration. Ann Intern Med. 2007;147(8):W163–94. ►https://doi.org/10.7326/0003-4819-147-8-200710160-00010-w1.

Verbeke G, Molenberghs G. Introduction to longitudinal data analysis. New York: Springer-Verlag Inc; 2000.

Voight ML, Hoogenboom BJ. Publishing your work in a journal: understanding the peer review process. Int J Sports Phys Ther. 2012;7(5):452–60. PMC: 3474310.

von Elm E, Altman DG, Egger M, Pocock SJ, Gotzsche PC, vandenbroucke JP, et al. The strengthening the reporting of observational studies in epidemiology (STROBE) statement: guidelines for reporting observational studies. Ann Intern Med. 2007;147(8):573–7. ►https://doi.org/10.7326/0003-4819-147-8-200710160-00010.

Walker E, Nowacki AS. Understanding equivalence and noninferiority testing. J Gen Intern Med. 2011;26(2):192–6. ►https://doi.org/10.1007/s11606-010-1513-8.

Wallwork A. English for writing research papers. New York: Springer; 2011.

Wehling M. Principles of translational science in medicine: from bench to bedside London: Academic Press; 2015.

Weinstein MC, Siegel JE, Gold MR, Kamlet MS, Russell LB. Recommendations of the panel on cost-effectiveness in health and medicine. JAMA. 1996;276(15):1253–8. ►https://doi.org/10.1001/jama.1996.03540150055031.

Wells GA, Shea B, O'Connel D, Peterson J, Welch V, Losos M, et al. The Newcastle-Ottawa Scale (NOS) for assessing the quality of nonrandomised studies in meta-analyses. 2013. ►http://www.ohri.ca/programs/clinical_epidemiology/oxford.asp. Accessed 9 Sept 2018.

Wold S, Martens H, Wold H. The multivariate calibration problem in chemistry solved by the PLS method. In: Kågström B, Ruhe A, editors. Matrix Pencils. Lecture Notes in Mathematics, vol 973. Heidelber: Springer; 1983. pp. 286–293.

World Medical Association. World medical association declaration of Helsinki: ethical principles for medical research involving human subjects. JAMA. 2013;310(20):2191–4. ►https://doi.org/10.1001/jama.2013.281053.

Zakharova IS, Zhiven MK, Saaya SB, Shevchenko AI, Smirnova AM, Strunov A, et al. Endothelial and smooth muscle cells derived from human cardiac explants demonstrate angiogenic potential and suitable for design of cell-containing vascular grafts. J Transl Med. 2017;15(1):54. ►https://doi.org/10.1186/s12967-017-1156-1.

288

Index